NURSING CONCEPTS
FOR
HEALTH PROMOTION

NURSING CONCEPTS
FOR
HEALTH PROMOTION

Ruth Murray, R.N.M.S.N.
Associate Professor of Nursing
School of Nursing
St. Louis University

Judith Zentner, R.N.M.A.

Mildred Heyes Boland, R.N.M.S.N.
Assistant Professor, College of Nursing,
University of Arizona, Tucson, Arizona

Mary Ellen Grohar, R.N.M.S.N.
Assistant Professor, School of Nursing
St. Louis University, St. Louis, Missouri

Beverly Leonard, R.N.M.S.N.
Assistant Professor, School of Nursing,
University of Texas, Austin, Texas

Mary Ann Lough, R.N.M.S.N.
Assistant Clinical Professor, School of Nursing,
St. Louis University, St. Louis, Missouri

Patricia Meili, R.N.M.S.N.
Instructor, School of Nursing,
Southern Illinois University, Edwardsville, Illinois

Sister Juliann Murphy, C.C.V.I., R.N.M.S.N.E.
Director of Nursing Service, St. Anthony's Hospital,
Amarillo, Texas

Norma Nolan, R.N.M.S.N.
Assistant Professor, School of Nursing,
St. Louis University, St. Louis, Missouri

PRENTICE-HALL, INC., *Englewood Cliffs, New Jersey*

Library of Congress Cataloging in Publication Data

MURRAY, RUTH.
  Nursing concepts for health promotion.

  Includes bibliographies and index.
  1. Nurses and nursing. I. Zentner, Judith, joint
author. II. Title. [DNLM: 1. Health education—
Nursing texts. 2. Nursing. WY100 M983na]
RT41.M9.   610.73   74-23439
ISBN 0-13-627653-9 pbk.

Nursing Concepts for Health Promotion

Ruth Murray, Judith Zentner et al.

© 1975 by PRENTICE-HALL, Inc.
Englewood Cliffs, New Jersey

10 9 8 7 6 5 4

Printed in the United States of America

PRENTICE-HALL INTERNATIONAL, INC., *London*
PRENTICE-HALL OF AUSTRALIA, PTY. LTD., *Sydney*
PRENTICE-HALL OF CANADA, LTD., *Toronto*
PRENTICE-HALL OF INDIA PRIVATE LIMITED, *New Delhi*
PRENTICE-HALL OF JAPAN, INC., *Tokyo*

This book is dedicated to:

Our students—for their inspiration

Our families—for their patience

Contents

To the Reader

We believe the nurse must consider the total health of the person and family. The physical, mental, emotional, sociocultural, and religious-moral needs are interrelated. Increasingly your emphasis must be on comprehensive health promotion rather than on patchwork remedies. This text, and the companion one, *Nursing Assessment and Health Promotion through the Life Span,* integrate material essential for such a nursing practice in any setting.

Often nurses study some of the topics presented, in isolated courses with little or no application to the care of the patient, his family, and the community. Therefore, an integral part of this book is the nursing application of such material, interwoven when appropriate, and emphasized in special sections at other times.

Your role in nursing is changing from that of working primarily for the physician or agency to that of being an advocate for the patient, client, or family. Today's physicians are often so specialized that the patient feels fragmented and unable to understand how a specific disease process—his avoidance, modification, or elimination of it—will affect his complete life. The person is afraid to ask. He thinks that the physician is too busy and too engrossed in medical terminology. The patient has been taught to seek the physician's help for illness and treatment; he rarely goes to maintain wellness. Thus *your* response to the person and to his family is crucial, whether they are well or ill. You are the one caring person who can interpret health care services, serve as a liaison between the physician, other health team members, and the person, and prevent fragmentation of health services.

Before reading any chapter, you should orient yourself by studying the organizational chart shown here, which illustrates the many facets that must be considered in nursing for health promotion. Next, read the Introduction. You can then gain a further orientation by (1) reading the table of contents, (2) looking at the objectives listed at the beginning of each chapter, (3) glancing at chapter headings, and (4) noting the terms in boldface italics which are followed by their definitions in italics.

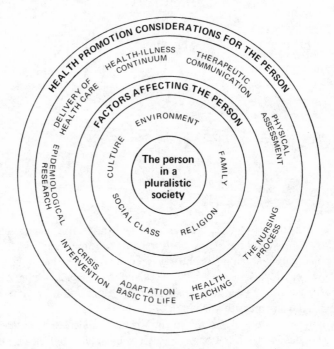

Organizational Chart

Consult the companion text, *Nursing Assessment and Health Promotion through the Life Span,* for a guide to physical and developmental assessment of each life era and for a study of death.

We invite you to be an active participant as you read. Our ideas are presented with conviction and directness, but we want you to integrate and modify our ideas into your specific circumstances. Each of you will have to adapt this information to your setting—be it independent practice, health maintenance organization, hospital, clinic, or home.

ACKNOWLEDGMENTS

The authors appreciate the support and assistance received from many friends.

We are especially grateful to Sally Lehnert for her conscientious assistance in preparing the manuscript, to John L. Boland, Jr., Dr. Takao Fujisawa, Mary Blanche Jordan, Edwin Murray, Hazel Nolan, and Alice Proctor for their assistance, and to Reid Zentner for his support and specific contributions.

We thank Prentice-Hall, Inc., especially Harry A. McQuillen, College Editor, and Margaret McNeily, Production Editor, who gave valuable guidance during the preparation of the text, and Roger MacQuarrie, who initially involved us in this adventure.

In addition, the following persons are acknowledged for reviewing the manuscript, partially or in total: Marietta Cohen, Northern Virginia Community College; Mary Dempsey, St. Louis University; Bernadine Hallinan, Howard Community College; Theodora Langford, University of Texas at Austin; Ray E. Miller and the staff of "Operation Survival through Environmental Education"; Sharon Roberts, University of California, Los Angeles; Sister Callista Roy, Mount St. Mary's College; Marilyn Rubin, St. Louis University; Louise Spall, Anderson College; Edna Dell Weinel, St. Louis University; and Dolores Zeis, St. Louis University.

Also, for help with final proofreading, we wish to thank Linda Niedringhaus, Hazel Nolan, Norma Nolan, Brenda Proebsting, and Anne White.

RUTH MURRAY

JUDITH ZENTER

Introduction

This text on nursing in a pluralistic society is divided into two units. Unit I (Chapters 1-8) establishes a framework for health promotion in a complex society. As society becomes more complicated, nursing increasingly requires a framework—a set of concepts and tools—that can be used in any setting with a variety of people. Chapters 1-8 present topics whose sequential arrangement does not necessarily indicate that one subject must follow another. Rather, these topics are just important components of nursing knowledge, gathered from various sources and placed together into one unit for convenient reference.

Chapter 1 introduces the reader to the concept of health and its many meanings, depending on the person's experience. Basic definitions of and variables influencing health and illness are examined.

Chapter 2 discusses the American health care system. You will get an overview of the system in which you work and suggestions on how to promote primary and comprehensive care, now and in the future.

Chapter 3 explores the meaning of therapeutic communication. Since you will observe and talk with persons and their families before, during, and after giving care, how you affect these people through your communication pattern will establish a basis for the nursing process, the topic of Chapter 4. Here the nursing process is described as a systematic method of providing health service to a person or group of persons, and the nurse-patient relationship is explored as the basic unit of interaction in this process. The changing role of the nurse is also examined.

To help you learn and teach more effectively as a nurse, health teaching is discussed in Chapter 5. Attention is given to the creative process, the difference between child and adult learning, and methods that you may employ in teaching others to maintain or regain health.

Chapter 6 considers concepts of epidemiology. Working directly with people who need health care, you are in a key position to use this research method to determine patterns of wellness and health care needs.

Chapters 7 and 8 provide two theories, along with suggestions for their practical application. The first, *adaptation theory*, considers how each aspect of the person or group must continually be adjusted to maintain wellness. The second, *crisis theory*, gives direction for helping the person and his family during crises, since many of the people you work with will be in some phase of crisis.

Unit II (Chapters 9-13) discusses factors influencing health development and use of the nursing process. In the past, the person's health status has usually been considered apart from the many factors that help define him—factors, moreover, that are an integral part of his health (or lack of it). The American health care system rips the person out of his environment, often disregarding his cultural and religious practices, social-class setting, and family life. Then we wonder why he seems disoriented in the health care setting.

Unit II takes a cosmopolitan view. Environmental pollution is considered as a world problem. Types of cultures and religions, in addition to those common in the United States, are examined. The individual's social class and family life are discussed. You need to understand the physical climate from which he comes and his working and living conditions. Knowledge of the person's background will help you better plan the environment in which to work with him and his family. You need to know whether his culture emphasizes trust or mistrust in the medical profession. You need to understand the basis for and importance of his religious rituals. You can better plan for his care if you know his social-class values. You can also work more effectively with the whole family if you are aware whether it is an extended or a nuclear family. A knowledge of all of these various background factors will enable you to treat each individual and his family with the special understanding that they deserve.

A FRAMEWORK FOR HEALTH PROMOTION IN A PLURALISTIC SOCIETY

CHAPTER 1

Basic Considerations in Health and Illness

Study of this chapter will enable you to:

1 Define *health* and *illness* and explain the meaning of the health-illness continuum.

2 Contrast the objective and subjective aspects of health and illness.

3 List and describe the environmental variables, internal and external, that influence the person's health status.

4 Discuss specific basic nursing measures that are conducive to health promotion.

"Al, are you ill?"
"No. Why?"
"Your face looks a little puffy."

Al, who thought he was well, suddenly decides he hasn't had his usual energy for several weeks. He thinks he'll make an appointment to see the doctor.

"I wish I really knew what you mean about being sick. Sometimes I've felt so bad I could curl up and die, but had to go on because the kids have to be taken care of, and besides, we didn't have the money to spend for the doctor—how could I be sick? ...How do you know when you're sick, anyway? Some people can go to bed most anytime with anything, but most of us can't be sick—even when we need to be"[56].

These expressions immediately portray the difficulty in defining health and illness. Each person's definition is affected by cultural concepts, economic level, the value system of self and others, ethnic background, customs, and past experiences.

Baumann intensifies the subjectivity by identifying three ways in which a person defines himself as ill: (1) if he feels "bad"; (2) if he has distressing symptoms, such as pain; and (3) if he cannot carry on his usual daily activities. Thus both illness and health are what the person says they are. Person *A* may have the same symptoms as person *B*; but while *A* says he is well, *B* says he is ill[1]!

The well person usually has some small degree of illness—physical or mental—such as minor aches, flares of temper, inappropriate forgetfulness, or overuse of certain defense mechanisms, such as denial. And the person who is physically very ill, even near death, may still have some health potential. Similarly, the emotionally ill person will manifest some health or appropriate behaviors.

Although *health* and *illness* are subjective and relative terms, Jourard believes that qualities such as hope, purpose, and direction in life can produce and maintain wellness, even in the face of stress. Likewise, demoralization through daily struggle for existence can help produce illness[31].

As a nurse, your concern, knowledge, and skill are directed to the health needs of persons from many different kinds of backgrounds and in various settings. It is essential, therefore, to understand the physical, mental, emotional, and social aspects of wellness and illness; the factors influencing health and illness; and the basic regulatory mechanisms in the human body which normally maintain a state of health. The use of this information will assist you in helping others to maintain as well as regain health.

DEFINITIONS
OF HEALTH AND ILLNESS

Working definitions of *health* and *illness*, although generalized, can give perspective. Traditionally they have been defined as opposites. An example is the definition given by the United Nations World Health Organization: *Health* is a "state of complete physical, mental, and social well being and not merely the absence of disease"[15]. The only option in the absence of complete physical, mental, and social well-being, according to such a definition, is illness. No allowance is made for degrees of illness and wellness.

Dunn defines *health* and *illness* on a graduated scale or continuum: Each person has neither absolute health nor illness but is in an ever-changing state of being, ranging from peak or "high-level" wellness to extreme poor health with death imminent[15].

Health/wellness and *disease/illness* are now thought of as complex, dynamic processes that include physical, psychological, and social components. They are adaptive or maladaptive behavioral responses to internal and external stimuli. Health is dependent on genetic and environmental influences that either help or hinder an individual in actively fulfilling his needs and reaching his highest health potential[3, 32, 48]. The emotionally healthy person generally shows behavior congruent with events within or around him[2, 57]. Key concepts in health/wellness include homeostasis, adaptation, dynamic nature of health-illness continuum, influence of internal and external environment, comfort, safety, social relationships, and prevention of disease, disability, and social decay.

The definition of "disease" has progressed through several stages. Primitive man saw disease as an independent force that dominates and eventually overtakes the victim. Next, the medical-physiological view interpreted man as an active being with ability to resist disease attack. The ecological definition looks at the environmental influence on health, while the equilibrium view emphasizes ineffective attempts to maintain homeostasis or adaptation. Last, the social approach defines illness in terms of whether the person is performing expected social functions[57].

Illness is an experience that exists when there is a disturbance or failure in the biopsychosocial development of a person. He experiences observable or felt changes in the body with discomfort or impaired ability to carry out minimal physical, physiological, or psychosocial behavioral expectations[57]. Sullivan's definition of mental or emotional illness corresponds to the above in that such illness is manifested as inappropriate or inadequate behavior in social contexts [52].

For use in this book, ***health*** *is a purposeful, adaptive response, physically, mentally, emotionally, and socially, to internal and external stimuli in order to maintain stability and comfort*; and ***illness*** *is a disturbed adaptive response to internal and external stimuli resulting in disequilibrium and inability to utilize the usual health-promoting resources.*

VARIABLES AFFECTING HEALTH

Health of the person, family, and community is affected by *external variables, factors or stimuli arising outside the body*, and *internal variables, characteristics or stimuli arising inside the body*. Although those factors are discussed separately, they obviously affect the person simultaneously. This ecological approach, which includes the interaction between man and his environment, is essential to solving the world's health problems[44, 47].

All men possess regulatory behaviors that either maintain or regain the homeostatic state when a need imbalance occurs in either the external or internal environment[10]. Stresses of any kind may upset the delicate balance. For example, maternal deprivation in infants may result in serious psychological problems, as may marital conflicts. Lack of water or oxygen may result in biochemical or physiological disorders. Excessive exposure to cold causes frostbite resulting in tissue damage.

Although responses to stressful situations vary, anxiety is a common one. *Anxiety, a state of mental discomfort or uneasiness related to a feeling of helplessness or threat to self-image,* occurs in everyone, well or ill. Often there is no objective cause. The ill or hospitalized person may experience anxiety because of environmental changes. He exhibits signs of anxiety about the unknown: the outcome of surgery, the stability of his job and family income, and possible death. This person may experience noticeable physical and behavioral changes. His heart and respiration rates increase; he may perspire excessively; he may cry, become angry and demanding, or have difficulty following directions. Other responses to stress include grief, mourning, and denial. These concepts will be covered in later chapters. Should the felt mental, emotional, or even physical disequilibrium become severe, mental or physical illness may result. Hence, the health of persons is directly related to and affected by their reactions to both the internal and external environment.

Environment outside the Body

External variables may be physical, biological, social, or cultural.

Physical Variables include climate. Thus a person with allergies may have to consider moving from a high- to a low-pollen-count area, or artificially control his home and work environment. Some physical factors affect persons because of their occupation. Coal miners are prone to develop anthracosilicosis, a disease which may result from excessive inhalation of coal dust. Smoke inhalation is a risk for firemen, while excessive exposure to radiation may affect X-ray technicians. Other physical variables are space, housing, and sanitation facilities. Tension and aggressive behavior increase in people when they are crowded together[29]. Even wild animals recognize their needs for living space and will fight to meet these needs[15]. Sunlight, fresh air, and adequate shelter from the weather are essential for health. In Chapter 9 environmental pollution as an external health variable is described in greater detail.

Biological Variables include use of drugs. Although drugs properly used— for example, in diabetes or venereal disease—can be and often are life-saving, the injudicious use of drugs, even those prescribed by a doctor, can be deadly. Television commercials testify to our self-medication practices. We wake up, go to sleep, eliminate pain, reduce swelling, gain or lose weight, and attempt to cope with emotions by taking various pills. Instead of treating physical warning symptoms (such as headache, heartburn, or backache) as reasons for investigating the cause of discomfort, we temporarily pacify them, perhaps extending beginning disease, rather than seeking medical help.

Drug-induced diseases are increasing. Drug addiction may have its start from the pressure exerted by television or peers, curiosity, emotional immaturity, or excessive use of over-the-counter drugs by parents. Even the indiscriminate use of antibiotics for colds or minor infections may cause hypersensitivity or other illnesses from side effects or toxicity.

Social Variables may include socioeconomic status, family-life patterns, and educational level. The socioeconomically deprived person has increased vulnerability to physical and emotional illness[19]. Although he learns his rights from television or others and is beginning to voice his opinion, he often is too involved in the day-to-day struggle for survival to think of future health. He also is afraid and ignorant in dealing with the sophisticated health care areas[27]. Even the middle class cannot meet the rising cost of medical care without hardship. Patients from the lower economic groups, as well as the middle class, are becoming more knowledgeable and may be expected to take a high priority within the national health system. More on life styles in various economic levels appears in Chapter 12.

Cultural Variables are also significant. Language, religion, family organization, child-care patterns, and food habits vary greatly. Health practices differ in various subcultures and classes. Mexican-Americans often consult and are treated by a recognized practitioner, not a medical physician. Upper- and middle-class Americans often consult a physician for specific symptoms, such as a fever or rash, while those in the lower class usually delay consultation[26]. These and other related topics will be discussed in greater detail in following chapters.

Environment inside the Body

Internal variables include personal structural characteristics, physiological processes, physical growth and development, body repair mechanisms, and behavior.

Personal Characteristics such as age, sex, race, intelligence, and motivation may affect a person's health. Certain diseases, such as rubeola, rubella, and chicken pox, primarily affect children, while cerebral vascular accidents and ulcers mainly affect adults. Senile osteoporosis, a condition involving softening of the bones from demineralization, is a potential hazard in any elderly person and can make him more prone to major fractures. However, the frequency of these conditions varies among groups of people[8].

Sex affects health status. Hemophilia is caused by an inherited defect in the clotting of the blood. The mother transmits the defective gene to her son, who develops hemophilia[5]. Lupus erythematosis, a chronic inflammatory disease, is systemic in nature and manifests itself dermatologically. It attacks young adults, chiefly females[8].

Race affects health. Sickle-cell anemia is a hereditary blood disease in which the red blood cells sometimes assume a strange shape—like sickles. These sickle cells cannot float through the body easily, and consequently the organs do not get enough oxygen. As a result, organs cannot function properly, causing pain and illness in the affected person. This disease affects primarily blacks, although people of Mediterranean, Arabian, or southern Asian descent, or offspring of Caucasians and blacks, may also be affected[8].

Intelligence and motivation, and other personal characteristics, help the individual take appropriate steps to follow hygienic or preventive measures or seek health care when necessary.

Physiological Processes, the next internal variable, maintain life and have a direct bearing on the health of an individual. These processes include biophysiological regulatory mechanisms, physical growth and development, and the repair of diseased or injured body tissues.

There are many biophysiological regulatory mechanisms described in anatomy and physiology texts. Most can be subsumed under one of three headings: (1) homeostasis, (2) biological rhythms, or (3) adaptation. These mechanisms, though intricate and highly interdependent, function silently unless they get out of whack. Most of us take them for granted.

Homeostasis is illustrated through a simple example. Repeatedly during the day we might move from a $72°$F air-conditioned building to the $98°$ outside environment. The change of $26°$ outside our bodies is in contrast to a very slight temperature change inside our bodies. Thus, *homeostasis describes the constancy of our internal environment in a changing external environment.* Our organ systems have automatic and coordinated responses to all outside environmental changes[11]. Some authorities instead call this mechanism *homeodynamics* or *homeokinetics* to designate an ever-active dynamic process[3].

Also *within our bodies are self-sustaining, repeating patterns called biological rhythms*, or inner clocks. They help explain why some people are mentally sharp at 6:00 A.M. while others work to full capacity at 10:00 P.M. The location of these automatic timing devices is unknown; each cell may contain its own. Biological rhythms may be *exogenous, dependent upon the rhythm of external environmental events* such as sunlight; or *endogenous, arising within the organism and uninfluenced by the environment*[12]. Biological rhythms are classified according to the length or occurrence of the rhythmic pattern (oscillation) as diurnal, circadian, ultradian, and infradian[12, 46]. The terms *diurnal* and *circadian* have been used in the past to mean a rhythm occurring once a day. However, the term *diurnal rhythm* is ambiguous when applied to diurnal animals; hence *diurnal rhythm is used to describe fluctuations in body processes confined to the working day*, while *circadian describes fluctuations occurring every 20 to 28 hours*. The terms *ultradian* and *infradian*, coined by Franz Halberg, *refer to rhythmic processes occurring less frequently than every 24 hours* and *on a weekly or monthly basis, respectively*[42].

The *constant adjustment of our homeostatic, biological-rhythm, and other internal mechanisms to the outside environment in order to survive better or change the environment is called adaptation*. Adaptation refers to change and permits forward movement by minimizing the effects of discord, deviance, or other adverse forces. There are many kinds of adaptation: biological, mental, emotional, social, and cultural[40]. A person who has a leg amputated, for example, must adapt in all these ways. Adaptation involves the whole person. He can adjust better when he is flexible, uses mechanisms which require the least effort possible, and when change is not sudden[3]. Chapter 7 extensively discusses adaptation and biological rhythms in relation to the nursing process.

Physical Growth and Development, the third internal variable, affects health in many ways, both positively and negatively. For example, genetically determined physical characteristics affect total personality. A tall, lanky, teen-aged girl may be very shy and self-conscious because of her physical appearance. A boy with a muscular physique may be forced to play football when he would prefer to play the clarinet. Physical abnormalities may elicit different personality responses in different persons, depending on their cultural norms, others' reactions, and the disabled person's perception of these abnormalities and of himself. One may develop self-pity; another shows courage to overcome the problem; while yet another manifests overcompensation intellectually to cope with the problem.

Body Repair Mechanisms, the fourth internal variable, consist of those processes involved in the repair of diseased or injured tissue, which require an accelerated cell reproduction to compensate for cell loss. For example, after a large amount of blood is lost, erythrocytes are replaced by rapid differentiation of precursor cells in the bone marrow[24]. The regulation of this process, though not completely understood, is controlled by the tissues. When the details of this problem are understood, scientists will also be able to explain more about embryonic development, organismic aging, and cancer.

Human Behavior, the last internal variable, encompasses a variety of inter-related activities. It is directed toward fulfillment of the basic needs of man and is an outward expression of the person's inner experience. The key to understanding behavior lies within the person himself. The observer can only guess at its meaning, and perhaps after the establishment of trust the person will share the meaning or the intent of his behavior with the observer[5, 6].

Some research studies utilizing prison inmates are being conducted to determine what predisposes a person toward socially unacceptable behavior, such as child molesting, robbery, or murder. *Temperament, an individual's outlook on life, his feelings, mood swings, and emotional reactions to stress*, is also being studied. Social scientists are trying to determine if heredity influences one's disposition. While the results of these studies have been inconclusive, the trend is to consider the possibility of a combination of inherited characteristics and environmental influences, both internal and external[5].

The internal and external environmental variables previously discussed relate to the quality of health and, possibly, to the quality of life. One final characteristic of behavior is a "zest for life." People who possess this trait exhibit gusto and exhilaration for living. Whatever they do is done wholeheartedly. This zest seems to enrich their entire life style; such persons truly live in a state of positive health[29].

ROLE OF THE NURSE:
PROMOTION AND MAINTENANCE
OF HEALTH

Personal Health Promotion

Today, most of the emphasis in health care is on disease and death, and only minimal information concerning how to achieve, measure, or maintain health is available. If each person is to reach the goal of optimum health, you must place more emphasis on the fulfillment of health for you and your client, through preventive measures, continuity of care, and health education. Since health is a purposeful, adaptive, total body response to internal and external stimuli to maintain stability and comfort, *health promotion includes those factors that aid the person in his attempt to maintain this necessary stability.* Langton suggests that the following be considered as factors that promote personal health for you and others:

1. Assessing present health status regularly through periodic health examinations, including dental checkups, and participating in mass screening programs in the community.

2. Learning preventive measures and warning signals of disease, such as those published by the American Cancer Society and the American Heart Association.

3. Caring for the body functions, including those factors affecting the skin, mucous membranes, teeth, elimination, and sensory organs.

4. Avoiding products harmful to health—for example, various pollutants, tobacco, drugs, ethyl alcohol, or excessive food.

5. Avoiding extreme stress, fatigue, or exhaustion and providing for adequate relaxation, rest, and sleep.

6. Maintaining essential nutrition.

7. Attending to any infection or injury that occurs[34].

In addition to these seven factors, observing the basic principles of good personal hygiene is necessary. For example, avoid such behavior as using other persons' drinking and eating utensils, eating leftover portions of their food, and sharing towels or combs.

You have a personal responsibility to promote your own health as well as that of persons under your care. Society has always expected contributions from its members commensurate with their educational background. Therefore, you are viewed as having more responsibility than the average citizen for personal health promotion.

Preventive Measures

Preventive measures enhance or promote health and may be primary, secondary, or tertiary[19]. *Primary prevention involves averting the occurrence of disease.* Immunizations and screening for early detection of disease, such as eye, diabetic, and cancer screening, are a primary means of preventing disease. If these tests are performed routinely, early detection of disease is possible, and consequently some of the disabling effects may be eliminated or minimized. Equally important is the development of coping behavior and a basic moral code and philosophy that enables the person to meet stresses and crises of living and still retain his equilibrium, emotionally and physically.

Secondary prevention involves early treatment to stop the progress of disease and thereby prevent complications. An example is initiating an immediate rehabilitation program for a person with a cerebral vascular accident. Taking prescribed medication for illness, rest of an injured body part, and surgery to prevent complications are other examples.

Tertiary prevention is aimed at avoiding further progression of sequelae from disease. For example, the person who has residual paralysis from a stroke is given treatment to avoid further deterioration of body or mind.

You will be involved with many different kinds of people in the prevention of disease, regardless of the nursing setting. School nurses are responsible for administering periodic vision and hearing examinations to children. Industrial nurses must help minimize occupational health hazards. Hospital nurses are engaged in prevention in several ways—for example, stopping the progress of disease, preventing spread of infection, implementing rehabilitation programs for patients, and doing health teaching. Community health nurses focus on prevention in some of the ways just mentioned as well as through responsibility for neighborhood clinics, home care, casefinding, and child-health conferences which provide health supervision for infants and young children.

Continuity of Care

Continuity of care, helping the person make a transition as he enters the health care setting or returns to his home, is an important health promotion responsibility. Your job will include planning, referral, and follow-up as you help the patient receive care which is his basic right.

Health Education

Health education is the learning process by which persons and groups learn to promote, maintain, or restore health. Burton says health education has two major objectives: (1) communication of information on the nature of disease, its causative factors, and the measures that are effective in preventing illness; and (2) motivation of people to want optimum health regardless of the expense of time, energy, or money [9].

Health education must be adjusted to learning levels and directed to situations of immediate interest for the particular age group. For example, a 10-year-old boy is more concerned with increasing his muscular prowess with proper food and exercise, while the 16-year-old boy is concerned with the effects of smoking, drugs, and alcohol consumption. Adults are increasingly concerned about the effects of stress, pollutants, smoking, and drugs on long-term health.

As a health educator, you must learn about the health and health needs of each person by determining his knowledge, attitudes, and practices related to personal health promotion, his plans for health protection, and his present mental and emotional health status. All of these points must be considered before the actual planning and during implementation of any health education program. Chapter 5 on health teaching discusses these points in detail.

You also play an important part in health education by promoting local and state control of infection and disease through mass screening or immunization and by supporting and promoting community projects for improved housing, adequate sanitation facilities, vermin control, slum clearance, and control of leaded paint and gasoline.

Teaching parents about child care, nutrition, normal patterns of development, how to manage given budgetary and other limitations, and realistic expectations for themselves and their children can promote adaptation to the ordinary stresses of family living and childrearing. Helping parents to feel "good" or positive about themselves and their children is basic to any teaching. By promoting the adaptive capacities of parents, you can help prevent child abuse. All of the above are interrelated to enhance the health—physically, mentally, emotionally, and socially—of the person and the family, and thereby, the community.

The remainder of this text will explore in greater depth the information that you can use to promote the well-being of yourself and of others in a *pluralistic society—a society containing groups of people distinctive in environmental setting, ethnic origins, cultural patterns, religion, and social class.* Information about developmental norms that will assist you in understanding people in a pluralistic society is also available [41].

REFERENCES

1. Baumann, Barbara, "Diversities in Conceptions of Health and Physical Fitness," in *Social Interaction and Patient Care*, eds. James Skipper and Robert Leonard. Philadelphia: J. B. Lippincott Company, 1965, pp. 206-18.

2. Beeson, Gerald, "The Health-Illness Spectrum," *American Journal of Public Health*, 57: No. 11 (1967), 1901-4.

3. Beland, Irene L., *Clinical Nursing: Pathophysiological and Psychosocial Approaches.* London: The Macmillan Company, 1971.

4. Benenson, Abram S., *Control of Communicable Diseases in Man.* Washington, D.C.: American Public Health Association, Inc., 1970.

5. Bowen, Eleanor Page, *Biology of Human Behavior.* New York: Appleton-Century-Crofts, 1968.

6. Bower, Fay Louise, *The Process of Planning Nursing Care: A Theoretical Model.* St. Louis: The C. V. Mosby Company, 1972.

7. Brinton, Diana Marion, "Health Center Milieu: Interaction of Nurses and Low-Income Families," *Nursing Research*, 21: No. 1 (1972), 46-52.

8. Brunner, Lillian Sholtis, Charles Phillips Emerson, L. Kraeer Ferguson, and Doris Smith Suddarth, *Textbook of Medical-Surgical Nursing* (2nd ed.). Philadelphia: J. B. Lippincott Company, 1970.

9. Burton, Lloyd Edward, and Hugh H. Smith, *Public Health and Community Medicine.* Baltimore: The Williams & Wilkins Company, 1970.

10. Byrne, Marjorie L., and Lida F. Thompson, *Key Concepts for the Study and Practice of Nursing.* St. Louis: The C. V. Mosby Company, 1972.

11. Cannon, Walter B., *The Wisdom of the Body.* New York: W. W. Norton & Company, Inc., 1939.

12. Conroy, R. T. W. L., and J. N. Mills, *Human Circadian Rhythms.* London: J. & A. Churchill, 1970.

13. Day, Sister Agnita Claire, unpublished lecture notes, 1969.

14. Dubos, Rene, *Mirage of Health.* Garden City, N.Y.: Doubleday & Company, Inc., 1959.

15. Dunn, Halbert L., *High-Level Wellness.* Washington, D.C.: Mount Vernon Publishing Company, Inc., 1961.

16. Engel, George L., "A Unified Concept of Health and Disease," *Perspectives in Biology and Medicine.* Chicago: University of Chicago Press, Summer 1960.

17. Felton, Geraldene, and Mary G. Patterson, "Shift Rotation Is Against Nature," *American Journal of Nursing*, 71: No. 4 (1971), 760-63.

18. Ferguson, Eugene S., "The Measurement of the 'Man-Day,'" *Scientific American*, 225: No. 4 (1971), 96-103.

19. Freeman, Ruth, *Community Health Nursing Practice.* Philadelphia: W. B. Saunders Company, 1970.

20. Frobisher, Martin, Lucille Sommermeyer, and Robert Fuerst, *Microbiology in Health and Disease*. Philadelphia: W. B. Saunders Company, 1969.

21. Goerke, Lenor, and Ernest Stebbins, *Mustard's Introduction to Public Health*. New York: The Macmillan Company, 1968.

22. Grollman, Sigmund, *The Human Body: Its Structure and Physiology*. New York: The Macmillan Company, 1969.

23. Guyton, Arthur, *Basic Human Physiology: Normal Function and Mechanisms of Disease*. Philadelphia: W. B. Saunders Company, 1971.

24. Handler, Philip, ed., *Biology and the Future of Man*. New York: Oxford University Press, 1970.

25. Hawker, Lilian, and Alan H. Linton, eds., *Microorganisms: Function, Form, and Environment*. New York: American Elsevier Publishing Company, Inc., 1971.

26. Irelan, Lola, *Low Income Life Styles*. Washington, D.C.: United States Department of Health, Education, and Welfare, 1966.

27. Jaco, E. Gartley, ed., *Patients, Physicians, and Illness*. New York: The Free Press, 1972.

28. Jahoda, Marie, *Current Concepts of Positive Mental Health*. New York: Basic Books, Inc., 1956.

29. Jamann, Joan, "Health Is a Function of Ecology," *American Journal of Nursing*, 71: No. 5 (1971), 970.

30. Johnston, Dorothy, *Total Patient Care: Foundations and Practice*. St. Louis: The C. V. Mosby Company, 1968.

31. Jourard, Sidney, *The Transparent Self*. New York: D. Van Nostrand Company, 1971.

32. King, Imogene M., *Toward a Theory for Nursing*. New York: John Wiley & Sons, Inc., 1971.

33. Kleitman, Nathaniel, "The Sleep Cycle," *American Journal of Nursing*, 60: No. 5 (1960), 677-79.

34. Langton, C. V., and C. L. Anderson, *Health Principles and Practice*. St. Louis: The C. V. Mosby Company, 1957.

35. Levine, Myra, "Adaptation and Assessment: A Rationale for Nursing Intervention," *American Journal of Nursing*, 66: No. 11 (1966), 2450-53.

36. Luce, Gay Gaer, *Body Time*. New York: Random House, 1971.

37. Maslow, A. H., *Motivation and Personality*. New York: Harper & Row, Publishers, 1954.

38. Mellot, Marion, "Patient Teaching Program," in *Continuity of Patient Care: The Role of Nursing*, eds. K. Mary Straub and Kitty S. Parker. Washington, D.C.: The Catholic University of America Press, 1966.

39. Miller, Benjamin F., and Claire Brackmen Keane, *Encyclopedia and Dictionary of Medicine and Nursing*. Philadelphia: W. B. Saunders Company, 1972.

40. Murphy, Juanita F., ed., *Theoretical Issues in Professional Nursing*. New York: Appleton-Century-Crofts, 1971.

41. Murray, Ruth and Judith Zentner, *Nursing Assessment and Health Promotion through the Life Span*. Englewood Cliffs, N.J.: Prentice-Hall, Inc., 1975.

42. National Institute of Mental Health, *Biological Rhythms in Psychiatry and Medicine*. Washington, D.C.: United States Department of Health, Education, and Welfare, 1970.

43. Nordmark, Madelyn, and Anne W. Rohweder, *Scientific Foundations of Nursing*. Philadelphia: J. B. Lippincott Company, 1967.

44. Payne, Anthony, *Environmental Determinants of Community Well-being*. Washington, D.C.: Pan American Health Organization, 1965.

45. Price, Alice L., *The Art, Science, and Spirit of Nursing*. Philadelphia: W. B. Saunders Company, 1965.

46. Richter, Curt Paul, *Biological Clocks in Medicine and Psychiatry*. Springfield, Ill.: Charles C. Thomas, 1965.

47. Rogers, Edward S., *Human Ecology and Health: An Introduction for Administrators*. New York: The Macmillan Company, 1960.

48. Romano, John, "Basic Orientation and Education of the Medical Student," *Journal of the American Medical Association*, 143: No. 5 (1950), 411.

49. Smith, Louise C., "Continuity of Nursing Education," in *Continuity of Patient Care: The Role of Nursing*, eds. K. Mary Straub and Kitty S. Parker. Washington, D.C.: The Catholic University of America Press, 1966.

50. Snively, William Daniel, and Donna R. Beshear, *Textbook of Pathophysiology*. Philadelphia: J. B. Lippincott Company, 1972.

51. Stein, Jess, ed., *The Random House Dictionary of the English Language*. New York: Random House, Inc., 1971.

52. Sullivan, Harry S., *Conceptions of Modern Psychiatry*. New York: W. W. Norton & Company, Inc., 1953.

53. "The Plight of the U.S. Patient," *Time*, 93: No. 8 (February 21, 1969), 53-58.

54. Ward, Ritchie R., *The Living Clocks*. New York: Alfred A. Knopf, Inc., 1971.

55. Wheeler, Margaret, and Wesley Volk, *Basic Microbiology*. Philadelphia: J. B. Lippincott Company, 1964.

56. Wilson, Robert N., *The Sociology of Health: An Introduction*. New York: Random House, Inc., 1970.

57. Wu, Ruth, *Behavior and Illness*. Englewood Cliffs, N.J.: Prentice-Hall, Inc., 1973.

58. Yamamoto, William S., and John R. Brobeck, eds., *Physiological Controls and Regulators*. Philadelphia: W. B. Saunders Company, 1965.

CHAPTER 2

Delivery
of Health Care

Study of this chapter will help you to:

1 Describe General Systems Theory and explain how knowledge of this theory relates to the individual as well as to the American health care system.

2 Define *voluntary agencies* and *official agencies* and differentiate between them.

3 Describe the four divisions in the American health care system and how people use them.

4 List the characteristics of a medical quack and discuss how you can help people avoid the hazards of medical quackery.

5 Discuss characteristics of the American health care system, including the hospital as a subsystem, modes of financing care, and differing roles of health workers.

6 Describe factors influencing the delivery of health care and trends in care.

7 Discuss the nurse's role in primary health care.

8 Collaborate, through appropriate referral, with the personnel of voluntary or official agencies to promote continuity of care.

UNDERSTANDING HEALTH CARE SERVICES

In every culture, care of the sick is undertaken by specified persons with a certain status or background who carry out a set of culturally determined practices. The care is given within a system. A theory to help you understand how health care is given as well as the person for whom you are caring, his family, and his community is General Systems Theory. This theory advocates that probably nothing is determined by a single cause or explained by a single factor. Taking a holistic view of man, General Systems Theory instead suggests that interrelationships exist among all elements of a society, institution, situation, family, or organism. [51] .

Characteristics of a System

A system is an entity consisting of definable interdependent parts that are in equilibrium. Two or more people interacting together constitute a social system,—for example, nurse-patient-family or nurse-doctor. Systems have specific characteristics. Change in one part causes change in other parts. A constant *exchange of energy and information* must exist with the surrounding specified *environment* if the system is to be open, useful, and creative. If this information or energy exchange, called *feedback*, does not occur, the system becomes closed and ineffective.

A system is organized, or structured, formally or informally, through *principles, policies,* or *norms,* which in turn maintain balance and control, change, flow of information, and behavior of people. Roles exist for the members and may shift, blur, or remain stable. All systems exist for a *purpose* and to achieve certain *goals* [3, 4, 45, 51] . A person belongs to a system as long as it meets his needs. For example, the public school is formally organized to teach students certain skills and behavior that will help them become self-supporting citizens.

Man as a Social System

Every person is an open social system, made up physically of a hierarchy of components such as cells, organs, and organ systems; emotionally of levels of needs and feelings; and socially of a relative rank in a hierarchy of prestige, such as boss, peasant, adult, or child. While internal stimuli are at work, such as those governed by the nervous and endocrine systems, outer stimuli also affect man— for example, the feelings of others, or the external environment. The boundaries or environment—such as one's skin, the limits set by others, one's status, home, and community—influence the person's needs and goal achievement. To remain healthy, the person must have feedback: the condition of his skin tells him about temperature; an emotional reaction signifies a job well done or a failure; a pain signifies malfunction or injury.

Man is an open system, receiving stimuli from the outer world and in turn influencing that world through his behavior.

Other social systems composed of man are the family, the church, political institutions, and health care agencies.

The American Health Care System

Many patients and most health workers are currently challenging traditional American health care practices and demanding change. Present practices are inadequate for the needs of people in a pluralistic society. The present health care system is closed, controlled by medical physicians, and does not distribute services equitably. There is little interchange among doctors, other health care professionals, and health institutions or agencies, on one hand, and the person, family, and community on the other. Health workers other than doctors of medicine cannot function in an independent, open manner, and thus have to work around the system to provide the kinds of services the public deserves and expects. Presently medical doctors control entry into and the pathway through the health care system.

The present health care system is the result of certain unrelated, independent, and divergently developing health care programs, services, and facilities that have managed to survive and expand. In general, the system grew without a plan. And since the system is organized and coordinated to stabilize and maintain existing facilities, services, and related enterprises, it does not support change.

People seeking preventive services or medical care and the practitioners of medical care may be seen as two components of the social system, often with divergent and conflicting interests. The people component consists of those who may be called patients or clients. *Patients are ill and are primarily concerned with their symptoms and how they feel*, rather than with organic diseases per se. They seek a return to normal functioning rather than physiological health as defined by the doctor. *Clients are not necessarily ill and seek health care workers for services which either maintain or regain health.* Being a client implies active participation in the treatment plan. The patient as a component of the health care system is too often seen as a passive observer rather than as an active participant in his treatment or inward life. As an increasingly enlightened consumer of care, the client will change this outlook unless the system retaliates by becoming even more mechanized and repressive. The medical component, the doctor, is often interested in illness or disease rather than the illness experience or the full social consequences of physical symptoms. The nurse is the liaison person, attempting to understand each aspect when working with the patient.

What about the workers in the health care system? They usually are separated by status levels, each eating and socializing with his own occupational levels. The equivalent of a caste system exists. Communication generally moves downward, deference upward. The worker may or may not feel a part of a specific unit. He is likely to stay employed if he feels a similarity between his attitudes and the philosophy of the agency and if there are pleasant working relationships and conditions. If the worker feels himself to be an outsider, if his competency or skill is higher than the norm, or if the situation is changing too rapidly, he won't remain employed. Job turnover is also influenced less directly by marital status, age, presence of children, and job history.

A registered nurse, even though unemployed, is often looked to or called upon to intervene with friends or relatives. With no specified status, however, it is difficult to break into the caste system and communicate with the health care hierarchy. Consider the following experience of such a nurse.

A Case Study

Mrs. S., a 78-year-old woman without relatives, lives alone on $170 a month Social Security benefits, and recently became a concern to a nurse friend. Mrs. S., while maintaining limited mental ability, became depressed and increasingly forgetful. She often forgot day and time, lost her way several times in the city, forgot that she had turned on the gas stove, ate rotten food, took her medicine too often or not at all, and was twice the victim of vandals.

The nurse friend wished to help Mrs. S. find a living arrangement where she would receive adequate personal and medical care. She called various nursing homes whose representatives said Mrs. S. would need a medical doctor's statement for admittance. The nurse explained the circumstances to Mrs. S.'s doctor, who told her that the only way he could admit Mrs. S. to a nursing home was through Medicare benefits via hospitalization. He said he would give her a complete physical examination and have a psychiatrist and social worker evaluate her condition.

Mrs. S. entered a hospital reputed to be one of the top ten in the United States. After 26 days of hospitalization, a $2500 hospital bill, a $250 physician's bill, a $50 X-ray bill, and $120 in consultation fees, Mrs. S. was *discharged to her home.*

What had happened? Not much. The physician said Mrs. S. initially resisted the nursing home idea, so he didn't pursue the matter. The nurse spoke repeatedly to the doctor of her friend's dire need. Finally he agreed to get a social worker to examine the case. But before the social worker appeared (if she was ever notified), the hospital's Patient Review Committee (composed of physicians who review patients' records and who are empowered to decide which patients will go home or have Medicare benefits terminated) informed Mrs. S.'s physician that her benefits were being canceled.

Mrs. S.'s physician then said he would—and did—send a nurse and social worker from a local religious health organization, who were to assess her home situation and help her make the proper move.

The nurse friend and a neighbor continued to see Mrs. S., who was now more depressed and confused than ever. The nurse friend tried to help her organize her medicines, check her supplies, find her lost items, and pay her bills. The neighbor fed her and did her laundry. Several weeks elapsed with no further plans made. Finally, the nurse friend called the religious health organization to determine the status of the case. The organization nurse had not been given complete background information by the physician, and was only planning to see Mrs. S. on a bimonthly or monthly basis to give an injection.

The nurse friend then called Mrs. S.'s minister and the director of a neighborhood ministry for the aged. Both were aware of some of her problems but had no comprehension of the overall situation.

The health care system had not worked! Unless all persons concerned, even peripherally, can work together, Mrs. S. will eventually destroy herself or be destroyed.

TYPES OF HEALTH CARE SUBSYSTEMS

Today's health challenge is no longer based on survival, but on the quality of being. What is the method of organization that will best enhance the pursuit of and opportunity for optimal health and increased longevity? Understanding the types of present health care agencies and health workers can help determine the changes that are needed.

In America, health care is big business, exceeded only by agriculture and construction in terms of expenditures for services rendered and increase in proportion of the gross national product[36]. As a business, it is organized in a variety of ways, depending on the goals of the particular organization and whether or not planning is through governmental or voluntary efforts. *Governmental or official agencies are tax-supported and are operated by federal, state, or local governments. Private, voluntary agencies function under a board of directors and are supported by donations, fees, membership dues, endowments, payments from insurance plans, and contracts[16].*

Voluntary Agencies

Voluntary agencies historically emerged first and have flourished in the United States because of a democratic society coupled with aggressive, interested persons. At the turn of the nineteenth century only the American Red Cross and a few tuberculosis societies existed, other than some private hospitals. However, increased knowledge from scientific and medical discoveries coupled with economic growth from industrialization stimulated the growth of voluntary agencies. Because government-sponsored programs were sparse, people volunteered their newly found financial resources and time[16].

Early organizations (unrelated to hospitals) were formed because of concern about specific health problems, including tuberculosis, venereal disease, mental health, child care, and maternal mortality. Interest in health problems continued, and during the 1920s and 1930s voluntary organizations were initiated to control cancer, diabetes, and heart disease; to prevent blindness; and to provide for maternal and child health and crippled children.

Present Contributions of voluntary agencies are considerable. Some agencies are concerned with prevention, eradication, or control of certain diseases. They conduct educational programs to improve the utilization of health services. Such organizations include the National Tuberculosis Association, American Cancer Society, American Diabetes Association, and the American Heart Association. These organizations are also concerned about the care people receive within various health facilities. Some contribute to nursing care indirectly; for example, volunteers from the American Cancer Society make dressings and donate them for appropriate use.

Promotion of local health programs is another function of voluntary agencies, particularly foundations. The Ford, W. K. Kellogg, and Rockefeller Foundations, for example, subsidize health programs, especially in rural areas. They also support research and public and professional education[16].

Professional associations are voluntary. Their activities vary but generally include provision for exchange of information and ideas among health professionals through local, state, or national meetings and conventions; promotion of improved standards for the organization's constituencies; and encouragement of research. Some of these include the American Nurses' Association, American Public Health Association, and American Medical Association.

You should become familiar with your professional organization, the American Nurses' Association. It is primarily concerned with fostering high standards of nursing practice and works continually to improve the quality of nursing care. It also promotes educational advancement of nurses, advises on legal aspects of practice, and has a strong lobby in the nation's capital.

Other voluntary organizations contribute primarily to improved health services. These are the private and nonprofit organizations: hospitals, visiting-nurses' associations, health insurance organizations such as Blue Cross and Blue Shield, privately sponsored clinics, and those health professionals who are in private practice.

Voluntary groups are also involved in setting standards and evaluating existing programs. For example, the Joint Commission on Accreditation of Hospitals makes recommendations concerning care given by hospitals and nursing homes. It is authorized to close those that do not meet established standards. These voluntary groups may need to make frequent revisions in their standards or changes in their programs to keep up with the fast changes in health care in the United States. Ideally there should be no duplication of services between two or more voluntary agencies or between a voluntary and an official agency.

But overlap obviously exists in the present system, a fact which has given rise to fragmentation and agency-hopping for patients and clients.

Organization of many voluntary agencies operates on the national, state, and local levels. Usually, these agencies (with the exception of the professional associations) are governed by boards of directors comprised of people from all walks of life—business, industry, politics, the arts, and the professions—who are civic-minded and work without pay in this capacity.

At the national level, general policies and programs are developed and reviewed, positive public image and the agency's cause is stressed, and money is raised. State functions include long-range planning, fund raising, and giving stimulation and guidance to local affiliates about program planning and administration. The local level works with immediate needs, develops and implements community programs, and determines priorities.

Voluntary agencies have financial problems. They have been criticized for conducting numerous campaign drives and questioned about their spending of publicly raised funds. Furthermore, people hesitate to donate to voluntary agencies because they are already paying taxes for government health and welfare programs. Constructive collaboration at the national, state, and local levels among all voluntary agencies is needed. Their primary goal should be to enhance the appropriateness, quality, and efficiency of programs and services within the country.

Official Agencies

Official agencies began after numerous epidemics in the 1800s when people realized that government should be responsible for safeguarding the health of the public. The population of the cities was rapidly increasing, adding sanitation and health to the ever-growing list of problems.

Hookworm infestation was a mounting problem in North Carolina. The voluntary Rockefeller Foundation recognized that its efforts in this area to control a single disease without other health services was in vain. So, in 1911, a health department was established in Guilford County, North Carolina. Shortly thereafter, another department began operations, and the growth of official agencies has continued ever since [8].

Present Agency Contributions are determined by federal and state laws and are operated by federal, state, or local governments.

At the federal level, concern is for national and international health and the health of special population groups. Provisions are made for international meetings and exchange of research findings and of students with other countries. The federal government is responsible for protection against hazards affecting large populations, such as flood relief programs, which cannot be provided by the states. Federal support is given to state and local governments to maintain health services and civil defense programs. Another responsibility is the collection and reporting of national vital and health statistics. Special populations that the federal government is responsible for include armed forces personnel and veterans, the aged, the economically deprived, and the physically and mentally handicapped, among others [16].

Official state agencies are usually concerned with policy, planning, legislation, consultation to local agencies, indirect services, financial support, organizational relationships, research, and evaluation.

Local agencies provide direct services to the public, including medical care, preventive services, nursing services, and environmental control. Medical and preventive services include treatment of venereal disease and tuberculosis, maternity and well child care, interest in school health problems, and services for crippled children. Nurses usually make home visits and provide nursing care in clinics and schools. Environmental health services include sanitation control and inspection, housing and urban planning services, air pollution control, and food and drug control programs [16].

Social service, laboratory services, and health education are supportive services in state and local health departments.

Organization of official agencies begins with the United States Public Health Service, one of eight agencies within the Department of Health, Education, and Welfare. The Office of the Surgeon General is its main governing body.

Both state and local health departments have a health officer, a board of health, and various numbers of divisions or bureaus to conduct programs and services, with advisory committees and consultants as necessary.

The official agencies are also witnessing the public demand for increased and better health care. Citizens are tired of lengthy bureaucratic proceedings and political power plays for funding. Citizens must increasingly speak up for needed services and vote on the issues. More combining of official and voluntary agencies, or at least more communication among them, might lessen duplication and fragmentation of services.

Additionally, the United States is a part of the World Health Organization (WHO), created by the United Nations in 1948 with the conviction that international health, peace, and security are simultaneous goals [54]. More than 120 countries belong to WHO and contribute to its budget. As an international health system, WHO engages in many activities: health education, research, and publication; statistical services; standardization of drugs, vaccines, and other biologicals; development of international quarantine measures; and care of people during endemics and epidemics [16, 56].

The Hospital as a Subsystem

Whether official or voluntary, each hospital (or health care facility) is a subsystem which defines the various functions and skills necessary to maintain the institution and establishes its own kind of social organization through a system of roles and statuses. The hospital is a bureaucratic organization with a hierarchy from the board of trustees on down to the maintenance or housekeeping employee. Increasingly more administrative persons are joining the hierarchy to manage and maintain the growing number of parts within a facility. The general hospital, with the many levels of nonprofessional and professional personnel each having its own values and ideologies, may have ineffective channels of communication and patient care.

The hospital seems to have conflicting goals within itself. To stay financially solvent, it must strive for maximum efficiency. But to provide expert patient care, education, and research, it must have time and money. It needs expert professional judgment from those highly trained in medical skill, but also needs obedience from lesser-trained personnel who are also, indirectly or directly, responsible for life and death. Citizens require that the hospital meet their health needs, yet they cannot afford the spiraling cost of these services.

Obviously, for effective organization and provision for the best patient care, communication and some agreement among *all* working members is essential. Establishing goals, priorities, and methods of achievement is an ongoing process with need of constant revaluation. Hospitals could benefit from industry's plan of considering and rewarding workers' suggestions, whether from doctor or housekeeper.

Not only does the hospital have its own culture exhibited through policies, attitudes, and relationships among workers. Patients, too, if allowed to get acquainted with one another, may develop a subculture of their own which may or may not have much in common with the overall hospital culture. This subculture is seen particularly in psychiatric, rehabilitation, chronic care, and geriatric divisions.

Four Divisions in the Health Care System

In addition to voluntary and official health agencies within the health care system, four divisions of medical health care have been delineated in the United States: two subdivisions of private health care; the charity system (although many Americans may not like to admit the existence of such care); and health professionals (other than medical doctors) who provide special services[46].

Within the Private Division, One Subdivision Is the Pediatrician-Internist Services, utilized by the upper and upper middle classes. Primary care for the family with children is assumed mainly by two physicians, the internist and the pediatrician. Inpatient care is obtained in private or semiprivate rooms in voluntary hospitals.

The Other Subdivision in the Private Division Is Care by the General Practitioner, used by the lower middle class and skilled laborers. Primary care is received from a single physician, and specialist services may be provided by the general practitioner himself or by qualified specialists. Inpatient care is usually obtained in semiprivate rooms in voluntary hospitals. Such care may be the only choice in rural areas and small towns, and the difficulty in obtaining such health care at all is compounded by the reduced numbers of general practitioners in the United States. Physicians have increasingly felt either that becoming a specialist is more prestigious or that trends in the health care system demand specialization. Presently, however, some renewed emphasis is being given to the training of family physicians.

The Charity Division serves the unskilled or unemployed, their dependents, and the elderly poor. Primary care in this division is provided in hospital out-patient departments by interns and residents or by internists and pediatricians, who also usually provide the specialist services. Inpatient care is usually obtained in the wards of city, county, or voluntary hospitals.

The Fourth Division Includes Several Services for obtaining health care. These are health professionals, like the medical doctors (M.D.), who follow a prescribed course of education and supervised experience, and must adhere to continuously updated standards prescribed by their professional organizations. Persons using these services may also use the other health services just described and may be a member of any social class.

A *dentist (D.D.S.) cares for teeth and surrounding tissue*, prevents and eliminates decay, replaces missing teeth with artificial ones, and prevents malocclusion. A dentist may specialize in *orthodontics, the correction and prevention of irregularities of the teeth and poor occlusion*, or in *oral surgery, surgical procedures involving structures of the mouth or the teeth.*

A *chiropractor (D.C.) employs a method of mechanical therapeutics based on the nervous system as the main determiner of health.* He gives specific adjustments to restore normal nerve function and does not use drugs or surgery. He refers the patient to an internist or surgeon when indicated.

An *optometrist (O.D.) examines eyes, measures errors of vision, and prescribes glasses to correct defects.* He does not treat eye disease or perform eye surgery but refers patients needing such services to an *ophthalmologist, a medical doctor who specializes in treating structures, functions, and diseases of the eye.* An *optician prepares and dispenses eyeglasses.*

A *podiatrist (D.P.M.) cares for the feet, preventing and treating foot disorders*, such as corns and ingrown nails. He prescribes medicine and performs surgery for such disorders. He refers those cases indicated to an *orthopedist, a surgeon who specializes in treating deformities, diseases, and injuries of bones, joints, and muscles.*

An *osteopath (D.O.) employs various methods of diagnosis and treatment, including skeletal manipulation, medicine, and surgery.* His practice is similar to that of a medical doctor. Originally his philosophy specifically emphasized the interrelationship of the musculo-skeletal system to all other body systems.

The four divisions, even with some provision for charity patients, points to the obvious but unfortunate fact that more money buys better care. The charity subdivision is underfinanced and does not begin to provide adequate health services. That charity patients receive better health care than others is a myth. Morbidity and mortality statistics show a strong correlation between level of income, on the one hand, and health and longevity on the other[16].

Quackery within the Health Care System

Self-styled health workers and "quacks" are also offering services. The self-styled health worker may emphasize certain herbs for healing or a special "hand-me-down" formula. He does not rely on professionally set standards. A *quack, one who makes pretentious claims about his ability to treat others with little or no foundation*, may be found representing any health profession. He raises false hopes and causes loss of money and time—often money and time that could be better used for proven treatment.

Perhaps just as much to blame as the quacks are those people who incessantly want a shortcut—a sure cure. They almost beg someone in authority to give them *the* answer.

You can help people avoid quacks by helping them set realistic health goals and by helping them recognize the following typical behaviors of the false practitioner:

1. Claims use of a special or secret formula, diet, or machine.
2. Promises an easy or quick cure.
3. Offers only testimonials as proof of his healing power.
4. Claims one product or service is good for a variety of illnesses.
5. States he is ridiculed or persecuted by health professionals.
6. Promotes his product through faithhealers, door-to-door health advisors, or sensational ads.
7. Refuses to accept proven methods of research.
8. Claims his treatment is better than any prescribed by a physician.

Reexamine your knowledge about and attitude toward the givers of health care in the four divisions. Remember that people think in terms of having symptoms and eradicating them. If the latter takes place to their satisfaction, they will place their trust in the health care worker who was responsible for their improvement, regardless of his credentials. After assessment, you can support those who find improvement and refer those who are dissatisfed into another direction, if that dissatisfaction is based on realistic expectations.

Application of Systems Theory for Nursing

Appreciating the complexity and interrelationships of the people, social institutions, and organizations giving health care will enable you to understand your role in giving health care. As a nurse, you will have a twofold purpose: to adjust at times to the system as it exists, and at other times to work with people to produce necessary changes. Increasingly the public expects you to do the latter to meet their needs.

Systems theory takes the major responsibility for change from you as an individual person and recognizes the importance of the total situation in creating and maintaining problems that hinder change and are beyond the power of the individual to correct. Each aspect of life is so interrelated and people are so interdependent that one person, for example, the nurse, is unlikely to make much change in a situation unless she works with others and considers many factors.

Fundamental changes come from within the individual or system. They cannot be imposed from without, although an outsider can be an influence. The push for maintaining the status quo and the push for change exist simultaneously. If you strive for better conditions in a health agency, you may find that they can only be achieved by pressures for policy and administrative change on a high level. Through your educational preparation and experiences as a nurse you will be in a position to promote changes in the health care system.

As a member of various health, education, welfare, and regulatory agencies in the community, you may function in the health care system in the following ways:

1. As an advocate for the person or family needing health services.
2. As a concerned, active community member.
3. As an expert in health affairs.
4. As a consumer of health services.

If you understand and are comfortable in the health care system, you can work more effectively for furtherance of health. Community surveys, assessments, and demographic and epidemiologic studies are tools that will help you use the nursing process in the social system of the community and specific health agency.

Intervention on the systems level includes talking with the nursing supervisor, clinical specialist, or dietitian about cold food at mealtimes, or getting a wheelchair for a patient so he can get out of the confining four walls of his room. You may be instrumental in creating a patient council that has at least some effect on improving the environment of a unit. Outside the institution you can participate in starting organizations for older or disabled persons that help to meet their individual needs as well as have an impact on the political life of their community.

While you will not always strive for big institutional upheavals, also avoid accepting the present situation as an unalterable fact. Often when you have worked at the same place for some time, you adapt to distressing situations so that you do not even notice them, even though they cause considerable discomfort or suffering for the patient. Periodically survey your work environment as if you were a stranger to it. You might keep a diary of your reactions to the work setting when you are first employed and then refer to it periodically to determine changes you wish to initiate. In that way you can better work as your patients' advocate.

You may not always be able to make constructive changes in the system. Some changes take longer than others, but you need to keep trying. Often an idea must be proposed several times before it gains acceptance by others.

MANPOWER IN THE HEALTH CARE SYSTEM

There appears to be a shortage of medical physicians, nurses, and other professional and nonprofessional health personnel in the United States today. However, measuring the full extent of the problem is difficult since manpower is unevenly distributed and inefficiently utilized, owing to lack of full cooperation among all health disciplines.

Medical Physicians

The number of physicians has increased in the last decade. Yet the increased number of physicians does not adequately meet the needs of the population because physicians tend to specialize, to concentrate on research, to remain in urban centers to practice, or to become full-time hospital staff with less time for office visits.

Physicians have increased their use of auxiliary personnel, the newest being physicians' assistants. The idea for such a person arose in response to the continuing problem of providing adequate medical services in nonurban areas of the United States. Some former military medical corpsmen have been trained as physicians' assistants. Their allegiance is to the physician they serve, and they may work in a clinic or hospital or assist the physician in his office practice or research. Some health professionals fear that physicians' assistants will usurp their jobs. Further concern is that they will not have adequate training and ability. Both professional and lay people will need further orientation about the functions of physicians' assistants, and certain safeguards need to be established to ensure their proper supervision and competency.

Nurses and Other Professionals

Nurses. The number of nurses has also increased over the past ten years, but this increase has not kept pace with the increasing demand for health services either[1]. There is an uneven distribution of nurses among the population, as well as limited opportunities for the professional nurse to fully use individual abilities, education, and skills. There are adequate numbers of technical and licensed practical nurses, while an inadequate number of nurses are prepared with baccalaureate, master's, and doctoral degrees.

Every nurse should examine his or her level of preparation for and role within the system for delivering health care to delineate more clearly the characteristics and qualifications needed for each level of prepared nurse. Transition from one level of preparation to another is increasingly available to nursing practitioners to allow preparation for clinical specialization, research, and family care positions[1].

With the movement toward improved health care for all, nursing needs dynamic leaders to help change the delivery system and to create and shape the character of nursing within the system. Nurses have moved away from complete dominance by the medical doctors. Yet they have not established themselves as a permanent force in the fourth system—as professionals from whom persons seek primary diagnosis and care. This trend is gaining impetus, however.

Other Professionals who perform important services in the health care system are the psychologist, chaplain, social worker, occupational therapist, physiotherapist, medical and X-ray technologist, dietitian, medical record librarian, and pharmacist, among others. Each member of the health team makes an important contribution to the well-being of the patient or family unit.

MODES OF FINANCING MEDICAL CARE

An increase in the numbers of subscriptions to various hospital and health plans has contributed to the increasing demand for medical care and the use of health facilities. However, the rise in the cost of living, including the cost of medical care and use of hospital facilities, has exceeded the ability of many people to pay, especially those in the middle-income range[47].

Some of the cost escalation has been expected. Inadequately paid hospital employees deserve better pay. Increased technology has provided more complex and costly equipment, along with the need for trained personnel to operate it. Finally, there are more aged persons in the population, and the prevalence of illness increases with age[46].

Often the person, no matter how ill, cannot be admitted to the hospital unless he has health insurance or can make a down payment of several hundred dollars. Workmen's compensation and private or government health insurance help defray medical costs.

Health insurance companies influence the health care system. In the past, most companies paid only for hospital care, thus encouraging people to enter hospitals for procedures or care which could have been accomplished on an outpatient basis. Thus the hospital subsystem expanded considerably. Today, more insurance policies cover outpatient costs, but other pressures are applied.

Insurance companies have special agents who investigate health benefit claims. Benefits are sometimes withheld until a special review board determines that treatment was necessary.

Privately Sponsored Health Insurance

Health insurance is a method for financing personal health service, but some plans are not adequate in the scope of services covered. One must read the fine print carefully when examining an insurance policy. The American public purchases health insurance from approximately 1800 organizations.

Blue Cross and Blue Shield are perhaps most frequently thought of when referring to insurance plans. Blue Cross pays for most of the cost of hospitalization; Blue Shield pays for physician's care.

Major Medical Plans are a recent addition to health insurance provisions. They may be supplemental to basic health insurance or may be the only coverage a person has. Such plans pay for hospitalization, physician's services, drugs, nursing care, and other related items. Most of these plans have reciprocal arrangements in that the insurance company will pay either the people and institutions giving care or the insured.

Indemnity Plans are offered at reduced rates which are determined by the cost of actual loss experience in past years to the group at risk. Premium rates are thus related to actual use of insurance. This plan might discourage over-utilization of insurance but also might keep the person from seeking early diagnosis and preventive health care to avoid using his insurance and increasing his rates. Predetermined benefits are paid to the insured in cash and he must pay for the remaining costs, another reason to delay care [44].

Independent Health Plans are another type of private insurance. These plans combine prepayment for medical care with *group practice, where a number of specialists work together in association, sometimes providing care to patients and families at a fixed annual rate.* Insured persons utilize the medical staff who are in the group practice and the specific facilities provided by the medical group and insurance company. Costs are spread among members over a period of time, and the total cost of medical care—prevention, cure, and rehabilitation—are included in the benefits. Disadvantages are that such plans are not available to people in all areas, reciprocal arrangements have not been completely worked out, and the insured must use the physicians and facilities affiliated with the plan [44]. Advantages are that independent companies watch closely the type of medical care rendered to their insured; the trend is thus toward decreased hospitalization, since preventive health measures are stressed [16]. The medical profession has not been too receptive to such plans, but recently some of the leading medical schools—Harvard, Yale, and Johns Hopkins—have started group practice prepayment plans [46].

Government-Sponsored Health Insurance

Medicare and Medicaid are federally sponsored insurance plans, the latter financed by federal and state matching funds. In 1965, Congress passed Title XVIII—Medicare—as an amendment to the Social Security Act for persons 65 and older. Medicaid (Title XIX) is a medical care program for all those declared eligible for public assistance by individual states, including the blind, those receiving Old-Age Assistance benefits, families with dependent children (ADC), and the permanently and totally disabled. If your patient is on public assistance, check whether or not he has a Medicaid card. If he does not, consult a social worker. Medicare and Medicaid are further discussed by Murray and Zentner in relation to the person in later maturity[38].

Workmen's Compensation

State workmen's compensation plans make legal provision for treating and rehabilitating workers injured on the job. The injury must be caused by the nature of the job itself, not by obvious negligence on the part of the employer or the worker. This requirement makes both employer and employee assume some responsibility for safety. For example, a mine cave-in would result in compensation for injuries to the victims. Laws related to workmen's compensation are continually being examined to determine that the worker and employer are being fair to one another and that the worker is receiving deserved benefits. As an occupational health nurse, you would be responsible for reporting job-related injuries and assuring that workers received proper compensation. In addition, you would work with management and labor to promote safe working conditions.

Projected Health Plans

The needs revealed by studies of Medicare and Medicaid payments along with other factors indicate that the delivery of health care must be improved. Medicaid has not begun to meet the needs of the medically indigent, and Medicare costs keep mounting for the federal government. Yet almost 46 percent of the population are either under 18 or over 65 years old and therefore need assistance with medical care costs because they are frequent users of health services[12].

Alternative health care plans that have been suggested include a national health service and health maintenance organizations (prepaid group practice).

Health Maintenance Organizations (HMOs), operative in some areas in the United States, are discussed in the section on current trends influencing the delivery of health care.

National Health Insurance is the payment method in several European countries and Great Britian. Various national plans have been proposed by politicians and organizations in the United States since the 1920s, but none has been adopted. Each suggested plan has certain distinct features, but some similarities do exist. Taxation, based on income and with a maximum ceiling, would pay for part of the insurance, while the consumer would directly pay the balance of medical care costs. Care for mental illness, dental care, long-term hospital care, and preventive services are generally excluded by these plans.

National health insurance still does not solve the problems of fragmentation of care, of proportionately greater payment by people with lower incomes, and of the need for preventive and comprehensive health services.

FACTORS INFLUENCING
THE DELIVERY OF HEALTH CARE

Social Changes

If, as estimated, 245 million people will be living in the United States by 1980, health care opportunity must increase. The birth rate has declined in the past decade, while the death rate has remained constant; yet the excess of births over deaths is still substantial[55]. Because people are living longer and thus are more likely to develop chronic disease problems, more and more people will need the services of better prepared doctors, nurses, allied health personnel, and service agencies. Technological advances in medical care have caused care to be increasingly fragmented and given more in hospital centers rather than at home or in the local community. However, these same advances, along with medical research, have permitted efficient and effective care and recoveries not possible in the past, in turn contributing to longer life spans and a growing population.

Consumer Involvement

Because of a growing belief that health and the services needed to maintain it are everyone's basic right, Americans now have higher health care expectations, which are being incorporated into their value system.

> The public has come to expect the right: to wellness; to receive adequate and qualified health care; to participate in decisions regarding their care; to be helped to understand their health and illness as well as the treatments undertaken in their behalf; to be cared for with concern when they are ill; to be accepted in a state of dependence when they are unable to care for themselves; to be kept as comfortable as modern science permits; to decline and die in reasonable dignity; to feel that someone cares and that they are not alone in their illness or dying[29].

Generally, the public is more health-conscious and knowledgeable about the nature of health, health care, and illness because such information is more readily available in schools, in popular literature, and on television. Along with increasing knowledge and sophistication is a tendency for the person to become more critical about his care (or lack of it) and to want to actively participate in planning his care. The practice of being "spoken for" is no longer accepted. To the shame of health professionals, legislative efforts were required to initiate consumer input into the health care system—through programs like neighborhood health centers, Model Cities, and comprehensive health planning that have consumer representatives on policy-making and planning boards[26].

One nursing organization, the National League for Nursing, includes consumers in its membership and on its advisory councils and works to improve health care delivery as well as the education of nurses.

Professional Response

Professional groups, including nurses, have responded and must continue to respond to the public's health care needs, rights, and expectations. Nursing has become aware of a broader spectrum of patient problems; trends in nursing education favor increased competence in perceiving care problems and better care planning. Nursing has determined that one of its roles is the coordination of health services because so many personnel, professional and nonprofessional, are utilized in providing patient care. Moreover, systematically identifying, analyzing, and planning the patient's nursing care needs along with the patient and family require the expertise of a professionally competent nurse.

Legislative Interest

Over the past decade Congress has exhibited a growing interest in health affairs. Legislators have been concerned about closing the gap between the knowledge people are acquiring and the care they are receiving. The Eighty-ninth Congress (1965-1967) was especially notable in this regard in that it passed 24 health or health-related bills[18].

Congress has attempted to encourage regional and comprehensive approaches to health care, with continued emphasis on planning and consumer involvement. Because some persons feel that the federal government should take a more active part in health care, pressure is continuously exerted for some type of national health insurance plan.

Nurses, individually and through membership in the nursing organizations, have lobbied and must continue to lobby for legislation that will assist the public in getting maximum health care.

Comprehensive Health Planning

As the concern about health problems and the delivery of health care increased during the 1960s, comprehensive health planning, enacted through federal legislation, had its origin. Federal grants, distributed to various designated state agencies, were the source of funding for the project. Certain stipulations were attached to the federal grants: (1) that a single state agency take responsibility for the grant, and (2) that a state planning council be established that included representatives from local and state governmental units and other agencies concerned about health and the consumer[12].

Nurses should be included as members of national, state, and local planning boards and advisory councils and active as citizens in promoting health standards.

If you discover a patient or family problem, regardless of your position or care setting, you can take positive action. Perhaps no organizational source of help exists, or a present source may be unable to meet the needs of the persons in question. What would you do? Your combination of creative ability and practical working knowledge can develop a program to meet the specific need. The following are proper steps to take should you find yourself in a position to make changes in organizational sources of help, and as a nurse in the primary care role you may indeed be in such a position.

Be very specific in identifying the problem. An epidemiological study may be needed. Note the number of people who are affected. If only a few isolated people are affected, redirect your plans to meet their needs within the existing care system. Once the problem is identified and found significant, write out the proposed solutions. Involve your supervisor throughout; perhaps that person can help you find unknown resources. Think about attaching the proposed program to one that already exists. If attachment is possible, costs can be cut drastically. Whatever your course—attachment or creation of a new program—inform your agency about your plans and ask for its support.

You are now ready to begin convincing others in the community that a new program is needed. Begin with the power structure of the community—the people known for "getting things done." Select people from various occupations and professions; get a cross section of the community. Visit each personally and ask for his advice, suggestions, and support. Get permission to mention the names of those who react positively when discussing the proposed program with others.

Plan the first group meeting. Invite those people with whom you spoke plus a variety of others from the community. Continue to look for support from valuable individuals or organizations. Don't forget the consumer! At the meeting, present your proposal verbally as well as distribute a written outline. A temporary chairman and interim steering committee need to be elected. The purpose of the committee is to review the proposed program in its entirety, determine cost details and ways to funding, investigate whether it is necessary to develop a new agency or if an existing one can be utilized, and, finally, prepare a written report of the findings.

At the second group meeting the findings of the steering committee are presented. A permanent board of directors should be elected. All involved people not on the board should be on the advisory council. The board is responsible for making policies, adopting bylaws, and writing a formal, detailed program proposal, including job descriptions of needed staff and facilities. The board must be prepared to state how the program will be financed if and when federal or state funds are discontinued. It should also solicit letters of commitment from organizations and agencies that will give free services. Program proposals may need to be written several times to meet particular funding requirements. Many meetings may be necessary to achieve your goal[56].

Convincing people that a new program is needed may take determination and fortitude. While keeping your goal in mind, you will constantly integrate new ideas that may change your direction somewhat. Worthwhile programs are created through this difficult process, but time and effort are needed. Such action is an extension of the nursing process described in Chapter 4.

Fragmentation of Health Care Services

Despite the growing interest and efforts of interested people, the health care system is still fragmented. People receive bits of treatment from various people and places. A given person may utilize a family doctor and several specialists, attend different hospitals for different purposes, maintain a number of insurers (or have no insurance), and rely on many health or health-related agencies. Not only is this pattern expensive, it also encourages duplication of services. No one assumes sole responsibility for the health of the person. Many times different health workers involved in giving care have no idea what the others are doing. When no single worker has a total picture of a person, the latter cannot receive comprehensive individualized care.

CURRENT AND FUTURE TRENDS
IN DELIVERY OF HEALTH CARE

Primary Health Care

Primary health care is a relatively new concept designed to provide comprehensive health services to a family. These include physical and psychological preventive, maintenance, and restorative services; general dental services; and sources for help related to social, economic, legal, and environmental problems. Care is individualized in order to prevent crises as best possible. The family has a long-term relationship with a small group of professionals who work closely with the family members and involve them in their own care. Ideally, primary health care settings are conveniently located, near or within the community being served, compatible with the life styles of the people served, and have some provision for 24-hour availability for emergencies[6].

The overall purposes of primary health care are to make care more accessible and equitable and to improve the quality of care delivered. The plan updates the family doctor concept with modern-day support services, in the form of specialists and technology, available on a continuing basis to a specific group of people.

Health Maintenance Organizations

A health maintenance organization (HMO) is a system for delivering primary health care with emphasis on adequate distribution and quality. If such a concept continues to be properly developed, it could drastically reduce the fragmentation, gaps, and duplication of the present system[35].

An HMO is designed to provide comprehensive health care for the whole person in its own ambulatory and inpatient care facilities. Financing is achieved by a fixed contract fee paid by subscribers each month, regardless of the number of times they use the services (or if they never use them). The plan encourages effective, personal treatment, and subscribers are likely to use the facility for preventive measures and to seek early treatment. The addition of hospital beds and the employment of too many specialists are discouraged, since health personnel and facilities are acquired according to the number enrolled in the HMO program, rather then according to the long-range projection of health care needs in the community. The goal is to give the best and most health care for the money available.

Designers of HMOs leave open the question of specific organizational form. They hope to encourage all kinds of organizational forms—public and private, profit and nonprofit. The consumer will be able to choose the type and level of health care he wishes. Competition will exist; those unhappy will leave if there is another available choice. Thus the HMO will be encouraged to establish and maintain a good reputation.

Problems have been cited with HMOs, and solutions have not been formulated. Cost competition could lead to a reduction in necessary care and hence a loss in quality of care. Physicians could determine their own fees, which would influence the corporate fee that the consumer pays monthly. Coexistence of two forms of practice within one organization could occur, one in the fee-for-service sector and another for those under the corporate fee[9].

HMOs are a threat to the individual practitioner. Under an HMO, the primary person responsible for an individual or family may not always be a physician, but may be a nurse or other health professional, depending on the needs of the person.

Nurses continue to constitute the largest group of health professionals and thus play a major role in all aspects of health care. In fact, nurses are currently functioning as the primary health care person in HMOs. They are defining problems, assessing needs, implementing and coordinating health care, educating patients and coworkers, and evaluating results. (These functions are discussed further in Chapters 4 and 5.) In general, nurses assume major responsibility for providing or securing all required primary health services. They are not substitute physicians or physicians' assistants. The nurses' functions are variously independent of, interdependent with, and dependent on those of other health team members[6].

Independent functions are performed legally, with the nurse being accountable for professional actions. Examples include health care coordination and implementation for a person with a stable chronic illness; complete history and physical assessment for well babies and adults; family planning counseling, health education, and patient counseling; and laboratory- and other diagnostic-test selection in illness situations. Interdependent functions, performed simultaneously with other members of the health team, include deciding whether to place patients in nursing homes or to maintain home care; planning for patient care with physicians; and dietary planning with nutritionists. Dependent functions are performed under the immediate supervision and guidance of physicians or other professionals. These functions include medical diagnosis; history and physical examination on an acutely ill or unstable chronically ill patient; psychotherapy and family counseling for patients with emotional or behavioral disorders; and performance of minor surgical procedures, such as uncomplicated suturing[6].

If nursing is to assume a major role in primary health care, more nurses must be graduated from baccalaureate programs that provide education and opportunity for clinical practice of the skills necessary to become a primary-care practitioner. More emphasis must be placed on such practitioners in planning for future health care delivery. Nurses can and should carry more responsibility than they have in the past, assuming they receive the necessary preparation. The nurse-practitioner is no longer a title for the future[21].

Directions for the Future

Exciting concepts and proposals are being discussed and enacted. Speculating about the outcome is difficult, but many hope for the development of an open system.

An open health care system would offer the client a choice of services from several health disciplines, not only physician services. He might not need to see a doctor at all if a nurse, social worker, physiotherapist, or nutritionist could effectively handle his problem. The person would get prompt care, possibly at less cost, without fragmentation and redundancy of services. The various health professionals would be fully contributing their skills and would be responsible to the client and accountable for their services, whether provided independently or in collaboration with other disciplines. The system would remain responsive to change. There would be an exchange of ideas among all health disciplines as well as consumer input. Consumer demand will hasten realization of this open system, although third-party insurance payments will have to be revised to accommodate the change.

Innovative health care models are few to date, but some suggestions for changes in the present health care system are:

1. Separating the well from the sick, using a multihealth screening plan to meet specific needs of clients.
2. Using interdisciplinary teams, including generalists, specialists, and the judicious use of paraprofessional workers.

3. Considering the cultural, social, psychological, and physiological aspects of the person.
4. Avoiding care that is hospital-based and physician-controlled, and instead delivering care in the community and focusing on the individual, wellness-behavior, and on ways to maintain or restore a healthy state.
5. Using health screening, health education, counseling, and referral more deliberately.
6. Encouraging health personnel to assume personal responsibility for their decisions and actions.
7. Encouraging social and natural scientists, humanists, health professionals, and consumers to become active participants in planning and evaluating care, distributing authority, and control.
8. Increasing emphasis on group approaches and on demographic planning in order to maximize individual potential and health-care services.
9. Avoiding hasty planning that creates situations demanding easy, quick, final answers and leads to abandoning problems too soon when immediate results are not forthcoming. Epidemiological data and scientific problem solving will help prevent the tendency to rely on such fast, unrealistic answers[5, 15, 27].

Some nurses are presently helping to create an open system of care by working as independent practitioners, performing many of the functions described as nursing roles in relation to HMOs but establishing their own offices or facilities for nursing practice. [For further information, see references 7, 24, 25, 30, 37, 41, 53.]

Changes must occur in order to build an open health care system, and health professionals, among others, must change to meet needs of the client. Educational preparation will have to include greater interdisciplinary study, increased understanding of and responsibility for primary care, and increased skill in caring for people of all ages and backgrounds. The rest of this text and its companion text[38] deal with the educational foundation needed to practice in such an open system.

REFERENCES

1. Armiger, Sister Bernadette, "Nursing Shortage—Or Unemployment?" *Nursing Outlook*, 21: No. 5 (1973), 312-16.
2. Bates, Barbara, "Nursing in a Health Maintenance Organization: Report on the Harvard Community Health Plan," *American Journal of Public Health*, 62: No. 7 (1972), 991-94.
3. Bell, Earl, *Social Foundations of Human Behavior*. New York: Harper & Row, Publishers, 1961.

4. Berrien, F. Kenneth, *General and Social Systems*. New Brunswick, N.J.: Rutgers University Press, 1968.

5. Brill, Naomi, *Working With People: The Helping Process*. Philadelphia: J. B. Lippincott Company, 1973.

6. Brunetto, Eleanor, and Peter Birk, "The Primary Care Nurse: The Generalist in a Structured Health Care Team," *American Journal of Public Health*, 62: No. 6 (1972), 785-94.

7. Burgess, Ann, and J. Burns, "Why Patients Seek Care," *American Journal of Nursing*, 73: No. 2 (1973), 314-16.

8. Coulter, Pearl, *The Nurse in the Public Health Program*. New York: G. P. Putnams' Sons, 1954.

9. Donabedian, Avedis, "An Examination of Some Directions in Health Care Policy," *American Journal of Public Health*, 63: No. 3 (1973), 243-46.

10. "Extending The Scope of Nursing Practice," *Nursing Outlook*, 20: No. 1 (1972), 46-47.

11. Fagin, Claire, and Beatrice Goodwin, "Baccalaureate Preparation for Primary Care," *Nursing Outlook*, 20: No. 4 (1972), 240-44.

12. Freeman, Ruth B., *Community Health Nursing Practice*. Philadelphia: W. B. Saunders Company, 1970, pp. 1-30, 74-108.

13. French, Ruth, *The Dynamics of Health Care*. St. Louis: McGraw-Hill Book Company, 1968.

14. Froh, R., and R. Galanter, "The Poor, Health, and the Law," *American Journal of Public Health*, 62: No. 3 (1972), 427-30.

15. Garfield, S. R., "The Delivery of Medical Care," *Scientific American*, 222: No. 4 (1970), 15-23.

16. Goerke, Lenor, and Ernest Stebbins, *Mustard's Introduction to Public Health* (5th ed.). New York: The Macmillan Company, 1968, pp. 43-80, 131-67, 436-60.

17. Greenidge, Jocelyn, Ann Zimmern, and Mary Kohnke, "Independent Group Nursing Practice: Community Nurse Practitioners—A Partnership," *Nursing Outlook*, 21: No. 4 (1973), 228-31.

18. Hanlon, John, *Principles of Public Health Administration*. St. Louis: C. V. Mosby Company, 1969.

19. Hazzard, Mary, "A Systems Approach to Nursing," *Nursing Clinics of North America*, 6: No. 3 (1971), 383-455.

20. Hulka, Barbara, and John Cassel, "The AAFP-UNC Study of the Organization, Utilization, and Assessment of Primary Medical Care," *American Journal of Public Health*, 63: No. 6 (1973), 494-501.

21. Ingles, Thelma, "Where Do Nurses Fit in the Delivery of Health Care?" *Archives of Internal Medicine*, 127: No. 1 (1971), 73-75.

22. Keller, Nancy, "The Nurse's Role: Is It Expanding or Shrinking?" *Nursing Outlook*, 21: No. 4 (1973), 236-40.

23. King, Imogene, *Towards a Theory For Nursing*. New York: John Wiley & Sons, Inc., 1971.

24. Kinlein, M. Lucille, "Independent Nurse Practitioner," *Nursing Outlook*, 20: No. 1 (1972), 22-24.

25. Kosik, S., "Patient Advocacy, or Fighting the System," *American Journal of Nursing*, 72: No. 4 (1972), 694-98.

26. Kramer, Marlene, "The Consumer's Influence on Health Care," *Nursing Outlook*, 20: No. 9 (1972), 574-78.

27. Leininger, Madeline, "An Open Health Care System Model," *Nursing Outlook*, 21: No. 3 (1973), 171-75.

28. Litman, Theodor, "Public Perceptions of the Physician's Assistant: A Survey of the Attitudes and Opinions of Rural Iowa and Minnesota Residents," *American Journal of Public Health*, 62: No. 3 (1972), 343-46.

29. Little, Delores, and Doris Carnevali, *Nursing Care Planning*. Philadelphia: J. B. Lippincott Company, 1969.

30. Logsdon, Audrey, "Why Primary Nursing?" *Nursing Clinics of North America*, 8: No. 2 (1973), 283-86.

31. Lynaugh, Joan, and B. Bates, "The Two Languages of Nursing and Medicine," *American Journal of Nursing*, 73: No. 1 (1973), 66-69.

32. Manor, Gloria, "The Berkeley Free Clinic," *Nursing Outlook*, 21: No. 1 (1973), 40-43.

33. Manthey, Marie, "Primary Care Is Alive and Well in the Hospital," *American Journal of Nursing*, 73: No. 1 (1973), 83-87.

34. Marram, Gwen, "Patients' Evaluation of Their Care: Importance to the Nurse," *Nursing Outlook*, 21: No. 5 (1973), 322-24.

35. McClure, Walter, "National Health Insurance and HMOS," *Nursing Outlook*, 21: No. 1 (1973), 44-48.

36. McNerney, W. J., "Personal Health Comprehensive Care Services: A Management Challenge to the Health Professions," *American Journal of Public Health*, 57: No. 10 (1967), 1717-27.

37. Murray, B. Louise, "A Case for Independent Group Nursing Practice," *Nursing Outlook*, 20: No. 1 (1972), 60-63.

38. Murray, Ruth, and Judith Zentner, *Nursing Assessment and Health Promotion through the Life Span*. Englewood Cliffs, N.J.: Prentice-Hall, Inc., 1975.

39. Nehring, Virginia, and Barbara Geach, "Patients' Evaluation of Their Care: Why They Don't Complain," *Nursing Outlook*, 21: No. 5 (1973), 317-21.

40. Paige, David, Edwardo Leonardo, Eve Roberts, and George Graham, "Enhancing the Effectiveness of Allied Health Workers," *American Journal of Public Health*, 62: No. 3 (1972), 370-73.

41. Rafferty, Rita, and Jean Carner, "Independent Group Nursing Practice: Nursing Consultants, Inc.—A Corporation," *Nursing Outlook*, 21: No. 4 (1973), 232-35.

42. Record, Jane, and Harold Cohen, "The Introduction of Midwifery in a Prepaid Group Practice," *American Journal of Public Health*, 62: No. 3 (1972), 354-60.

43. *Report of the National Advisory Commission on Health Manpower*, Vol. 1. Washington, D.C.: U. S. Government Printing Office, November 1967.

44. Report of the National Commission on Community Health Services, *Health is a Community Affair*. Cambridge, Mass.: Harvard University Press, 1967.

45. Sutterly, Doris, and Gloria Donnelly, *Perspectives in Human Development*. Philadelphia: J. B. Lippincott Company, 1973, pp. 3-24.

46. Terris, Milton, "Crisis and Change in America's Health System," *American Journal of Public Health*, 63: No. 4 (1973), 312-17.

47. "The Plight of the U.S. Patient," *Time*, February 21, 1965, pp. 53-58.

48. Tinkham, Catherine, and Eleanor Voorhies, *Community Health Nursing, Evolution and Process*. New York: Appleton-Century-Crofts, Educational Division, Meredith Corporation, 1972.

49. United States Department of Commerce, Bureau of the Census, *Pocket Data Book, USA, 1967*. Washington, D.C.: U. S. Government Printing Office, 1967.

50. United States Department of Health, Education, and Welfare, *Health, Education, and Welfare Trends, 1965*. Washington, D.C.: U. S. Government Printing Office, 1967.

51. von Bertalanffy, Ludwig, *General System Theory*. New York: George Braziller, 1968.

52. Wagner, Dorris L., "Issues in the Provision of Health Care for All," *American Journal of Public Health*, 63: No. 6 (1973), 481-85.

53. Walker, A., "PRIMEX: The Family Nurse Practitioner," *Nursing Outlook*, 20: No. 1 (1972), 28-31.

54. Walsh, Margaret, "On Nursing's Role in Health Care Delivery," *Nursing Outlook*, 20: No. 9 (1972), 592-93.

55. Wilner, Daniel, Rosabelle Walkley, and Lenor Goerke, *Introduction to Public Health* (6th ed.). New York: The Macmillan Company, 1973.

56. World Health Organization, *The First Year of the WHO*. Geneva: The World Health Organization, 1958.

57. Yankauer, Alfred, Sally Tripp, Priscilla Andrews, and John P. Connelly, "The Outcomes and Service Impact of a Pediatric Nurse Practitioner Training Program: Nurse Practitioner Training Outcomes," *American Journal of Public Health*, 62: No. 3 (1972), 347-53.

58. Zentner, Reid, personal directives on project establishment, May 1973.

CHAPTER 3

Therapeutic Communication: Prerequisite for Effective Nursing

Study of this chapter will enable you to:

1 Define *communication* and describe the elements in the communication process.

2 Identify the levels of communication and use this knowledge in nursing.

3 List and describe the tools used in communication.

4 State the definition of an interview and list its purposes.

5 List and discuss interviewing methods.

6 Interview a person, well or ill, using the correct methods, and analyze the effectiveness of the interview.

7 List and describe methods of therapeutic communication and the rationale for each method.

8 Practice therapeutic communication with a patient and analyze the pattern of communication, using knowledge of rationale.

9 Discuss barriers to and ineffective methods of communication, identify personal use of these, and analyze why they are ineffective.

10 Explore how use of effective communication methods is basic to nursing care and contributes to health.

> My Spanish friend looked puzzled when I said, "Let's keep in touch." I meant, "Let's talk to each other periodically."
>
> He heard the literal meaning. Often we don't communicate because we use words symbolically rather than literally, as further illustrated by the following statement:
>
> "I know you believe you understand what you think I said, but I am not sure you realize what you heard is not what I meant."—Anonymous

The ability to communicate should not be taken for granted; it is not a simple process but rather a complex means by which the world's work gets done.

Communication is the matrix for all thought and relationships between persons and is bound to the learning process. Early sensory experiences shape subsequent learning abilities in speech, cognition, symbol recognition, and in the capacity for maturing communication. Perception of the self, the world, and one's place in it results from communication. Verbal and nonverbal communication is learned in a cultural setting, and if the person does not communicate in the way prescribed by his culture, many difficulties arise, for he cannot conform to the expectations of society. Disordered thinking, feeling, and actions result, along with mental anguish, and perhaps even physical illness.

Communication is the heart of the nursing process, since it is one of the primary methods used to accomplish specific and general goals with many different kinds of people. It is used in assessing and understanding the patient and family as well as in nursing intervention. Communication helps people express thoughts and feelings, clarify problems, receive information, consider alternate ways of coping or adapting, and remain realistic through feedback from the environment. Essentially the patient learns something about the self, how to identify health needs, and if and how he wishes to meet them.

DEFINITIONS

The word *communication* comes from the Latin verb *communicare*, "to make common, share, participate, or impart." *Communication establishes a sense of commonness with another and permits the sharing of information, signals, or messages in the form of ideas and feelings.* A series of messages exchanged between persons forms an interchange or communication[30]. Communication is a continuous dynamic process by which one mind may affect another through written or oral language, gestures, facial expressions, music, painting, sculpture, drama, dance, or other signs.

Communication pattern refers to the relatively consistent network of messages sent and received in short- or long-term exchanges, the habitual way of interacting with others. Part of this pattern is the **social amenities pattern**, the interaction that uses socially prescribed rules, ceremonies, or customs according to the situation and usually results in superficial communication. The social pattern includes **small talk**, social chitchat that encompasses mundane topics and is used to kill time, to test the reactions of others, to avoid involvement, or to serve as a bridge to significant conversation. The **information pattern** differs in that it involves a request for or giving of information or orders but is not likely to establish intimate understandings because there is little disclosure of self. Neither the social nor the informational pattern is adequate by itself in the nursing process. The communication pattern in the nurse-patient-family relationship should be a **dialogue**, involving *purposeful, reciprocal, close expression between the participants* and focusing on the here-and-now problems of the one seeking help rather than on the helper. Yet there should be an openness which contributes to the growth of all participants involved[66].

THE COMMUNICATION PROCESS

Every communication process includes a sender, a transmitting device, signals, a receiver, and feedback, as shown in Figure 3-1. The sender attempts to convey a message, idea, or information through the appropriate use of symbols or signals directed to another specific person or group. That the message is sent does not guarantee that it will be received at all, let alone by the person for whom it is intended.

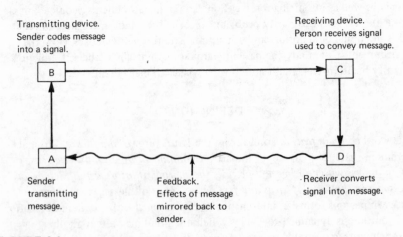

Transmitting device.
Sender codes message
into a signal.

Receiving device.
Person receives signal
used to convey message.

Sender
transmitting
message.

Feedback.
Effects of message
mirrored back to
sender.

Receiver converts
signal into message.

FIGURE 3-1
Elements in the Communication Process

Many factors influence how the message is sent and whether, how, and by whom it will be received: the needs and condition of both the sender and the receiver, emotionally, physically, and intellectually; the occasion or setting; and the sender's knowledge about and relationship with the receiver. Other factors include the content of the message, or the vocabulary to be decoded; the mood or attitude present in the situation; and the communication experience already in operation.

The receiver in turn perceives, interprets, and responds to the message. Through some process, he gives feedback to the sender, confirming that the message has been sent. The receiver at that point himself becomes the sender of a message. If the original message sent does not result in a response or feedback, there is no official interchange.

Communication involves feedback, and each message sent, including feedback, affects the next message sent and its feedback. The process is circular; communication from *A* affects *B*, and *B* in turn affects *A*.

Communication and related behavior can be studied only in context. Studying only the information, the command, the question—the words—is not enough. Behavior and the way of communicating are not static, but vary with the specific situation. In certain situations, seemingly inappropriate responses may be highly appropriate behavior. For example, the apparently senseless talk of an emotionally ill person may be the only feasible reaction in an absurd or untenable family communicational context—his only way of achieving family equilibrium. Or a child's aggressive behavior may be his only way of maintaining initiative and self when his mother communicates overprotection or "smothering" nonverbally.

In the strictest sense, all behavior in the presence of others is communication, and all communication affects behavior[70]. How you gesture, posture, dress, move, speak, behave, or fail to carry out certain behaviors will provide an understandable signal for someone. For example, two persons sitting side-by-side on a plane may neither speak nor look at one another. Yet there is a communication process present, for each by his behavior conveys to the other that he does not wish to engage in an interchange of words, for whatever reason. Contrast this with two persons sitting side-by-side who do not speak but occasionally look at one another and smile. Then a few words are exchanged. The initial nonverbal expressions encourage the eventual verbal exchange. Thus anything perceptibly present or absent can serve as a signal of communication that need only be decoded to be meaningful.

Levels of Communication

Communication can be divided into three areas: (1) syntactics, (2) semantics, and (3) pragmatics. *Syntactics refers to the problems of transmitting information and to the statistical properties of language apart from its users and its context. Semantics refers to the message and its meaning that is agreed upon by* the persons involved. *Pragmatics refers to the behavioral outcomes of the meanings, the results of communication,* and includes nonverbal concomitants, the context of the communication, the words, and their meanings[70]. Each of these three areas must be considered as you talk with others.

Communication occurs on several levels because of the perceptions of each person involved in the communication, and each level becomes increasingly abstract, as demonstrated in Figure 3-2. When two persons are communicating, the following levels may occur:

1. This is how I perceive me.

2. This is how I perceive you.

3. This is how I perceive you seeing and hearing me.

4. This is how I think you see me seeing you.

In a nurse-patient dialogue, on level 1, you are thinking only of the self while talking to the patient. Self-awareness is important, but awareness must include more than that. Level-1 communication would not be very helpful to the patient. On level 2, you are thinking of the self but also observing the patient's behavior and hearing what he has to say. This level of dialogue is more appropriate for the communication of the patient's needs. On level 3, you are aware of how the patient might be perceiving you in addition to being aware of what both you and the patient are saying, doing, and feeling. Thus you can better consider the effect of yourself on the patient and the behavioral cues from the patient, and respond to them. In addition, you may ask for validation of personal perceptions—whether or not the patient is actually perceiving you as you believe. For level-4 communication to occur, you must be very alert, feeling energetic and attuned to the situation. Now, in addition to the above, you consider how the patient thinks you are perceiving him—your feelings and attitudes toward the patient as *he* perceives them[70]. Level 4 takes considerable empathy, but will allow you to be most helpful in communicating with the patient. These levels increase in complexity with increasing numbers of people. If you understand the levels of communication, you can anticipate the communication process, hear "hidden meanings," and recognize your impact upon the process.

TOOLS OF COMMUNICATION

The tools of communication—language, observation and perception, nonverbal behavior, silence, and listening—are closely interrelated and are used simultaneously, although they are discussed separately in the following pages. Knowledge of these tools is essential before appropriately using the nursing process discussed in Chapter 4.

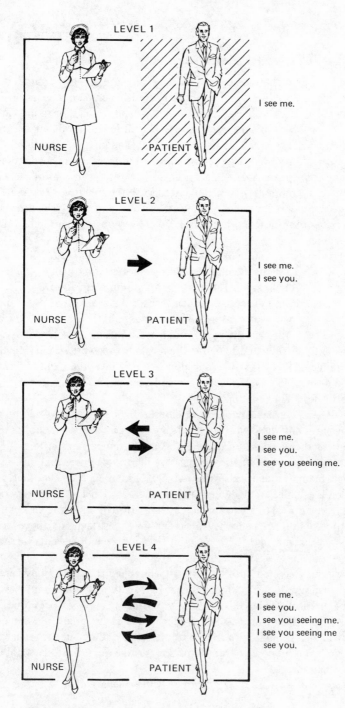

FIGURE 3-2
Levels of Communication

Language

Language is basic to communication. Without language, the higher-order cognitive processes of thinking, reasoning, and generalizing could not be attained. Words are tools or symbols used to express ideas and feelings, or to indicate objects; they are *not the same as the experience*, although words shape experience, communicate facts, convey interpretations, and influence relationships.

The functions of language can be classified in three categories: expressive, arousal, and descriptive. A speech act is *expressive* if it informs us of a speaker's state of mind or emotions; it is also likely to serve the function of *arousal*, triggering an emotional response in the receiver of the message. The *descriptive* function serves to inform another person, to convey observations, memories, ideas, or inferences.

Visual images are more likely to serve the function of arousal than is language. Viewing a picture can arouse strong emotion, for much of the self can be projected into the image. Yet the visual image is unable to show the many contexts of description or tense of which verbal language is capable, for in listening, the personality of the speaker more easily strikes us.

The same words have different meanings for different people, and you must constantly be prepared to define the meaning of a word or phrase. Also, word meanings change over time in response to new inventions and to developments and changes in travel, mass media, and occupations. Thus, language is a map of behavior and communication.

You select, consciously or unconsciously, the part of the world you wish to experience at any time. No two people are in exactly the same spot at exactly the same time; therefore, all our experiences are to some extent different. Many problems in communication arise because we fail to remember that individual experiences are never identical. When two persons talk with one another, communication is established by determining mutual experiences. If the experience being discussed is new to a person, he may have difficulty making sense out of it. Much difficulty in introducing new ideas and much resistance to change arise from the fact that we have to learn *what* to experience in the events we live through.

Words may be used both to express feelings and to avoid expressing them. When a person says he feels "fine," he may be functioning at optimum level—or he may be physically ill but wish to stop your further inquiry by responding with the word "fine." Words may also be used in deliberately obscure ways in order to convey hidden meanings, to test your interest in finding out such meanings, or the degree of your concern for the person, or to express hostility without fear of retaliation.

Besides the language of words, there is the language of time, space, and color.

The Language of Time conveys feelings not expressed by words and may depend on the culture and one's concept of time. The nurse who frequently looks at her watch, who walks too fast for the patient to stay abreast, or who keeps a person waiting past the hour of an appointment may be conveying rejection, neglect, or lack of concern.

The Language of Space—the distance between you and another—helps determine the nature of the communication. Physical distancing varies with the setting and is culturally learned. Placing a person near the center of a group is one way of telling him he is important. The amount of space given a person—the size of a desk or office, the size of the hospital room or ward cubicle—conveys differential importance or status to the person. The distance you maintain between the patient and yourself must be carefully determined, depending on the situation and the needs of the patient, for it may convey feelings to the patient varying from concern to rejection.

The Language of Color elicits fairly specific responses. In American culture, warm colors such as yellow, red, and orange stimulate creative, outgoing, happy responses. Cool colors such as blue, green, and gray tend to encourage meditation and deliberation and have a dampening effect on quality of communication. Color in the environment can be better planned to be therapeutic and to enhance communication in nursing if you are aware of what is being conveyed to the patient through the colors in his surroundings[6]. You should also be aware of what the color of your uniform (or other dress) and hair means to the patient. For example, white clothing may arouse fear in children with past illness experiences. Or the patient may perceive any redheaded nurse as quick-tempered or "sexy" until he can learn otherwise through observation.

Observation and Perception

The second tool of communication is observation and perception. *Observation is the act of noting and recording facts and events. Perception is the personal interpretation of observations.* Rarely do observations exist alone. Frequently one attaches meaning to or makes judgments about observed events based on his knowledge, experience, and/or bias. The observer is part of the observed. What you communicate depends upon the quality of your observations and your interpretation of them. Observations are made because of curiosity, a desire to understand others, a need for security or self-preservation, or any combination of these. In nursing, each patient's needs vary and constantly change. Since you are the one health team member who has continuous contact with the patient, and since the diagnosis, treatment, and prognosis frequently are determined by your observations, your keen perception will help guide the other team workers in their services.

Factors influencing observation and perception are similar to those influencing the communication process generally, and include the following:

1. Physical, mental, and emotional states and needs of the person.
2. Cultural, social, and philosophical background.
3. Number and functioning ability of the senses involved.
4. Past experiences associated with the present situation.
5. Meaning of the observed event to the self.
6. Interests, preoccupations, preconceptions, and motivational level.
7. Knowledge of or familiarity with the situation being observed.
8. Practice in purposeful observation.
9. Environmental conditions and distractions.
10. Availability of technical devices.
11. Presence, attitudes, and reactions of others—for even if observations and perceptions are accurate, if they do not agree with group consensus the person is likely to conform to the group.

You perceive best what you are prepared to perceive and that to which you direct your attention unless other stimuli are exceedingly unusual, intense, or compelling. Some stimuli are admitted to the nervous system in whole, some in part, and some are turned away—not received at all. Thus you must consciously attend to sensory stimuli—visual, auditory, tactile, olfactory—and identify, group, sort, separate, and combine those entering the mind in order to communicate significant observations.

One aspect of communication to remember in patient care is that when two sounds are presented simultaneously to both ears, any verbal signals, such as words, nonsense syllables, and separate speech sound, are more readily heard and identified by the right ear; whereas music and environmental noises are better recognized by the left ear—if the person hears equally well with both ears[35].

In nursing, observations must fulfill certain criteria. They must be purposeful, planned, objective, accurate, complete, and orderly. In *purposeful* observation, you decide what to observe, which are the general and which the specific factors, and why the observation is important. The *planned* observation considers timing, duration, interval between observations, and kind and location of observations. An observation is *objective* when it can be validated directly, indirectly, or through replication by others and is not based on personal bias. *Accuracy* involves use of knowledge, concentration, memory, and problem solving. A *complete* observation meets the purposes for which it is made. *Orderly* or systematic observation permits relating parts of data gathered, observing the commonplace and general data, and then focusing on minute details[53]. Whenever you make an interpretation, it should be stated as such.

Perception of the same event varies from person to person and within the same person at different times, depending on his feelings and what he is prepared for or wishes to see. In addition, the person often simplifies things not understood, so that he may leave out important facts or substitute others, even if distortion results. Recognize this in relation to yourself, the patient, the family, and coworkers, because perception of the event determines action.

Peplau describes four types of relationships between the observer and the observed in nursing:

1. The spectator relationship, where the person is not aware he is being observed and the nurse is outside his focus of attention. This could occur when you observe the sleeping or critically ill patient.

2. The interviewer relationship, where the person is more or less aware he is being studied and that you are taking notes of what he is saying in response to a situation or question. This could occur during the admission procedure or nursing rounds.

3. The collector relationship, where you use records or reports prepared by other health care workers to learn what has happened to the patient. This occurs in the change-of-shift conference, team conference, or when reading the chart to assist in planning care.

4. The participant-observer relationship, where you engage in ordinary acts connected with nursing, such as morning care, and at the same time observe the relationship between the patient and self. The patient is aware he is getting care but not necessarily aware that his response to a situation and your attitudes about giving care are being observed and studied[53].

Action or Nonverbal Behavior

Movement or action is the third tool of communication—for example, finger pointing, head nodding, and other gestures; eye contact, a wink, smile, and other facial expressions; a touch or a slap on the back, general posture, and body sounds such as belching, knuckle cracking, and laughing.

Body Language. Through body language, moving or positioning the body or some portion of it, a person conveys what he cannot or will not verbalize, although this body language may be used simultaneously with verbal activity. Expression of self through movement is learned before speech, so that under stress the person often reverts back to preverbal communication. Thus, this individual may overtly manifest the expression he feels is expected in the existing situation—for example, the smile that is only a facade—rather than show what he really feels. Nonverbal behavior is nevertheless more likely to express hidden meanings, although these must be interpreted with extreme care. Laughter is not always a sign of humor or happiness; it may be a device to cover anxiety, show ridicule, or seek attention.

Body language is often a reliable index of the real meaning of what is being said or communicated because the person is generally unable to exert as much conscious control over this aspect of his behavior as over the words he uses. But knowledge of the person's sociocultural heritage is essential here, since various body parts are used differently in different cultures to enhance conversation. Thus, in India and Greece, the use of the eyes is all-important, while in Africa the torso is frequently moved. And in America, head nodding is common. The amount of movement also varies culturally.

You must observe the nonverbal behavior of the whole person in order to interpret his communication correctly, for an isolated gesture or expression may require a completely different interpretation in proper context. In addition, you must also validate your impressions with other health team members who have observed the person, as well as with the person himself, for the same nonverbal behavior can be interpreted differently by different people. Also look for inconsistencies between nonverbal and verbal behavior. For example, a person's eyes may be cold even though his words are affectionate. And the meaning of words may be altered or even contradicated by the way the words are said.

Touch is an important nonverbal tool in communication, for touching another with some part of the body or an extension of it is an outside event that stimulates a response. Touch, like movement, precedes speech as a form of communication; thus the relationship between touch and communication begins in infancy and remains throughout life as a means of returning to direct experience.

In some cultures, touch is considered magical and healing. In American culture, however, there is still a considerable taboo on casual touching, in part due to residual Victorian sexual prudery. In the health care context there is also the desire to be very scientific, to divorce religion and magic from healing[17].

Once the child reaches school age, he or she is touched less and less even by his own parents. Americans teach their children not to touch themselves unnecessarily and to keep their hands off grown-ups' objects and others' possessions in general, thereby dampening their natural curiosity and desire to explore. There is a recent surge of interest in touch—almost a compulsive one—as a result of the general movement toward exhibitionism (for example in dress), and the "encounter group" movement.

Certainly touch must be used judiciously and not forced on anyone. But a great deal of communication, closeness, mutual encouragement, and caring can be conveyed between two people in rapport when they touch. Touch may of course also convey either physical or psychological assault and the invasion of personal territory and privacy[13, 18, 29]. The message conveyed through touch depends on the attitude of the people involved and the meaning of touch both to the person touching and to the person touched. In general, the need for intimacy and touch is so strong that the satisfaction of that need is a greater influence on behavior than is the fear of closeness or of possible rejection.

When another human being reaches out to you, hopefully you will be there as a fellow, caring human being. Between people who care about one another, touch can communicate feelings where words would fail. In the healing professions, the therapeutic use of touch is indispensable. Touch is, thus, an important tool in the nurse-patient relationship and in the healing art of communication. The back rub, the hand on the shoulder, the squeeze of a hand—each encourages closeness and communication between you and your patient.

Silence

Silence is the fourth tool of communication, even though silence may also interfere with communication. Since one of your essential tasks is to encourage verbal description, you need to intervene effectively into silence. There are different types of silence.

The Blank, Empty, or Blocked Silence occurs when the patient says he has nothing to say while his nonverbal behavior reflects anxiety. In this type of silence you initiate speech and somewhat structure the interchange. You might ask, "What are thinking?" or "What is going on with you now?" A comment can be made about the patient's daily routine. You may even suggest that the patient think of something to say as a way to break the impasse.

The Stubborn, Resistive Silence occurs when a feeling of anger is present. The person is trying to set up a power struggle to gain control over you, a ploy that can stimulate reciprocal anger in you unless you understand the basis for the anger. A response of impatience perpetuates the power struggle. Sit out the anger; be undemanding but interested. Ask, "I wonder what is going on with you?" or "What are you feeling?" When the person recognizes he is angry and understands the possible causes of his anger, he is more likely to give up his resistive silence.

Fearful Silence occurs when a person's previous experiences in similar or identical situations were excessively intimidating. Perhaps other people or hallucinations threatened him if he talked. Staying with him, recognizing efforts to talk, showing a kind, positive approach, and accepting what is said will help to reduce such fears.

A Thoughtful Silence, when the person is resolving difficulties or doing problem solving, is productive. Do not interrupt unless the silence is prolonged. Then suggest that he share his thoughts with you.

Do not cut off silence prematurely because of your own anxiety. Much can be learned from the silence by examining the data preceding the silence and observing the person during the silence.

Listening

Listening is the fifth tool of communication. We have two ears and one mouth, which should give us a clue! Everyone loves a listener, but few persons are skilled listeners.

Because listening gives no chance for self-assertion, instruction, or giving opinion, most people think listening is a passive act requiring no special talent. The evidence is to the contrary. You have to learn to listen attentively and curb the desire to speak.

The act of listening consists of more than just hearing. Listening occurs only when the mind is purposefully attentive to what is being said or communicated. The mind is a selective organizer and responder to experience. On the average, we receive thousands of exteroceptive and proprioceptive impressions every second. Thus a drastic selective process is necessary to prevent the brain's higher centers from being overwhelmed by irrelevant data. Decisions concerning what is relevant and essential and what is irrelevant vary from person to person and are determined by processes and criteria outside the person's awareness. A person may say something that another does not hear because of the latter's selective response, his selective inattention. Selective hearing and listening are influenced considerably by past experience and associations as well as by the need to decrease anxiety over what is being said in the present situation.

Listening is a faster process than speaking. No matter how fast the speaker's mind is racing, he cannot articulate more than about 200 words per minute, whereas the listener can take in words as quickly as he can think. The endings of most sentences can be guessed before they are completed. In fact, a person may hear the end of the sentence inaccurately due to the false sense of security and selective inattention caused by this phenomenon. In the nursing situation you should listen attentively throughout the length of each sentence rather than guess or assume what will be said.

A message is not a spear of thought thrust into the listener's mind by a speaker or writer. Meaning is transferred only when the listener rearranges his mind in accordance with the speaker's voice or printed word signals. Your attitude while listening to another person is an important form of feedback. Realize that you may have no control if a patient, because of illness or particular feelings, blocks your efforts at communication. But learn to adapt and to control your own behavior in order to listen attentively and to stimulate the communication of others.

INTERVIEWING AS PART
OF THE COMMUNICATION PROCESS

In nursing, all activities involve communication, and verbal communication with patients often involves interviewing.

Definition and Factors Involved in Interviewing

An *interview is a transitory relationship between two persons, one seeking information from another without gaining personal advantage, and the other giving information without suffering disadvantage.* The interview is a conversation directed to a definite purpose other than satisfaction in the meeting itself. Interviewing in the nursing situation involves the following five factors:

1. The interview is usually conducted in connection with other nursing activities where you do something for the patient so he can see and feel

the immediate effect of nursing efforts; or you use interviewing to determine how best to give care or to evaluate effectiveness of care given.

2. Either you or the patient can initiate the interview.
3. The situation of the interview is flexible in regard to the setting, interruptions, and availability of time for patient and nurse. The setting may be the waiting room, home, office, factory, or bedside. Interruptions may occur from other health team members, other patients, or visitors. Time limits may be beyond your control, due to intervening demands, so that you may have to return several times to the patient to achieve the purpose of the interview.
4. The patient is usually physically and emotionally confined or restricted and relatively dependent upon you and the climate created by you.
5. There is a continuum of people who represent "the nurse" over a 24-hour period. Each nurse, in the process of continuity of care, participates within the framework of the total plan of care. Thus each nurse may achieve a portion of the purposes of the interview—for example, teaching or gathering information—and the entire nursing team together achieve or work toward the total purpose.

Purposes of the Interview

In nursing, the following purposes can be achieved through an interview:

1. Establishing rapport to convey to the person that he is important, that someone cares; developing or maintaining his feelings of self-esteem; diminishing his feelings of isolation.
2. Establishing and maintaining the nurse-patient relationship.
3. Listening in order to provide release of tension or allow expression of feelings.
4. Obtaining information; identifying and clarifying needs.
5. Giving information or teaching.
6. Counseling to clarify a problem; encouraging self-understanding and constructive problem solving in the person.
7. Referring the person to other resources of help as necessary.

Your Role as Interviewer

Your self—your personality—is the principal tool of the therapeutic interview or communication. Your character structure, values, and sensitivity to the feelings of others influence your attitude and helpfulness toward people.

As a beginner you are more likely to have certain problems in interviewing and therapeutic communication than your more experienced colleagues. Often there is a strong fear you will do something wrong or be criticized by others. Defense mechanisms used to control your anxiety reduce your sensitivity to the emotional responses of others. Fear of being inadequate can be projected onto the patient. You may feel competitive toward professional peers and wish to perform better than they. You may feel guilty about "using" or "practicing on" the patient. With experience, you will learn to overcome or cope with these feelings and become increasingly aware of relationships and subtleties.

At first you may bombard the patient with questions. Later you will learn when a patient has completed the answer to your question or when he needs some slight encouragement to go on. As competence grows with experience, you will be able to hear the content of his words and simultaneously consider how he feels, deduce what he is inferring or omitting, and gauge your emotional response to him. In addition, you will be able to actively intervene when necessary rather than sit and passively listen.

In order to gain this competence, careful notes must be taken during or after each interview. And regular sessions should be held with a teacher or supervisor who can guide you, promoting self-understanding.

Techniques of Interviewing

Prepare for the interview as much as possible, through use of records, by application of general knowledge to the specific situation, and by being alert and observant to the situation. Know or define what information is needed to achieve the purpose of the interview. What you ask or say is dependent upon the purpose of the interview. Avoid, however, the "self-fulfilling prophecy," setting up the interview situation in such a way that the person tells you (or *seems* to tell you) only what you have predetermined he will or can tell you. If selective inattention causes you to see or hear only what you wish to, much information will be missed or misinterpreted and you will not be fully helpful to the person.

The personality and attitude of the interviewer influences the interviewee's responses. The emotional climate and immediate conditions surrounding the interview also affect you and the other person. The following techniques will help promote productive interviews:

1. Establish rapport. Create a warm, accepting climate and a feeling of security and confidentiality so that the person feels free to talk about that which is important to him.
2. Arrange comfortable positions for both yourself and the person so that full attention can be given to the interview.
3. Control the external environment as much as possible. This is sometimes difficult or impossible to do, but try to minimize external distractions or noise, regulate ventilation and lighting, and arrange the setting to reduce physical distance.
4. Consider wearing casual clothing without excess adornment instead of a uniform when working in the school, home, or occupational setting. Consider what expectations the interviewee may have of you. In some cases, he will respond more readily to your casual dress; other times he may need your professional dress as part of the image to help him talk confidentially.

5. Use a vocabulary on the level of awareness or understanding of the person. Avoid occupational jargon or words too abstract for the interviewee's level of understanding or health condition.

6. Avoid preconceived ideas, prejudices, or biases. Avoid imposing personal values on others.

7. Begin by fully exploring the purpose of the interview. Either you or the interviewee may introduce the theme. You may start the session by expressing friendly interest in the everyday affairs of the person or by discussing unimportant events to warm the person up, but avoid continuing trivial conversation. Maintain the proposed structure.

8. Be precise in what you say so the meaning is understood. Ask questions that are well-timed, open-ended, and pertinent to the situation. This pattern allows the person to stamp his own style, organization, and personality on the answers and on the interview. Getting unanticipated data can be as useful in an interview as in giving care. Meaningless questions get meaningless answers. Questions that bombard the person produce unreliable information. Open-ended sentences usually keep the person talking at his own pace. Carefully timing your messages, verbal and nonverbal, and allowing time for the interviewee to understand and respond are essential in nursing.

9. Avoid asking questions in ways that get socially acceptable answers. The interviewee often responds to questions with what he thinks the interviewer wants to hear, either to be well-thought-of, to gain status, or to show that he knows what other people do and what is considered socially acceptable.

10. Be diplomatic when asking questions about home life or personal matters. What you consider common information may be considered very private by some. Matters about which it would be tactless to inquire directly can often be arrived at indirectly by peripheral questions. If a subject you suggest meets resistance, change the topic; when the anxiety is reduced, you can return to the matter for further discussion. Remember, what the person does not say is as important as what he does say.

11. Be an attentive listener. Show interest by nodding, responding with "I see" or "uh-huh." Remain silent and control your responses when another's comments evoke a personal meaning and thus trigger an emotional response in you. While the person is talking, find the nonverbal answers to the following: What does this experience mean for him? Why is he telling me this at this time? What is the meaning of the choice of words, the repetition of key words, the inflection of his voice, the hesitant or aggressive expression of words, the topic he has chosen? Listen for his feelings, needs, and goals. Recognize the levels of meaning in communication previously discussed. Do not answer too fast or ask a question too soon. If necessary, learn if the words mean the same to you as to the interviewee. Explore each clue as you let the person tell his story.

12. Observe carefully nonverbal messages for signs of anxiety, frustration, anger, loneliness, or guilt. Look for feelings of pressure hidden by the person's attempts to be calm. Encourage the free expression of feelings, for feelings often bring facts with them.

13. Encourage spontaneity. Provide movement in the interview by picking up verbal leads, clues, bits of seemingly unrelated information, and nonverbal signals from the patient. If the person asks you a personal question, redirect it to *him*: that may be the topic he unconsciously (or even consciously), wishes to speak about in relation to himself. Only occasionally will it be pertinent for you to answer personal questions.

14. Ask questions beginning with "What...," "Where...," "Who...," and "When..." to gain factual information. Words connoting moral judgments should be avoided; they are not conducive to a feeling of neutrality, acceptance, or freedom of expression. The "How..." question may be difficult for the person to answer, for it asks, "In what manner...?" or "For what reason...?" and the individual may lack sufficient knowledge to answer. The "Why..." question should also be avoided, for this asks for insights which the person should not be expected to give.

15. Indicate when the interview is terminated, and terminate it graciously if the interviewee does not do so first. Make a transition in interviewing or use a natural stopping point if the problem has been resolved, if the information has been obtained or given, or if the person changes the topic. You may say, "There is one more question I'd like to ask...," or, "Just two more points I want to clarify...," or, "Before I leave, do you have any other questions, comments, or ideas to share?"

16. Keep data obtained in the interview confidential and share it only with the appropriate and necessary health team members, leaving out personal assumptions. If you are sharing an opinion or interpretation, state it as such rather than have it appear to be what the other person said or did. The person should be told what information will be shared and with whom.

17. Evaluate the interview. Were the purposes accomplished? Recognize that not everyone can successfully interview everyone. Others may see you differently than you see yourself, thus preventing you from being helpful or obtaining information. Evaluate yourself in each particular situation.

You must be sincere, knowledgeable about the purpose of the interview, and skillful in using tools of communication during the interview as well as in establishing and maintaining a climate conducive to successful data collection. The effective interview takes a great deal of energy and attention.

THERAPEUTIC COMMUNICATION

Analysis of your communication pattern will help you improve your methods. Realize that you cannot become skilled in therapeutic communication without supervised and thoughtful practice. However, as you talk with another, don't get so busy thinking about a list of methods that you forget to focus on the person. Your keen interest in the other person and use of your personal style are essential if you are to be truly effective.

To be effective while communicating with the patient or family, use simple, clear words geared to the person's intelligence and experience. Develop a well-modulated tone of voice, especially with the sick person, since auditory sensitivity is increased during illness. A number of authors have described principles, attitudes, and methods essential in therapeutic communication that are useful with individual persons as well as with groups[26, 33, 53, 54, 55].

Effective Methods

The following are basic methods for conducting purposeful, helpful communication with a person, well or ill, along with their rationale. Some elaborate on earlier suggestions for interviewing.

Use Thoughtful Silence to Encourage the Person to Talk. Silence gives you and the person time to organize thoughts. It directs the person to the task at hand but allows him to set the pace, aids consideration of alternative courses of action and delving into feelings, conserves energy if he is seriously ill, and gives time for contemplation and relaxation. There is a time not to talk. Focus on the person, even if he is silent.

Be Accepting. This is a difficult task at times. Realize that *all* behavior is motivated and purposeful. Indicate that you are following his trend of thought. Encourage him to continue to talk while you remain nonjudgmental, but not necessarily in agreement.

Help the Person Strengthen His Self-Identification in Relation to Others. *Always* use *you, I,* and *we* in their proper context. Do not say, "We can take a bath now," but rather, "You can take a bath now."

Suggest Collaboration and a Cooperative Relationship. Offer to share and work together with the person for his benefit; offer to do things *with*, and not *for* or *to* him. Encourage him to participate in identifying and appraising problems and involve him as an active partner in treatment. Tell the person you are available to help him. "I'll stay with you" or "I'm interested in your comfort" are examples of statements that can help reassure him that you will stay and care regardless of his behavior.

State Open-Ended, Generalized, Leading Questions to encourage the person to take the initiative in introducing topics and to think through problems. Examples include: "Is there something you'd like to talk about?" "Tell me about it." "Where would you like to begin?" "Go on." "And what else?" "Would you like to talk about yourself now?" "After that?" Avoid conventional pleasantries after initial greetings, as these constrict the patient's expression of feelings and ideas. It is important for the person to talk about his mental turmoil and questions, for often he can't think about his feelings until he says them.

State Related Questions. Do not let a subject drop until it is adequately explored. Peripheral or side questions help the person work through larger issues and engage in problem solving. Explore by delving further into the subject or idea without seeming to pry. Many patients deal superficially with a topic to test if you are truly interested. Avoid questions that call for a yes or no answer. Explorative questions call for answers that elaborate, thereby helping the person to increase his understanding and do further problem solving or clarifying.

Place Events Described in Time Sequence. In order to clarify relationships associated with a given event, determine how it happened, place it in perspective, determine the extent to which one event led to another, and seek to identify recurrent patterns or difficulty or significant cause-and-effect relationships. Ask questions such as "What happened then?" or "What did you do after that?"

State Observations That You Perceive about the Person. Statements such as "You appear...," "It seems to me that...," "I notice that you are...," and "It makes me uncomfortable when you..." encourage mutual understanding of behavior. Such observations offer something to which the person can respond without your having to probe, and they call attention to what is happening to help him notice or clarify his own behavior. In this technique, you and the other person can compare observations, and you can encourage him to describe self-awareness. In addition, when you openly acknowledge that another's efforts at a task or behavior are appropriate to the situation, you reinforce the behavior and add to the person's self-esteem.

Encourage Description of Behavior or Observation through statements like "What did you feel?" "Tell me what you now feel," "What does the voice seem to be saying?" and "What is happening?" You can better understand the person when you observe and understand things as they seem to him. He will not have to act out impulses and feelings if he feels free to state them.

Restate or Repeat the Main Idea Expressed to convey that it was communicated to you effectively, thereby encouraging the person to continue, or restate until he does clarify. Reformulating certain statements, using different words, brings out related aspects of material that might otherwise have escaped his (or your) attention.

Reflect by Paraphrasing Feelings, Questions, Ideas, and Key Words to encourage further talking. Indicate to the person that his point of view is important; acknowledge that he has a right to his own opinions and decisions. Encourage his acceptance of his own feelings and ideas as a part of himself. Show interest in hearing as much as he wishes to tell you. Emphasize the word *you* while conversing, as in "*You* feel...," in order to reflect what he has said. (However, do not just mindlessly parrot his words.)

Verbalize the Implied or what the person has hinted at or suggested in order to make the discussion less obscure, to clarify the conversation, and to show that you are listening and interested, and that you accept what he says. Questions can be used as a subtle form of suggestion. For example, you might ask, "Have you ever told your wife how you feel?" or "Have you ever asked your boss for a raise?" Regardless of the answer, you have indicated that such an act is conceivable, permissible, and perhaps even expected.

Attempt to Translate Feelings into Words. Sometimes what the person says seems meaningless when taken literally. Hidden meanings of verbal expressions as well as their actual content must be considered.

Clarify when necessary through statements like "I don't understand what is troubling you," or "Could you explain that again?" The person is usually aware if he is not being understood and may withdraw or cease to communicate. It is not necessary to understand everything he says as long as you are honest about it and do not pretend to understand what you don't. Attempting to discover what the person is talking about can help him become clearer to himself.

Reintroduce Reality by voicing doubt, or calmly presenting your own perceptions or the facts in the situation when the person is being unrealistic. Indicate an alternate line of thought for him to consider, but do not attempt to convince him of his error by arguing. Such action only provokes resistance and a determination to maintain his idea. Encourage him to recognize that others do not necessarily perceive events as he does nor draw the same conclusions. Encourage reconsideration and revaluation (even though it may not change his mind) through statements like "What gives you that impression?" "Isn't that unusual?" and "That's hard to believe." Expressing your doubts may reinforce doubts he already has but which he has discounted because no one else shared them before. A doubting tone of voice can be as effective as any specific statement.

Offer Information, making facts available when the person needs or asks for them. Well-timed teaching builds trust, orients, and gives additional knowledge from which to make decisions or draw realistic conclusions. Inappropriate or partial information or advice may cause alarm or needlessly suggest problems to the person. Give the person information concerning what he can expect and what he can do to help himself.

Seek Consensual Validation. Search for mutual understanding; words should mean the same thing to both of you. Therapeutic communication cannot take place if both you and the other person attach autistic (private) meanings to the words you both use. Always ask yourself if what you heard could have a meaning other than what you think. As a person defines himself for his listener, he also clarifies in his own mind what he means. Avoid words and phrases that are easily misinterpreted or misunderstood, and encourage the person to ask whenever he is in doubt about what you mean.

Encourage Evaluation of the Situation by the Person. Help him to appraise the quality of his experience, to consider people and events in relation to his own and others' values, and to evaluate the way in which people affect him personally as well as understand how he affects others. A simple query may help him understand feelings in connection with what happened to him and discourage him from uncritically adopting the opinions and values of others.

Encourage Formulation of a Plan of Action by asking the person to consider examples of behavior likely to be appropriate in future situations. He can then plan how to handle future problems or how to carry out necessary self-care.

Summarize. Bring together important points of discussion and give particular emphasis to progress made toward greater understanding. Summarizing encourages both you and the person to part company with the same ideas in mind, provides a sense of closure at the end of discussion, and promotes a grasp of the significance of what was said.

The quality of any response depends on the degree of mutual trust in the relationship. Techniques can be highly successful, or they can misfire or be abused, depending on how they are used, your attitude at the time, and the other's interpretation. There must be a feeling of caring, of safety and security in your company, and a feeling that you want to help the person help himself. The more important or highly personal a feeling or idea is, the more difficult it is to say. This situation causes hesitancy in revealing thoughts, feelings, or intimate needs. By using therapeutic principles such as those previously listed, you will help the person and his family identify you as someone to whom ideas and feelings can be safely and productively revealed.

Barriers to Effective Communication

Various authors have written about communication patterns to be avoided by persons in the helping professions and the rationale for their avoidance [28, 33, 34, 46, 54]. The following approaches and techniques will interfere with helpful communication with the patient and family, whether you are conducting an interview or communicating in any other nursing situation. Continually study your personal pattern of communication, verbal and nonverbal, to make sure you *avoid* these practices.

Using the Wrong Vocabulary—vocabulary that is abstract or intangible, full of jargon, slang, or implied status; talking too much; or using unnecessarily long sentences or words out of context can be interpreted by the person as your unwillingness to communicate. But words alone do not block. Perhaps even more crucial can be your attitudes and prejudices resulting from personal and cultural background and your failure to understand the receiver's background. Think about what the message will mean to him, depending on his age, sex, personality, socioeconomic status, cultural background, occupation, religion, and degree and nature of illness.

Conveying Your Feelings of Anxiety, Anger, Strangeness, Denial, Isolation, Lack of Control, or lack of physical health negatively influences your initial and continued responses to another. Such feelings also interfere with your ability to listen and will certainly cause the other person to withdraw, since rapport cannot be established. The appearance of being too busy, of not having time to listen, of not giving sufficient time for an answer, or apparently not really wanting to hear are equally forceful in "cutting off" another. Establishing contact on a social rather than on a therapeutic basis also limits communication to the superficial issues.

Failing to Realize That the Person's Reluctance to Make a Message Clear (resulting from his feeling that what he needs to express is socially unacceptable or inappropriate) can prevent therapeutic communication. He may be afraid to ask questions for fear of getting an obscure answer or of being reprimanded for his questioning. This fearful silence can cause a sense of futility and a closure of communication. Lack of dialogue prohibits evaluating the effectiveness of any message and blocks further attempts at communication. Also avoid interpreting cooperation or passivity as understanding. Sometimes the person answers yes to please you but really does not understand you at all.

Making Inappropriate Use of Facts, Introducing Unrelated Information, offering premature explanation or counseling, wrong timing, saying something important when the person is upset or not feeling well and thus unable to hear what is really said—all these provoke anxiety and prohibit problem solving on the part of the person.

Making Glib Statements, Offering False Reassurance by saying, "Everything is OK," or unfairly indicating that there is no cause for anxiety—these are dishonest ways of evaluating the patient's personal feelings and communicate a lack of understanding and empathy. You cannot foretell the future accurately, so you cannot honestly say there is nothing to worry about. Such verbal behavior belittles the person who feels he has legitimate problems, and it discourages further expression of feelings and trust, although it may relieve your own anxieties.

Using Clichés, Stereotyped Responses, Trite Expressions, and Empty Verbalisms stated without thought, such as "It's always worse at night," "I know," "You'll be OK," or "Who is to say?" makes the person uncomfortable and prohibits you from maintaining objectivity. Such statements, unfortunately common, do not allow expression of feelings or show understanding. You cannot understand a person as he really is if you respond to him automatically. Also, do not jump to conclusions based on initial impressions.

Being Too Strongly Opinionated in any aspect of your conversation with another presents a barrier, since you do not allow for a different response. Neither can you be totally neutral; recognition should be given for accomplishments. However, approval or agreement, and disapproval or disagreement carry overtones of judgment about the person.

Expressing Unnecessary Approval, stating that something the person does or feels is particularly good, implies that the opposite is bad and limits freedom of the patient to think, speak, or act in ways that may displease you. Excess praise arouses undue ambition, competition, and a sense of superiority, closing off possible learning experiences because the person may continue to speak and act only in ways that will bring approval. This approach does not allow the person to live up to his potential. Similarly, *excessive agreement*, indicating the person is right, can be equally inhibiting, for you leave him little opportunity to modify a point of view later without admitting error. Do not take sides with another, but use the time to help him gather data so he can draw his own opinions and conclusions.

Expressing Undue Disapproval, denouncing another's behavior or ideas, implies that you have the right to pass judgment on his thoughts and feelings and that he must please you. This moralistic attitude diverts your attention away from his needs and directs attention to your own. *Excessive disagreement*, opposition to another's beliefs or values, implies he is wrong and you are right, and puts him on the defensive. Disagreement usually results in resistance to change and shows lack of respect. Likewise, *rejection*, refusing to consider, or showing contempt for, the person's ideas and behavior, closes off the topic from exploration and also rejects him as an individual. Every person has no doubt experienced some degree of disapproval, disagreement, and rejection in the past; but such responses from others reinforce loneliness, hopelessness, and alienation, and may even contribute to illness. This person may then avoid help rather than risk further disapproval, disagreement, or rejection.

Giving Advice, Stating Personal Experiences, Opinion, or Value Judgments, Giving Pep Talks, Telling Another What He Should Do—such behavior emphasizes yourself, elevates your self-esteem, and relieves your anxiety, but implies that you know what is best and that the person is incapable of self-direction. Such behavior inhibits spontaneity, prevents him from struggling with and thinking problems through, and may unnecessarily keep him in a state of prolonged dependency. Certainly talking about yourself is of no interest or relevance to the person or family in need of help. Remember that when a person asks for your advice, opinion, or judgment, he has frequently already made a decision and is actually seeking a sounding board or validation for his idea. (Instead, such queries should be met with questions like: "What have you been told to do?" "What would you like to do?" "What do you plan to do?" Then you can facilitate the person's problem solving by using the effective methods of communication previously described.)

Probing or Persistent, Pointed Questioning places the person on the defensive and makes him feel manipulated and valued only for what he can give. Often the data obtained will not be accurate because he will give the answers he feels you want to hear or, to protect himself, will give no answers.

Requiring Explanations, Demanding Proof, Challenging or Asking "Why...?"—when the person cannot provide a reason for his thoughts, feelings, and behavior and for events—forces him to invent reasons, to give partial answers, to expand delusions, or to rationalize since he feels "on the spot." Emotionally charged topics will be avoided. If he knew the "whys," the reasons, he could handle the situation himself.

Belittling the Person's Feelings (equating intense and overwhelming feelings expressed with those felt by everyone or yourself) implies that his feelings are bad, that he is bad, or that his discomfort is mild, temporary, unimportant, or self-limiting. Such statements indicate a lack of understanding and no constructive assistance is offered. When someone is concerned with his own misery, he is not concerned about nor interested in the misery of others; but he does expect you to be concerned and interested in his feelings and problems. Don't say, "Everyone feels that way."

Making Only Literal Responses or asking questions related only to practical matters cuts off exploration of feelings. Persons often cannot state feelings directly or in conventional phrasing but must use symbolism or statements with hidden meanings. If you respond to symbolism on its literal level, you may be showing a lack of understanding. For example, if the person says, "I'm a real doll," he may mean that he feels likable, less than human, or conspicuous. Similarly, a statement such as "It's a gray day" may have no reference to the weather.

Interpreting the Person's Behavior or Confronting Him with analytical meanings of his behavior may cause great anxiety, denial, or withdrawal, and indicates your limited confidence in his capacity to cope with, work through, or understand his own problems. Self-understanding does not come directly from someone else but rather through assistance from another.

Interrupting or Abruptly Changing the Subject takes control of the conversation, often to escape from something anxiety-provoking. The new topic may be of no interest or relevance to the patient. Such verbal behavior is rude and shows a lack of empathy. The other's thoughts and spontaneity are interrupted, the flow of ideas is cut off or becomes confused, and you will get inadequate information or be unable to do effective counseling or teaching. The relevance of what is being said may not be immediately apparent, but you should remain hopeful for later understanding.

Defending or Protecting Someone or Something (nurses, doctors, hospital) from verbal attack by the patient is unnecessary and implies that the patient has no right to express impressions, opinions, or feelings. Stating that his criticism is unjust or unfounded doesn't change his feelings because his feelings are valid to him. Moreover, what he is saying may be true. Genuine acceptance, understanding, and competent care of the patient make defense unnecessary.

IMPLICATIONS FOR HEALTH PROMOTION

Applications to Nursing

The first communication problem that you must control is that of personal emotions in the nurse-patient-family relationship. Since the main barrier to communication is emotions, you must develop skill in building bridges over these barriers. The basic bridge to effective communication is feeling. Everyone seeks *warmth, security, assurance,* and *appreciation.* When these qualities are present, tough problems can be taken in stride, particularly when commitment is combined with skillful use of the methods described in this chapter.

Study yourself to discover those points at which you could be responsible for blocking communication through your own shortcomings. Know your likes and dislikes; recognize them for what they are; and keep them under control. For you to accept another person, you must first accept yourself. You must be aware of your own needs in order to help another meet his needs.

Cultivate an understanding of the part played by body language in human interactions and be as aware of what you are saying with your body movements as you are of what others say with theirs. Feelings are frequently expressed by gestures, attitudes, gait and body posture, and facial expressions. Refer to LaMeri, Mahl, and Christoffers[40, 43, and 14, respectively] for more information on the science of body language.

For the person to make full use of therapeutic communication, he must feel safe with you, respected by and trusting of you. Revealing one's innermost thoughts and feelings to someone one scarcely knows is difficult for any individual, even when he needs and expects help. Use of communication techniques in counseling makes no attempt to influence the speed or direction of the person's problem-solving efforts; be a facilitator rather than a doer or a teller.

The nurse is in a key position to apply an understanding of the communication process and to carry out therapeutic-communication methods in nursing—while conducting routine procedures, teaching, counseling, or giving support. Thus you can enable the person and family to achieve optimum wellness and to prevent future health problems. In addition, through communication, you will learn of the effectiveness of care you have given.

Application to Daily Living

Although this chapter has centered around nurse-patient-family interaction, the discussions of the communication process, of interviewing, and of techniques and blocks to communication apply equally well to associations with your colleagues and other health team members. In fact, application of all information in this chapter to your everyday relationships with family and friends will promote an increasingly appropriate, harmonious living pattern.

Appropriate, realistic, constructive communication between persons is a basic step toward mental, emotional, and, indirectly (but no less significantly), physical health. Communication patterns that block or restrict the other person reduce his feelings of autonomy and equality and increase his feelings of being misunderstood. The resultant emotions—frustration, anger, depression, and the like—will eventually affect the relationship between the persons involved as well as the physiological functioning of the body.

As a nurse you will find yourself refining your personal pattern of communication, practicing therapeutic communication with others, and teaching others patterns of communication that promote health individually, within the family, and within community social groups.

REFERENCES

1. Aasterud, Margaret, "Explanation to the Patient," *Nursing Forum*, 2: No. 4 (1963), 36-44.

2. Allport, Floyd, *Theories of Perception and the Concept of Structure.* New York: John Wiley & Sons, Inc., 1955.

3. "Anxiety: Recognition and Intervention—A Programmed Instruction," *American Journal of Nursing*, 65: No. 9 (1965), 130-52.

4. Asch, S. E., "Effects of Group Pressure on the Modification and Distortion of Judgments," in *Groups, Leadership, and Men*, ed. H. Geutzkow. Pittsburgh: Carnegie, 1951.

5. Ball, Geraldine, "Speaking Without Words," *American Journal of Nursing*, 60: No. 5 (1960), 692-93.

6. Bartholet, M., "Effects of Color on Dynamics of Patient Care," *Nursing Outlook*, 6: No. 10 (1968), 51-53.

7. Bender, R. E., "Communicating With the Deaf," *American Journal of Nursing*, 66: No. 4 (1966), 757-60.

8. Bermosk, Loretta, "Interviewing: A Key to Therapeutic Communication in Nursing Practice," *Nursing Clinics of North America*, 1: No. 2 (1966), 205-14

9. Bigham, Gloria, "To Communicate with Negro Patients," *American Journal of Nursing*, 64: No. 9 (1964), 113-15.

10. Bird, Brian, *Talking with Patients*. Philadelphia: J. B. Lippincott Company, 1965.

11. Burkhardt, M., "Response to Anxiety," *American Journal of Nursing*, 69: No. 10 (1969), 2153-54.

12. Burton, Genevieve, *Personal, Impersonal, and Interpersonal Relations* (3rd ed.). New York: Springer Publishing Company, 1970.

13. Cashar, Leah, and Barbara Dixson, "The Therapeutic Use of Touch," *Journal of Psychiatric Nursing*, 5: No. 5 (1967), 442-51.

14. Christoffers, Carol, "Movigenic Intervention: An Expanded Dimension," *Journal of Psychiatric Nursing and Mental Health Services*, 6: No. 6 (1968), 349-60.

15. Cohen, M., "Easy to Listen to," *American Journal of Nursing*, 66: No. 9 (1966), 1999-2001.

16. Davis, Anne J., "The Skills of Communication," *American Journal of Nursing*, 63: No. 1 (1963), 66-70.

17. DeThomaso, Marita, "Touch Power and the Screen of Loneliness," *Perspectives in Psychiatric Care*, 9: No. 3 (1971), 112-17.

18. Durr, Carol, "Hands That Help—But How?," *Nursing Forum*, 10: (1971), 392-400.

19. Dye, Mary C., "Clarifying Patients' Communication," *American Journal of Nursing*, 63: No. 8 (1963), 56-59.

20. Elder, R., "What Is the Patient Saying?" *Nursing Forum*, 2: No. 1 (1963), 25-37.

21. Eldred, S., "Improving Nurse-Patient Communication," *American Journal of Nursing*, 60: No. 11 (1960), 1600-1602.

22. Evans, Frances, *Psychosocial Nursing: Theory and Practice in Hospital and Community Mental Health*. New York: The Macmillan Company, 1971, pp. 103-41.

23. Flynn, G., "The Nurse's Role: Interference or Intervention?" *Perspectives in Psychiatric Care*, 7: No. 4 (1969), 170-76.

24. Freund, H., "Listening With Any Ear at All," *American Journal of Nursing*, 69: No. 8 (1969), 1650-53.

25. Gibran, Kahlil, *The Prophet*. New York: Alfred A. Knopf, Inc., 1953, p. 21.

26. Goldin, P., and B. Russell, "Therapeutic Communication," *American Journal of Nursing*, 69: No. 9 (1969), 1928-30.

27. Gombrich, E. H., "The Visual Images," *Scientific American*, 227: No. 3 (1972), 82-96.

28. Greenhill, Maurice H., "Interviewing With a Purpose," *American Journal of Nursing*, 56: No. 10 (1956), 1259-62.

29. Gunther, Bernard, *Sense Relaxation*. New York: Collier Books, 1968.

30. Guralnik, David, ed., *Webster's New World Dictionary* (2nd College ed.). New York: The World Publishing Company, 1972.

31. Haggerty, Virginia, "Listening: An Experiment in Nursing," *Nursing Forum,* 10: No. 4 (1971), 382-91.

32. Hardiman, M., "Interviewing or Social Chit-Chat?" *American Journal of Nursing,* 11: No. 7 (1971), 1379-81.

33. Hays, J., and K. Larson, *Interacting with Patients.* New York: The Macmillan Company, 1963.

34. Hewitt, H., and B. Pesznecker, "Blocks to Communicating with Patients," *American Journal of Nursing,* 64: No. 7 (1964), 101-103.

35. Jakobson, Roman, "Verbal Communication," *Scientific American,* 227: No. 3 (1972), 73-80.

36. Johnson, B., "The Meaning of Touch in Nursing," *Nursing Outlook,* 13: No. 2 (1965), 59-60.

37. Juzwiak, M., "How Skilled Interviewing Helps Patients and Nurses," *R.N.,* 29: No. 8 (1966), 33ff.

38. King, Imogene, *Towards a Theory for Nursing.* New York: John Wiley & Sons, Inc., 1971.

39. Kron, Thora, *Communication in Nursing.* Philadelphia: W. B. Saunders Company, 1967.

40. LaMeri, Russell, *Dance Composition: The Basic Elements.* Lee, Mass.: Jacobs Pillow Dance Festival, Inc., 1965.

41. Little, D. E., "The Say-Something-Tell-Nothing Concept of Nursing," *Nursing Forum,* 2: No. 1 (1963), 38-45.

42. MacKinnon, Roger, and Robert Michels, *The Psychiatric Interview in Clinical Practice.* Philadelphia: W. B. Saunders Company, 1971, pp. 1-64.

43. Mahl, George, *Gestures and Body Movements in Interviews.* Paper prepared for the Third Research in Psychotherapy Conference, Chicago, June 1-4, 1966.

44. Manthey, M., "A Guide for Interviewing," *American Journal of Nursing,* 67: No. 10 (1967), 2088-90.

45. Mattes, Norman, "Are You Listening?" *American Journal of Nursing,* 58: No. 6 (1958), 827-28.

46. Meadow, Lloyd, and Gertrude Gass, "Problems of the Novice Interviewer," *American Journal of Nursing,* 63: No. 2 (1963), 97-99.

47. Meyers, M., "The Effect of Types of Communication on Patients' Reactions to Stress," *Nursing Research,* 13: No. 2 (1964), 126-31.

48. Mickens, Patricia, "The Influence of the Therapist on Resistive Silence," *Perspectives in Psychiatric Care,* 9: No. 4 (1971), 161-66.

49. Muencke, M., "Overcoming the Language Barrier," *Nursing Outlook,* 18: No. 4 (1970), 53-54.

50. Muller, Theresa, "Dynamics of Communication in Nursing," *American Journal of Nursing,* 63: No. 1 (1963), 9-16.

51. Murray, Jeanne, "Self-Knowledge and the Nursing Interview," *Nursing Forum,* 2: No. 1 (1963), 69-79.

52. Paynich, Mary, "Cultural Barriers to Nurse Communication," *American Journal of Nursing,* 64: No. 2 (1964), 87-90.

53. Peplau, Hildegarde, *Interpersonal Relations in Nursing*. New York: G. P. Putnam's Sons, 1952.

54. ——, *Basic Principles of Patient Counseling* (2nd ed.). Philadelphia: Smith, Kline and French Laboratories, 1969.

55. ——, "Talking with Patients," *American Journal of Nursing*, 70: No. 7 (1970), 964-66.

56. Pirandello, L., "Language and Thought," *Perspectives in Psychiatric Care*, 8: No. 5 (1970), 230ff.

57. Prange, A., and H. Martin, "Aids to Understanding Patients," *American Journal of Nursing*, 62: No. 7 (1962), 98-100.

58. Rodger, B., "Therapeutic Communication and Posthypnotic Suggestion," *American Journal of Nursing*, 72: No. 4 (1972), 714-17.

59. Ruesch, Jurgen, and Gregory Bateson, *Communication*. New York: W. W. Norton and Company, Inc., 1951.

60. Skipper, James, "Communication and the Hospitalized Patient," in *Social Interaction and Patient Care*, eds. James Skipper and Robert Leonard. Philadelphia: J. B. Lippincott Company, 1965, pp. 61-82.

61. Skipper, J., D. Tagliacozzo, and H. Mauksch, "What Communication Means to Patients," *American Journal of Nursing*, 4: No. 4 (1964), 101-3.

62. Suhrie, Eleanor Brady, "The Importance of Listening," *Nursing Outlook*, 8: No. 12 (1960), 687.

63. Tarasuk, M., J. Rhymes, and R. Leonard, "An Experimental Test of the Importance of Communication Skills for Effective Nursing," in *Social Interaction and Patient Care*, eds. James Skipper and Robert Leonard. Philadelphia: J. B. Lippincott Company, 1965, pp. 110-20.

64. Taylor, M. "The Process Recording: Aid to Interviewing," *Canadian Nurse*, 64: No. 10 (1968), 49.

65. Thomas, M., J. Baker, and N. Estes, "Anger: A Tool for Developing Self Awareness," *American Journal of Nursing*, 70: No. 12 (1970), 2586-90.

66. Travelbee, Joyce, *Intervention in Psychiatric Nursing*. Philadelphia: F. A. Davis Company, 1969.

67. Underwood, P., "Communication Through Role Playing," *American Journal of Nursing*, 71: No. 6 (1971), 1184-86.

68. Veninga, Robert, "Communications: A Patient's Eye View," *American Journal of Nursing*, 73: No. 2 (1973), 320-22.

69. Ward, Anita, "My Silent Patient," *Perspectives in Psychiatric Care*, 7: No. 2 (1969), 87-91.

70. Watzlawich, P., J. Beavin, and D. Jackson, *Pragmatics of Human Communication*. New York: W. W. Norton and Company, Inc., 1967.

71. Wilson, L., "Listening," in *Behavioral Concepts and Nursing Intervention*, coord. C. Carlson. Philadelphia: J. B. Lippincott Company, 1970, pp. 153-70.

72. Wu, Ruth, *Behavior and Illness*. Englewood Cliffs, N.J.: Prentice-Hall, Inc., 1973.

CHAPTER 4

The Nursing Process: A Method to Promote Health

Study of this chapter will help you to:

1 Define the *conceptual approach* and describe some concepts used in nursing practice.

2 Define *holistic* and describe the importance of this approach in nursing.

3 Contrast the scientific method with the nursing process.

4 List and discuss essential attributes for professional practice.

5 List the steps of the nursing process, and define *assessment* and the actions involved in assessment.

6 Discuss the purpose of an assessment tool and construct an assessment tool appropriate for patients in each life era with various health problems.

7 Differentiate nursing diagnosis and nursing history and write a nursing history on a patient.

8 Define *intervention* and explain the importance of identifying scientific rationale for intervention.

9 Define *evaluation* and relate this step of the nursing process to accountability.

10 Use your knowledge of the total nursing process to formulate a nursing care plan for an assigned patient and describe the use of nursing care plans in patient care.

11 Use the process recording and analysis of care to evaluate your effectiveness in patient care.

12 List and describe the phases of the nurse-patient relationship and the effect of each person's feelings upon each phase.

13 Differentiate between a social and helpful nurse-patient relationship to describe the feelings that promote a positive interaction.

14 Compare the schools of thought that have influenced the direction of nursing.

15 Discuss the potential impact of the clinical nurse specialist upon the health care system.

16 Project how your role in nursing will differ from current nursing roles and describe the components of nursing practice that serve to maintain flexible, patient-centered care.

17 Compare problem solving and research and explore the importance of each to nursing.

Most nursing in the past, and even today, has been practiced on an empirical basis. Care patterns established by early nurses, such as Florence Nightingale and Clara Barton, were chiefly concerned with procedures and aimed at providing an environment of cleanliness, comfort, and safety. Nursing's responsibility was to foster solely a reparative process, and functions toward this end have accompanied the growth of technology in nursing—a tradition that is almost holy[22]. However, in recent years this limited approach has proved inadequate. Thus a conceptual approach to care has emerged, essential in order to care for a diverse population in a complex society.

The *conceptual approach is the uniting, combining, modifying, and utilizing of many theories or ideas from various disciplines into a new form; it is a holistic, dynamic approach.* Thus for resources or inspiration you might draw upon methods or approaches of medicine, religion, education, psychology, sociology, or business. Your approach will be refined as you constantly look for ideas from other fields which are applicable to nursing. For example, learning theories that have been successful in psychotherapy can be translated to nursing and adapted to patient teaching. The conceptual approach does not isolate procedures. Instead it fits these aspects of nursing into a health-promotion emphasis, using whatever knowledge is applicable, such as basic human needs, and levels of wellness, stress, and adaptation. While the conceptual approach is concerned with repair, it is also concerned with prevention of breakdown; while it is concerned with practical measures, it is also concerned that sound scientific principles underly these measures.

This chapter discusses concepts basic to the nursing process, the systematic method of nursing practice, ways to evaluate effectiveness of the nursing process, the use of a helpful nurse-patient relationship as one of the unique functions of nursing, and the changing role of the nurse. As you study this chapter, keep in mind that besides acquiring a mastery of skills and knowledge necessary for your clinical area, you will also need to possess a zeal for continuing your learning and a commitment to the good of mankind rather than to self-aggrandizement. Moreover, you should view nursing as an art, a systematic but compassionate way of applying knowledge and skill to achieve clearly defined goals [40].

BASIC CONCEPTS

The Holistic Approach to Man and His Needs

At all times man is striving to maintain optimal balance by means of discharging and conserving energy. Your goal is to assist persons in maintaining or restoring this balance, to help them remain adaptive; thus you will need an understanding of the nature of man and his needs.

Man is a part of all that is within and around him—whether it be a cell, organ system, family, or society. He is more than the sum of all his parts. This view, called holistic or total, will provide a foundation for considering all the areas that affect health.

Man's *behavior, his observable characteristics and responses,* can help you recognize his needs. Although man usually seeks to meet his physical and psychosocial needs simultaneously, preservation of physical integrity is basic. Man must maintain an optimal level of oxygen-carbon dioxide exchange, fluid and food intake, rest and activity, elimination of waste products, temperature regulation, and participation in sex in order to guarantee the species' survival [6, 26]. Next in order are needs for safety, belonging and love, self-esteem, and self-actualization (realizing the best of one's potential) [26]. In nursing, you help the person meet the basic needs that he is unable to meet by himself. Knowing man's priority of needs will help you set your priorities of care. For example, you would not expect a person to concentrate on job safety while he is suffering from excessive hunger.

A Systematic Approach to Nursing Practice

You will be systematic in your nursing practice through use of the scientific method, long a part of research in other disciplines. The scientific method must also be an intricate part of nursing if goals of health care are to be effectively met.

The *scientific method* begins with identifying the problem through repeated *observations* from which *generalizations* are made. Next a *hypothesis, a tentative theory or statement of why relationships occur between particular phenomena,* is formulated. The validity of the hypothesis must be tested through data collection and analysis.

You cannot use just one person in data collection or testing, so the *universe of the investigation, the group to be studied,* is established. Rarely is it possible to study the entire population affected by a problem, so *a smaller group, a sample,* must be selected according to a sampling design. There are many sampling procedures, but the principle to remember is that the sample must be representative of the specified universe if the results are to be applicable to the total considered population. Another consideration at this stage is determining sources and methods of data collection as well as frequency of collection. Sources may include clinical records, government records, personal interviews, laboratory tests, clinical examinations, questionnaires, and written tests.

Next, you must gain a thorough understanding of the data in order to formulate conclusions. Statistics are employed to *tabulate, classify,* and *analyze the data,* although in nursing this has not been done as frequently as in other professions. In essence, analysis consists of making the data "talk." Finally, appropriate statistical computations and tests are performed to *assess the significance of data collected.*

Your hypothesis now becomes either a proven theory from which you and others can base sound working practices or a soundly disproved statement. Be aware, however, that circumstances continually change these results and further testing is necessary.

As you work with patients, you may not always follow these exact steps in a sophisticated manner. But any assumptions you make concerning problems, trends, or health promotion and care should be subjected to this basic objective process.

THE NURSING PROCESS

The steps of the nursing process are assessment *(identifying needs),* intervention *(ministering to needs), and* evaluation *(validating the effectiveness of the help given).* In this sequence of operations, using the scientific method, your knowledge plus available resources will combine with your personality, compassion, and commitment to produce an effective art of nurturing. Thus the nursing process is unique and creative. Understanding this circular process is the key to the formulation of a nursing care plan, which will be discussed later in the chapter.

The nursing process is what you as a nurse do. Every decision for action is carried out within the context of one of these three steps, whether it be an instantaneous decision in an emergency or a long-range plan that grows out of a team conference. Only the time factor varies. The process can be as simple as deciding to sit with a lonely elderly patient or as complicated as intensive-care nursing. After you engage in a knowledgeable, purposeful series of thoughts and actions, you then evaluate their effectiveness.

Assessment

The first step in the nursing process is *assessment, an appraisal of the whole person to establish a baseline and determine the person's potential and his need for help*. Once established, this baseline is fluid and your assessment is a continuous process. As changes in the patient yield new data, nursing problems and objectives may require restatement or may no longer be relevant for his care.

Assessment is done through observation, the use of knowledge and resources, and communication.

Observation includes recognizing objective signs in the patient, family, or community; watching their interactions with one another; determining the response of the patient to you; and discerning the way in which the patient arranges his personal belongings and speaks of himself. Observation and perception are closely related and are more fully described in Chapter 3.

Knowledge from previous experiences and courses of study must be used in assessment. Knowledge of normal physiology and anatomy and of growth and development provides a basis for understanding pathological states and enables you to predict patient responses and plan care accordingly. Sociology, psychology, and philosophy are also examples of large areas of information you must use to enhance your conceptual approach to care. Both units of this book, as well as other texts, present theory and facts upon which to base assessment. Essential to assessment is a sound knowledge of the developing person[31].

Other Resources include data gathered from the patient's chart and health history. The literature pertinent to his condition must be explored—including information about his medical regimen, such as treatments and drugs—and the implications of these for nursing care must be considered. A word of caution is advisable regarding the use of literature in assessment. Do not attempt to fit the patient completely into a textbook pattern. Everyone's adaptational response is unique, and information you gather is to be used only as a guideline.

Communication as part of assessment involves a goal-directed approach to the patient, his family or significant others, the physician as your colleague, and other members of the health team. Verbal and nonverbal exchanges take place between you and the patient, ideally leading to a meeting of the minds—a sharing of the same meanings as each sees the other's point of view. Clarification of meaning is necessary when any doubt exists so that needs can be met in a way acceptable to the patient.

Methods of effective communication and interviewing and barriers to communication are discussed in Chapter 3 and must be used for thorough assessment.

Assessment Tools

Each calling has its tools, and nursing is no exception. Nursing tools are not the devices with which treatments are carried out, but rather the methodology through which assessment of needs is compiled. These tools include nursing diagnosis, nursing history, and systematic assessment of the patient's functional areas, using a specific format.

Nursing diagnosis consists of recognizing and labeling commonly recurring patient conditions or behavior related to health and amenable to nursing care. Nursing diagnosis results from nursing assessment and covers problems not specifically analyzed or prescribed for by the physician, including not only the patient's functional disabilities but also his most important functional abilities[8]. The term *nursing diagnosis* has been controversial and the concept misunderstood, but its use has led to successful organization of the factors involved in determining the need for nursing care, delineating the nursing process, and obtaining nursing histories. Examples of nursing diagnoses are lack of understanding, anxiety, and decubitus ulcer.

The **nursing history** *is distinct from a medical history in that it focuses on the meaning of illness and health care to the patient and family as a basis for planning nursing care,* whereas the medical history is taken to determine or rule out pathology as a basis for medical care[30]. Instead of recommending a specific format or a list of steps to follow, the following discussion explains the kind of data a nursing history provides and the ways in which you can make use of this tool.

An initial interview with the person upon his entrance into a health care agency—hospital, clinic, physician's office—must be done by the professional nurse if personalized care is to be planned effectively. Systematically collecting data will help you make maximum use of your limited time with the person.

Whether you use a standard form or an unstructured interview will depend on agency policy, your own ability to collect data, the effectiveness of your communication, and the time available. Techniques for this initial assessment are the interview, direct observation, and inspection. Subjective as well as objective data are collected and recorded. Analytical thinking and the knowledge you bring from the contributing sciences permit you to make judgments and decisions for care[28].

To be of practical use, *a nursing history should reflect the patient's perception of his illness, his need to seek care, and his expectations regarding the care he hopes to receive. The history must provide clues about his personal needs and his ability to deal with his health problems.* These areas can be covered in an interview guide that includes:

1. The meaning of illness and agency care to the person and to the important family members with whom he lives; his interests; and his projected care plans after discharge.
2. His specific needs and the extent to which nursing intervention will be required to help satisfy basic needs: hygiene, rest, sleep, relief of pain, safety, nutrition, fluids, elimination, oxygen, and sexuality.
3. Additional data that can be labeled "other," such as allergies, language barriers, and educational level (prerequisites for successful communication and health teaching)—and *anything* the patient thinks would be helpful to you in caring for him.
4. Your impressions and a summary of the initial assessment. If a questionnaire is used, this last area could be completed away from the patient.

The entire form can be the first nursing entry on the patient's record and serves as a complete admission note, either on the traditional nurses' notes or in the Problem Oriented Medical Record[30].

Systematic assessment of the patient's functional areas, using a specific guide, is basic to on-going understanding of the patient and the development of a nursing plan. This assessment tool is distinct from the nursing history, which focuses on relatively unchanging information that identifies potentials, strengths, attitudes, efforts, and weaknesses present on admission. The assessment focuses on areas that change, depending on the patient's position on the illness-wellness continuum.

All working guides that have been developed by nursing leaders address themselves to the primary areas of the patient's physiological and psychosocial needs. Several typologies are in use and variations are emerging. Well known to nursing are the 21 problems suggested by Abdellah[2], the functional-abilities tool devised by McCain[28], and Henderson's activities of daily living[16]. Geitgey describes a guide that makes use of the acronym SELF-PACING to identify needs and to emphasize the patient's right to be as self-directing as possible[12]. The letters stand for the past and current status of Socialization and special senses; Elimination and exercise; Liquids and factors influencing fluid balance; Foods and dietary modification; Pain, personal hygiene, and posture; Aeration; Circulation; Integument; Neuromuscular control and coordination; and General condition. Geitgey's format is cited as just one you may wish to use in making a care plan.

You will be using a conceptual approach, regardless of the assessment tool used, if you combine the following questions with other nursing, psychosocial, and pathophysiological content:

1. What are the constants for those in the situation: age? sex? education? culture?
2. What are the potential problems and resources: the patient's view of himself? his priorities as he sees them?

3. What is the person's adaptive capacity as shown by behavioral cues? by energy allocation? by position on a wellness continuum?
4. What are the stressors or the sources of stimuli? To what degree is the person motivated? Do the patient and you share priorities so that he may use his adaptive capacities to the fullest?
5. What consequences can be anticipated? Who will be most affected and in what ways? [6]

Figure 4-1 is an example of a patient assessment using McCain's assessment tool as a guide [28]. Although your assessment may vary in length and thoroughness, strive to be as systematic and comprehensive as possible in order to understand the patient or client as a person, establish nursing diagnoses, and plan and give care which meets his needs.

On the basis of your systematic study of the patient, decide which functional area is presently in most need of your help. The problems of care must be determined before you can set priorities. Then you will be able to state the objectives for the patient's return to wellness—the priorities for today, this week, and for eventual discharge to his usual life with optimum health *for him.*

Setting Priorities of Care is an essential part of the step of assessment. It deserves special attention because it is often the stumbling block encountered by the beginning nurse. Although armed with a broad data base culled from the patient and his records, the literature, and your own knowledge, you may find sorting out the priorities difficult.

As in all problem solving, start with the general and move toward the specific. First consider the person as an open system in his present situation but influenced by the socioeconomic and cultural climate from which he comes. Next consider his most urgent need and identify it in terms of a comparison between the actual state and the desired state.

You still may not be able to see through the maze of data. The patient's most urgent need may be restoration of fluid balance, but when asked what the priorities are, you may reply: "To measure his intake and output." Do not confuse priorities of care and objectives with the mechanical tasks that you will carry out, important as they may be. Use your data to set short-term and long-range goals based on the *response you expect to foster* through your nursing actions.

Consider Mr. Denton, age 62, who sustained a cerebral vascular accident and has been in the hospital 24 hours prior to your being assigned to care for him. He has a right hemiplegia and is on complete bedrest. What are the immediate priorities of care? You might select his bath, or the monitoring of his intravenous fluids. These are important, but they are not ends in themselves; rather they are ways of meeting the needs of those functional states that are in varying degrees of maladaptation.

Assuming that you know Mr. Denton's age, occupation, social-cultural background, and general response through a nursing history, you can correlate

FIGURE 4-1

Example of a Patient Assessment

PATIENT: Mrs. K. L.	ROOM: 106	CONDITION: Thyroiditis

I. *Social Status:*

    A. Age: 45

    B. Sex: Female

    C. Ethnic origin: American

    D. Race: Caucasian

    E. Marital status:
       Chart indicated separation but not confirmed through conversation with her.

    F. Living relatives:
       Eight living relatives in the immediate family: mother, two brothers, two sisters, one
       daughter, and two sons.
       Brothers and sisters all married and living with their families in the Des Moines area.

    G. Religious affiliation:
       Catholic

    H. Occupation:
       Secretary for several professors at local university.

    I. Housing accommodations:
       Owns home in same city where hospitalized.

    J. Financial status:
       In a semi-private room at the cost of $55 daily and has Blue Cross-Blue Shield Insurance.

    K. Pattern of hospitalization:
       Previously hospitalized for evaluation of colitis, a hemorrhoidectomy, proctosigmoid-
       oscopy, and repair of a cystocele.

II. *Mental Status:*

    A. State of consciousness:
       Quite alert and quick to respond to stimuli.

    B. Orientation:
       Aware of time, place, and person: for example, spoke of Halloween, the length of her
       illness, the various hospitals in which she has been a patient, and mentioned several of
       the nurses on the division.

    C. Intellectual capacity;
       Besides discussing present employment, hospitalization, etc., discussed her childhood
       in Arkansas. Moved from Arkansas approximately 30 years ago. Uses complex,
       technical words: for example, stated she had jaundice as a child and was diagnosed
       with mucoid colitis a few years ago. When discussing job, spoke of typing papers for
       publication by the various professors. Was able to talk at length on the various subjects
       mentioned.

    D. Insight into health status and/or problems:
       Easily recalled and related information given to her by the doctors.
       Explained diet for mucoid colitis in detail, listing foods allowed on the diet.
       Emphasized that "he" (the doctor) thought she had a problem with her thyroid.
       Did not answer when asked what she thought was wrong.
       Questioned the nurses and doctor about various statements she overheard while in
       X-ray and was also worried about some questions that the technician asked.

FIGURE 4-1 (cont.)

III. *Status of Special Senses:*

    A. Auditory perception:
       Able to distinguish low sounds with most of conversation taking place with a distance of approximately 3 feet between the two participants.

    B. Visual perception:
       Did not wear glasses, even for reading.
       Pupils equal in size and symmetry, and responsive to light during assessment.

    C. Speech perception:
       No speech abnormalities noted, but spoke rapidly.

IV. *Motor Ability Status:*

    A. Current mobility status:
       When seen on 11/1, up as tolerated and quite active, walking back from X-ray.
       When seen on 11/2, confined to bed because of an I.V. infusing in left arm.

    B. Posture:
       Stood and walked in an erect posture.
       No evidence of a spinal deviation.
       When seated in a chair, crossed her legs and then pulled one leg up underneath her.

    C. Range of joint motion:
       Had full range of motion in her shoulders, elbows, wrists, and ankles. (No other joints assessed.)

    D. Muscle and nerve status:
       No atrophy noted.
       Movements were coordinated.
       On 11/2 complained of slight weakness when she walked to the bathroom; no such complaints offered on 11/1. On 11/1, even with nausea caused by the barium, did not have problems with equilibrium.
       Has small frame with well-developed arm and leg muscles.

V. *Body Temperature Status:*

    A. Range:
       Prior to hospitalization, had a fever for 2 weeks.
       Since hospitalization, body temperature has ranged from $97.2°$ to $101°$ F.
       Pyrexia intermittent in character. Precipitating factor for pyrexia an inflamed thyroid and pharynx.

VI. *Respiratory Status:*

    A. Character:
       Since hospitalization, respirations ranging from 18 to 32 per minute, are regular, and of moderate depth.
       Breathes with ease, and quietly.
       Lungs clear without evidence of any infiltrate according to chest X-ray.

    B. Interference with respirations:
       No sneezing, coughing, expectoration of sputum during the interview.
       No complaint of respiratory problems.
       Has thyroid mass which was observed and outlined through palpation.
       Enlargement on the right side, involving inferior and superior portion of the gland, indicated by thyroid scan.

FIGURE 4-1 (cont.)

VII. *Circulatory Status:*

    A. Character of arterial pulse:
Radial pulse 130, regular and strong at the time of the assessment; had ranged from 88 to 140 since her admission.
Normal sinus rhythm with tachycardia indicated by EKG.
Possible factors precipitating tachycardia: inflamed thyroid, elevated body temperature; excessive smoking and drinking of coffee observed during the interview, and anxiety noted during the interview.

    B. Apical-radial pulse:
Apical and radial pulses 130; no pulse deficit.

    C. Character of blood pressure:
Systolic range 100 to 130 and diastolic range 70 to 80.
Blood pressure reading taken on left arm while she was lying down, 100/80.
Heart within normal size indicated by chest X-ray.

    D. Movement of fluids:
Drank 2 pots of coffee during the interview on 11/1.
On 11/2, 1000 c.c. of 5% D/W infusing at a slow, "keep-open" rate.
No evidence of edema or dehydration.

VIII. *Nutritional Status:*

    A. Condition of buccal cavity:
Wore upper and lower dentures; had chipped tooth on the upper plate.

    B. Ability to masticate:
Had no difficulty chewing toast which was on her breakfast tray or eating candy provided by her roommate.

    C. Ability to swallow:
Had no difficulty swallowing coffee, toast, or medicine.
Denied dysphagia.
Normal esophagus without evidence of narrowing shown by upper GI X-ray.

    D. Appetite:
Stated has had a decreased appetite since her illness, that gains weight easily, and must watch her weight all the time.
During interview no opportunity to discuss food preferences, but did note that she did not like the diet prescribed for treatment of her colitis.

    E. Ingestion of nutrients:
Stated she does most of her cooking for the week on Sunday and then warms up the leftovers for the rest of the week.
Unable to assess adequacy of her food intake except to note that she ordered only toast and coffee for breakfast on 11/1.
Some food restrictions on certain religious holidays because of Catholicism.
Also a restriction because of her previously diagnosed colitis.
However, does not follow any special diet at home unless her colitis begins to produce symptoms.
While in the hospital, is on a bland diet.
On 11/2, questioned the doctor about reason for diet since she does not adhere to one at home.

    F. Digestion of nutrients:
Experienced slight nausea without vomiting following X-rays with barium.
U.G.I. X-ray normal.

FIGURE 4-1 (cont.)

   G. Weight:
     121 pounds (5'½'' tall). States she recently lost weight because of anorexia.

IX. *Elimination Status:*

   A. Bowel:
     Had some diarrhea before hospitalization but has not complained of any since admission.
     Lomotil ordered if diarrhea returns.
     Diarrhea possibly caused by colitis or hyperthyroidism.

   B. Bladder:
     Not on intake and output.
     Numerous WBCs, mucous threads, sp. gr. of 1.017, and acidic pH shown on admission
     urinalysis.
     Voiding in adequate amounts.

X. *Female Reproductive Status:*

   A. Age of menarche:
     13 years

   B. Pattern of menses:
     According to chart, periods regular, every 3 weeks.
     Menstruating at the present time.

   C. Pregnancies:
     Three full-term.

   D. Breasts:
     Small, symmetrical, and without masses.

XI. *State of Skin and Appendages:*

   A. Skin:
     Clean skin, dark complexion, with a distinct flushing of the neck and face.
     No abnormal pigmentation or lesions noted.
     Dark circles and many wrinkles under her eyes.
     Small scar on her lower lip.
     No evidence of dry skin or perspiration.

   B. Hair:
     Wore her black, gray-frosted hair in a medium length, neat shag with a bouffant top.

   C. Nails:
     Finger- and toenails were manicured.

XII. *State of Physical Rest and Comfort:*

   A. Sleep and/or rest pattern:
     Stated she sleeps "well" but is still tired.
     Rubbed her eyes frequently during the interview.
     Took a nap following the X-rays.
     Usually sleeps 6 hours nightly.

   B. Presence of pain, discomfort, or restlessness:
     Did not complain of actual pain but had tenderness in region of thyroid.
     On 11/2, stated that the tenderness had decreased, probably because of the I.V. admin-
     istration of Solucortef.
     Has not required any pain medication.

FIGURE 4-1 (cont.)

C. Use of supportive aids:
Has been taking Dalmane at bedtime for sleep, and has been resting during the night without problems.
Also receiving Valium, a tranquilizer, and Stental, a sedative.
After observing her rapid talking and frequent change of position on 11/2, would be accurate to state that desired results apparently not attained.

XIII. *Emotional Status:*

Shows anxiety through frequent questioning of everything that takes place; for example, questioned the presence of the interviewer three times during the interview, each time wanting reinforcement that interviewer's presence did not mean she was seriously ill.

Her mother also a patient at same hospital and recently had surgery for cancer of the colon. No verbalization about fear of cancer, but earlier statement made by her: "He [the doctor] thinks it is an inflammation of the thyroid gland," indicating she might think otherwise.

Several times during the interview, laughed and stated, "The doctor wants to know what I am worried about." Also denies being nervous or worried.

Also of interest in the assessment of this patient are the results of some of the diagnostic studies on the thyroid function.

Patient	Normal
PBI 11.4μg/100ml	4.5-9μg/100ml
Radioactive Iodine Uptake	
1.4%	15-35%
T3 Resin Sponge Uptake	
33%	27-37%
Serum Thyroxine	
19.7μg/100ml	5.3-14.5μg/100ml
Free Thyroxine Index	
6.5	1.2-5.00

Notes:
As seen in these results, there is some uncertainty whether the patient is experiencing hyper- or hyposecretion of the thyroid gland.

The McCain's assessment tool was used to assess this patient. Information was obtained from the patient, team leader, charge nurse, doctor, and by observing the patient and studying the chart.

This example is based on an assessment done by Miss Norma Nolan, R.N.M.S.N., for an assignment during graduate studies.

theoretical knowledge to his situation and use an assessment guide to determine his present response. What do you hope to accomplish? Immediate priorities may be to establish rapport and guide his understanding of the situation, preserve musculoskeletal function, prevent skin breakdown, assist the family in the crisis situation, and establish adequate elimination and nutrition. Long-range goals may include rehabilitation to optimum physical function, a return to work, or help with the acceptance of a disability. The physical and intellectual means for meeting, in an individualized manner, those priorities of care most in need of adaptive help are the components of the next step.

Intervention

All actions that you carry out to promote the patient's adaptation comprise intervention, the second step in the nursing process. You *intervene* (from the Latin meaning "come between") *when you modify, settle, or hinder some action* in order to prevent harm or further dysfunction.

"Ministering" to patients, carrying out "comfort" measures, or "caring" for the sick are terms often equated by lay people with conserving the ill person's energy by waiting on him. But your interpretation of *care* and *comfort* should encompass the overall goal of professional nursing: to assist the person to function as effectively and efficiently as the limits of his illness permit, and to encourage him to react to the situation in his own unique way. Care that is limited to energy-conserving measures on the patient's behalf may be very detrimental to his progress.

Without the foundation of assessment your actions will be mechanical, meaningless, detached, and often inaccurate. In addition, you must know the *scientific rationale, the reasons, either physiological or psychosocial, for performing any action.* For example, do you bathe the patient because of a rigid schedule or because of physiological and psychosocial principles involving (1) increased circulation and aeration, (2) care of the integument, (3) preservation of musculoskeletal function, and (4) opportunity for communication, further assessment, and health teaching?

Nursing actions may comprise either dependent or independent functions: those depending on the medical regimen as outlined by the physician, or those derived from nursing judgments. Through nursing intervention you execute all those ministrations that help meet needs the individual cannot meet for himself. Intervention includes all comfort and hygiene measures; safe and efficient use of medical techniques and skills; planning and creating an environment conducive to wholeness, including protection from risk and injury; and health teaching, formal and informal. It also includes the offering of self for strength and courage in coping with problems through counseling, listening, and socializing; and utilizing information for referrals wherever indicated, either for in-agency care or as discharge planning.

The concept of rehabilitation could be considered as almost synonymous with intervention, since from the very beginning of your relationship with the patient, intervention must be geared to restoration of the person's potential for optimum functioning.

Since the nursing process is a problem-solving mode of action using the scientific method, your nursing actions are hypotheses to be tested in practice. When they are shown to be effective and can be validated, specific actions or ways in which needs are best met become a part of the on-going individualized nursing care plan. The third step of the nursing process, evaluation, is used to determine the validity of these actions.

Evaluation

Evaluation, determining immediate outcomes and predicting long-range results, cannot be entirely separated from intervention or assessment. The nursing process moves continually in a circular path with constant reassessment, redefinition of priorities, and reevaluation of the effects of your care. Nursing objectives based on priorities of care establish the criteria for evaluation. These criteria must be observable or measurable, indicating that the care given was or was not effective. The hypotheses tested during intervention are thus proved or disproved as achieving the desired effect. Validation must include feedback from the recipients of care, patient or family, and from members of the health team who are objective observers. Subjective symptoms such as pain and results of intervention are best evaluated by the patient. Observable signs may be evaluated best by the health team.

The goal of your chosen action within the nursing process is always to objectively minimize the negative consequences to the greatest degree possible and to capitalize on those outcomes that are positive. In evaluating results of intervention you will seek to duplicate the positive effects and to determine the cause of unexpected outcomes, whether positive or negative. In a negative outcome, attempt to control or help the patient control the events responsible so that the outcome does not recur.

Recognizing that an act may have more than one consequence, you must evaluate who will be affected by the act, what results can be anticipated, and what will be the value of the consequences to those involved [6]. Being aware of this evaluation process will help you appreciate that even the simplest activity is a means of achieving the goals you have set for the patient in his striving toward wellness. Emptying a bedpan then becomes not an isolated menial task, but a part of your intervention for carrying out some of the priorities of care, such as provision of needed rest and maintenance of elimination and fluid balance.

Evaluation of care is directly related to what is termed *accountability, the state of being responsible for one's acts and being able to explain, define, or measure in some way the results of decision making*. Accountability involves evaluating the effectiveness of care on the basis of "how," "what," and "to whom" [24]. Just believing that your care makes a difference is not enough. You must have criteria that justify both the need for and the effectiveness of your nursing actions.

The "how" is measuring your effectiveness against a set of criteria—a predetermined outcome to be observed. Noting that an immobile patient to whom you have been giving daily prune juice is now able to have a normal stool at reasonable intervals without requiring enemas or cathartics is one example of observing a predetermined outcome. You can evaluate the care of an individual patient, care given within a nursing unit, or care delivered by an entire community health agency or clinic[35].

The "what" of accountability involves intervention measures and intangibles, such as attitudes and subtle nuances. The nursing measures you carry out are important, but equally important is the meaning of care to the person.

In order to decide "to whom" you are accountable, you must first clarify for yourself the nature and the purpose of your care. You will be accountable to the patient, client, family, group, doctor, nursing staff, agency administration, and community[24].

By being accountable and sharing evaluations with the health team through team conferences, you help assure optimum health promotion, especially if there is joint agreement on results expected and a willingness to try new approaches.

FORMULATING A NURSING CARE PLAN

A nursing care plan is a record summarizing all information required to carry out appropriate nursing care for an individual patient or a family at a given time. The plan is built upon the nursing assessment of health needs and indicates specific goals to be reached with the patient and family through designated nursing actions[13].

You can establish an effective plan by using information derived from the nursing history and the current assessment data and by communicating with other health care personnel to set priorities, to establish goals, and to decide on a common approach to the individual patient's or family's care.

Formulating a care plan can thus be considered as assessment, but it is discussed separately because knowledge of the entire nursing process is necessary before you can formulate a plan.

Historical Background

Nursing care plans have been discussed and written about for over 20 years, yet in actual practice they are seldom used as originally conceived. Nursing care plans grew out of the team-nursing concept. As the professional nurse became a leader of a small group of ancillary nursing personnel with limited expertise, developing a means of communicating a plan for patient care became necessary. Many writers in the 1960s emphasized that nursing care plans should reflect the goals of nursing care and be the means of setting priorities and stating objectives[10]. Recently, care plans have been used more comprehensively by including input from other disciplines as well as from nursing goals, priorities, and objectives. Psychosocial as well as physical needs are included in today's plans, and more patient and family participation in formulating a plan is encouraged.

Purposes of the Nursing Care Plan

Properly formulated and executed, nursing care plans improve care and minimize wasted efforts.

Harris gives a poignant account of a patient for whom a nursing care plan would have provided comfort and relief from uncertainty[15]. Ms. Harris shared a two-bed room with an elderly patient who was almost totally deaf, who nodded agreement and replied, "Fine," to whatever any staff person said. When she did push her signal button, the ward clerk's "May I help you?" was never heard. Consequently her mechanical bed controls remained a mystery to her. Cartons of milk and the strange packets on her food tray often remained unopened. Almost in rebuttal is the statement by Palisan that "nursing care plans are a snare and a delusion." She gives examples of situations in which poorly written or nonupdated care plans were used to the detriment of patient or family care and the wasting of staff's time[34].

Both of these experiences point to the importance of the "who" in relation to care plans as opposed to the "why." There are two sides to the "who." One refers to the patients and families who stand to benefit from the use of written care plans. They are the patients or families who cannot communicate their needs either because of disability, communication barriers, or psychological reasons. Many persons on self-care units may have little or no need for a written plan. But some patients or families with few physical problems may have so many emotional needs that nursing intervention should be more extensive for them than for a patient who requires only physical help.

The other "who" refers to those persons who make the decisions for care and write the plans. Nurses must be responsible for practical plans that are kept current with the patients' changing conditions. The communication of relevant patient information from one nurse to another and from one shift to another is not new. Formerly, the head nurse used a notebook, a "day sheet," or some such method whereby she communicated instructions for patients' care to the students and staff. At no time was word-of-mouth used exclusively. Whether written communication can be refined into effective care plans thus depends on who uses it and how it is used.

One of the most important reasons for devising a nursing care plan is to provide consistent, up-to-date care to the patient and family in the face of a constantly changing staff. But keeping information current applies to other Kardex* data, such as the person's diagnosis. You should take a personal interest in keeping this accurate as new findings appear on the patient's record. When a patient is admitted to a hospital, his doctor gives the business office an admitting diagnosis. Check the spelling and accuracy of terms when this information is

---

*Kardex refers to a holder with card(s) for each patient, providing space for summary of treatments, medications, and specific approaches to nursing care.

received in your unit, as the typist is not expected to know medical terminology as well as you do. She may also have had difficulty differentiating between similar terms when spoken quickly on the phone by the physician. After the patient is admitted his diagnosis may change, and unless noted on the Kardex, your approach to his care could be wrong.

Consider the experience of a nurse who was admitted as a patient to the hospital with a diagnosis of acute enteritis. The next day the cause of her illness was found to be pyelonephritis. During the ensuing 12 days, certain new team leaders who talked with the patient on their "walking rounds" approached her in the context of the diagnosis of enteritis. She was questioned about her bowel pattern to the exclusion of any concern for urinary function. The team leader would consult her Kardex and ask such things as, "Why are you still on I & O?" or "Don't you think this cranberry juice you asked for will irritate your bowel?" The patient explained her revised diagnosis, but apparently no one had ever changed it on the Kardex. If she had been a lay person rather than a nurse, this situation could have been most confusing and even serious in terms of possible errors in intervention.

Format for the Nursing Care Plan

The format used for the written care plan will vary from agency to agency, but in any situation the plan must be simple to use and capable of being readily understood by all workers. Figures 4-2 and 4-3 show a simple Kardex form designed as a double card for an individual patient's plan. One card usually contains spaces for basic information: age, activity, type of bath, and directions regarding intake, output, and vital signs (see Figure 4-2). Note the section for indicating communication barriers: If the patient is blind, aphasic, hard of hearing, or speaks a foreign language, it should be noted in a prominent place. The space for indicating diet information runs the width of this card; stating several modifications of or exceptions to basic diet orders is frequently necessary. Spaces for writing in the patient's treatments and medications also appear on this card, as well as a space for special instructions in administering them. Each person administering treatments should be aware of special modifications and of the patient's wishes regarding particular treatments. The size and number of dressings to be used, any special way equipment should be arranged, and difficulties to be anticipated and avoided should also be noted in the space under "Special Instructions." The Kardex card may also have a space for indicating ordered diagnostic tests and special procedures.

Figure 4-3 illustrates the companion card in the Kardex. In actual practice this card is often without any entry, or contains a few facts that more properly belong under "Treatments" on the other card. Frequently a laboratory report or a date of a diagnostic test is written here erroneously. This card, devoted to the actual plan of nursing care, should receive your most critical attention. It sepa-

FIGURE 4-2
Sample Kardex Card

NAME		AGE	BATH	Tub	Shower	Bed
RELIGION				Complete	Assist	
ACTIVITY			COMMUNICATION BARRIERS			

I & O	V.S.
DIET	

TREATMENTS	SPECIAL INSTRUCTIONS FOR PATIENT

MEDICATIONS	

rates the *nursing orders* (needs, problems, and goals and how to meet them) from the *medical orders* (treatments).

Figure 4-4 illustrates the kinds of entries that might appear on a nursing care plan. Notice that the patient's needs (in parentheses) are exemplified by the stated problems. This plan is for an elderly man with diabetes, arteriosclerotic-heart disease, and tuberculosis. (Needs relating to physiological or psychosocial problems are not usually written on the plan, but are illustrated here to help you understand the basis for the problems.) Whenever you list special problems and the ways in which they may be helped, be sure you can identify the need from which they stem. This step will strengthen your conceptual approach to nursing care and provide a way for validating your nursing actions on the basis of scientific rationale. Glibly stating problems without seeing the underlying need

FIGURE 4-3
Sample Kardex Card, continued

NEEDS – PROBLEMS – GOALS	HOW TO MEET
DIAGNOSIS	SURGERY
RM. NO. NAME	DOCTOR

reflects a lack of awareness of the adaptation occurring in the person's progress toward health and will result in a limited approach to care.

Teaching begins at the time of the patient's admission and should appear in your care plan from the beginning. It may appear as a part of intervention aimed at a current need, such as explaining the importance of elevating the legs, or of using foam pads (as shown in Figure 4-4). Or it may be geared to discharge arrangements, as is the plan for teaching a diabetic. Whatever the need, include it in your plan in such a way as to insure teaching which can be carried out easily and consistently by everyone. Writing instructions is not enough. Conference discussions and individual help to team members in interpreting the need for teaching are necessary if instruction is to be productive.

The example in Figure 4-4 represents only one common form for writing a nursing care plan. Nothing prevents you from creating your own or from using a form that is particularly suited to the setting in which you work. One such form is a nurse's order sheet. It may be kept in the chart and the orders transcribed onto the Kardex by the ward clerk in the same way as are physicians' orders. This procedure provides a permanent record of nursing intervention while keeping the Kardex current. It might well serve in a long-term facility or as a part of a patient's clinic record.

A different approach to care plans, the *standard care routine*, has emerged

FIGURE 4-4
Example of Entries for Nursing Care Plan

PROBLEMS	HOW TO MEET
(Need for increased aeration)	
Dyspnea.	Head of bed 45°.
Mouth dry.	Frequent mouthwash and mouth care.
Tends to slide down in bed.	Check position frequently.
	Keep footboard in place.
(Need for improved circulation and skin integrity)	
Generalized edema.	Monitor flow of I.V. fluids carefully—15 gtts./min.
Tends to sit on edge of bed.	Explain to patient importance of elevating legs.
	Prevent dependence of extremities when up in chair.
Pressure on edematous areas.	Change position q. 2h.
	Frequent skin care to back and extremities with lotion.
	Use foam pads on heels.
(Need for improved GU function)	
Incontinent of urine at night.	Offer urinal at 2-hour intervals.
	Check condition of bed frequently.
Anxious and embarrassed when wet.	Reassure—keep bed dry—urinal at close reach.
(Need for patient teaching)	
Lacks understanding of his diabetes and dietary management.	Encourage discussion and questions.
	Refer to literature he has been given—check with dietician at intervals to keep current on her plans for him.
Should be able to give own insulin several days before discharge.	Check with Mrs. R. (clinical specialist) re her plans and how we can cooperate in his learning.

in the last few years[27]. In this type of plan, similarities as well as differences among patients are recognized (see Figure 4-5).

Under this system, the most frequently occurring types of patient problems are identified, and routine standards of care for each are developed and pre-printed onto cards. The effectiveness of these routines is based on the assessment of the patient to determine whether or not his problems are "usual" or "unusual." If the former, this is noted on the printed form placed in the Kardex, and the standard routine for that particular illness, surgery, or disability is followed. "Usual Problems" are listed under that heading and accompanied by appropriate "Expected Outcomes" and "Nursing Directions" in adjoining columns on the form.

FIGURE 4-5

Standard Nursing Care Form for Preoperative Care

USUAL PROBLEMS	EXPECTED OUTCOMES	NURSING DIRECTIONS
Date 1. Anxiety due to impending surgery and unfamiliar environment.	1. Verbalize questions and concerns. Verbalize: "I know what to expect now." Restful preoperative night.	1. (a) Evening or afternoon before surgery, explain unit and pre- and postoperative routines. (b) Explain specific procedures relating to patient's type of surgery: prep. sleeping medication. preoperative medication. time of surgery. visitors can be present. when doctor will visit. time in recovery room and what to expect. when first ambulate postoperatively. general postoperative management. usual length of hospital stay.
2. Potential complications or injury while medicated or anesthetized.	2. (a) No injuries, falls, or accidents. (b) No physical complications.	2. (a) Routine prep. (b) See preoperative checklist: no jewelry. no dentures. no hairpins. no contact lens. no prosthesis. (c) Patient to void before preoperative medication given. (d) Preoperative medication as ordered (will not put patient to sleep). (e) Stay in bed after preoperative medication given.

UNUSUAL PROBLEMS	EXPECTED OUTCOMES	NURSING DIRECTIONS

Dr. _____ Patient Name _____ Addressograph _____

Note: Modification of plan developed by nursing staff, St. Mary's Health Center, Tucson, Arizona.

If, however, the patient is assessed to have "unusual" problems, these are written into a space left blank at the bottom of the sheet for that purpose and matched with Expected Outcomes and Nursing Directions in the other two columns.

The success of the plan depends on making an appropriate individualized assessment of each patient in order to determine his "usual" and "unusual" problems. Having printed cards in readiness saves writing time and yet ensures that routine measures will not be forgotten. The danger of a standard care routine is that the "unusual" will not be noticed, and robot-like care will be given to every patient, negating the original intent of individualized care.

Use of the Nursing Care Plan

One recent study that reviewed over 1000 nursing care plans revealed that over 70 percent of the notations related to medications, treatments, monitoring of vital signs, intake and output, and diagnostic studies. Less than 10 percent related to the prevention of harmful sequelae. And nursing orders related to preservation of body defenses, elimination, comfort measures, emotional support, rehabilitation, and discharge planning comprised only about 5 percent of the total—a sad commentary on nursing's ability to translate ideas into action. Even worse, 15 percent of the information was really irrelevant[10].

What can you do to change this ratio? Only when you and your colleagues can concentrate your efforts as individual nurse practitioners will you be able to create an impact on the struggle of nursing for professionalism and for an accumulation of a body of knowledge unique to itself. The forms you use for nursing care plans may not spell out the differences between sections for medical orders and those for nursing orders as clearly as the forms illustrated here. But if you follow the suggestions and examples given, you and your coworkers should be able to compile a nursing care plan that is clear and helpful enough to inspire its faithful use for the benefit of patients' and families' care as well as for increased efficiency of the staff.

A nursing care plan is everyone's responsibility. If the aide is capable of admitting the patient, taking his vital signs, weighing him, and writing the results, she is capable of beginning a care plan by writing other information: "says he often feels faint" ... "has an artificial left leg" ... "likes to sleep with the window open" ... "requires kosher food". These observations can then be sorted out and used by the professional nurse to begin the written plan in a more formal sense. Much of the potential success of written plans lies in the ability of the professional nurse to involve team members on all levels in the task of keeping the plan current. If ancillary personnel are never consulted about the plan or coached in its use, it will never become a viable part of the scheme of care.

Implementing a nursing care plan should follow these guidelines:

1. Keep it simple.
2. Keep it on-going.
3. Encourage and help every team member, whatever his or her level of ability, to take responsibility and pride in amending, adding to, and improving the plan.
4. Meet periodically with the whole team on your shift to evaluate the outcome of care and to revise the plan.
5. Include the patient and the family in the planning.
6. Communicate your ideas to teams on other shifts and encourage them to make suggestions or changes as needed.
7. Include patient teaching as an integral part of the plan.

Even if the nursing administration issues edicts requiring the use of care plans, their potential will not be realized unless there is support from each team member. Additionally, time must be allocated for the writing of care plans. It cannot be an activity "tacked on" to the daily work or sandwiched in between other tasks.

You can help create interest in systematic and continued care planning wherever you work by utilizing such written care plans, by exploring ways in which to implement them, and by encouraging your coworkers to do the same. Keeping the nursing care plan consistent and accurate, eliminating conflicting information, and updating pertinent data will take little time if done daily. Your personal commitment plus an interested administration will make nursing care plans a realistic adjunct to improved care.

TOOLS FOR
EVALUATING YOUR EFFECTIVENESS

The Process Recording

Communication is essential to the nursing process and thus will be repeatedly emphasized throughout the book. One tool for analyzing your communication pattern with patients is the process recording.

The *process recording is a written account of the responses of patient and nurse and the analysis of these responses*, providing for the reconstruction of a nursing incident in order to identify and examine the elements in it. It may be written during the time the conversation or interview is occurring or from recollection.

The reconstruction of an interview or conversation with a person is valuable for picking out clues to his behavior and for determining inconsistencies in your response to him. The process recording allows you to evaluate your responses in relation to communication principles and methods, improve communication, more accurately focus on the patient's needs, and make predictions about nursing intervention. In addition, you provide the patient a seldom-available opportunity to express himself to someone who listens in a nonjudgmental way. Thus you help him sort out his thoughts and feelings. The process recording is also a teaching tool. When you share with other team members what you have told the patient and his reaction to his illness, they can use this information as a guide in further therapeutic communication.

The forms used for process recordings are various, but all should provide columns in which the responses or perceptions of the nurse are separated from the responses of the patient. A third column is used to analyze the responses of either the nurse, or the patient, or both. Figure 4-6 is an example.

You should get the person's consent if you plan to take notes during an interview. A stenographer's notebook is sufficient—one column for the patient's responses and one for yours. The success of this approach depends on your writing down the first few words spoken by you or the patient in each exchange and leaving these thoughts as incomplete sentences. Also, jot down nonverbal clues. (You will need to devise your own "shorthand" system.)

Although you may initially feel self-conscious when writing, most patients agree to this system when you tell them it will help you give better care. The interview you analyze through a process recording may occur in a variety of settings and may last from five minutes to an hour, depending on your purpose and the patient's needs and condition.

You will build on the foundation of interviewing and therapeutic communication studied in Chapter 3. Generally you will make use of open-ended questions beginning with "Who...," "What...," "When...," or "Where...," as well as statements that encourage the patient to talk freely about his concerns. The patient must be able to sense your regard for him and your interest in his ideas, hopes, and fears. Your nonjudgmental attitude is essential to help the patient sort out *his* ideas and reach the solution he sees as most feasible for him.

As soon as possible after the interview, reconstruct it from your brief notes and make an analysis of the verbal and nonverbal dialogue. This expansion can help you gain insight into yourself and the patient and provide data for planning care. If your approach to the patient seems to be unproductive, a process recording in which incidents are reconstructed may help identify the problem. Clues can be analyzed for their meaning by writing out what preceded certain of your or the patient's responses. You can better realize ways in which you could have intervened in a more direct or helpful manner, perhaps by rephrasing or refocusing your portion of the dialogue.

Written Analysis of Nursing Care

Another tool for evaluating your effectiveness in the nursing process and nurse-patient relationship is a *written analysis of nursing care*. This provides a way of looking at your assessment of needs, your intervention, and the scientific rationale upon which your intervention was based, and of evaluating the care you gave.

FIGURE 4-6

Process Recording

PATIENT'S VERBAL AND NONVERBAL COMMUNICATION	NURSE'S VERBAL AND NONVERBAL COMMUNICATION	ANALYSIS OF COMMUNICATION PATTERN, THOUGHTS, AND FEELINGS
	I knock and enter the room to do preoperative teaching. I sit down on a chair near the bed and look at her with a serious expression and say, "Mrs. Jones, have you been told you're going to surgery tomorrow?"	Wanted to make sure she knew about surgery before I began teaching and to check her level of readiness for teaching. Sat down to show her I had time and was interested in her.
"Yes, that's what they told me." Facial expression is serious as she looks at me. She clenches the sheet; restlessly moves legs. Chin quivers as she speaks.		
	I pause briefly to let her continue talking if she wishes.	Noted her movements and that her pupils are dilated in a well-lit room, indicating anxiety.
She looks down.	"What are you feeling about going to surgery?" I lean slightly forward and maintain eye contact.	Asking open-ended question to encourage her to talk about feelings. Must relieve anxiety before she will be able to hear or utilize my teaching.
"Oh, honey, I'm scared to death!" She shifts position toward me. "You know, they're cutting on me for my gall-bladder. The doctor told me it was nothing, but I know of a person who died after gall-bladder surgery."	I nod as she talks to show acceptance of her feelings and to encourage further talking. I maintain silence.	Noted the use of words "cutting on me"—surgery can mean mutilation and be a threat to body image. Need to talk about feelings to resolve them.
	"You're afraid you'll die?" Speak softly, with acceptance.	Reflect back main idea to encourage further talking.
"Yes, I just might not wake up. People *die* with surgery." Pauses.	Silence.	Let her continue talking about this if she needs to. Nothing I say right now would make a difference.
"I keep telling myself that it's unlikely that I'll die, that my doctor is right saying I won't die, that I am in good hands."		

FIGURE 4-6 (cont.)

PATIENT'S VERBAL AND NONVERBAL COMMUNICATION	NURSE'S VERBAL AND NONVERBAL COMMUNICATION	ANALYSIS OF COMMUNICATION PATTERN, THOUGHTS, AND FEELINGS
	"Yes, facing surgery is frightening, although your ideas about not dying and being in good hands are true. It takes courage to go to surgery, but in this case it is for your ultimate comfort.	Restate feelings, recognize and validate feelings, but also try to reinforce ideas so she can feel less worried.
She smiles, clenched hands relaxed. "You do understand! I thought maybe I was abnormal."	Look toward her with a slight smile. "Your feelings are not abnormal. Tell me more about how you're feeling."	Noted she is beginning to relax. Being accepted and listened to as she talked helped reduce anxiety. Validate with her about her feelings; show acceptance. Use open-ended question to encourage further talking if she needs to.
Stretches in bed, smiles, "Oh, I feel better just being able to tell you and having you understand."		
	"Do you feel ready to discuss the preparation you'll be having for surgery?"	Question phrased to get "yes or no" response. Want to check readiness for teaching.

You may at first have difficulty delineating the steps of the nursing process. These steps can be made clearer by answering the following questions: What did you see that required your help? What did you do about it and why? What happened or is likely to happen as a result of what you did? These are essentially *assessment, intervention and rationale,* and *evaluation* expressed in elementary terms.

Assessments may be put down in a sequential order if you wish, or they may be sorted out according to functional areas. Figure 4-7 gives an example of analyzing care according to functional areas.

Intervention, Together with the Reason for Your Action, is placed in a second column. A stumbling block in this portion of your analysis is often the confusion of medical intervention with that of nursing. For example, if the patient has an intravenous pyelogram done in X-ray, that is medical intervention. If you explain the test to the patient, allay his fears through communication and teaching, and prepare him for the test by administering prescribed medication or treatments, these are nursing interventions.

You should justify or give the rationale for action on the patient's behalf, validating your rationale with the literature. Therefore, familiarity with the

FIGURE 4-7

Analysis of Care, Sample Form

Name _____ Mrs. S. _____ Age __56__ Date __2-1__

Diagnosis __Arthritis – R. total hip replacement – 2nd postop day__

Nurse __Mr. J._____

ASSESSMENT	INTERVENTION AND RATIONALE	EVALUATION
8:30 A.M. Obese female—appears in pain—has Buck's traction on R. leg. Foot plate is resting against foot of bed.	Had aide help me move patient up in bed to release pressure on footplate which interferes with efficiency of traction. Checked chart to see when pain medication was given last. Most pain medication is given no oftener than q. 3–4 hours to avoid oversedation and respiratory embarrassment.	Should help alleviate some of her pain by allowing a more even pull from traction. Must remember after this to check on time of last medication before seeing patient.
No pain medication given since 2:00 A.M.	Gave injection of Demerol 100 mg. IM before beginning bath to promote relaxation, relief of pain, and more ease in moving.	Mrs. S. more relaxed after about 20 minutes.
Has perspired during night. Breath is somewhat fetid—mouth dry.	Gave oral care (preserves integrity of gums, prevents dental caries, and heightens enjoyment of food). Gave complete bed bath to refresh, provide chance for observation, stimulate circulation and aeration, and cleanse skin. Removed traction for skin care and gave back care q. 2h. to prevent pressure areas by stimulation of areas over bony prominences. Did ROM exercises with unaffected extremities to maintain joint mobility, muscle tone, enhance circulation, prevent thrombus formation. Bath and exercises aid maintenance and reintegration of body image.	Appeared more comfortable after bath and is in proper body alignment.
Talked during bath about fear of crutch walking.	Encouraged Mrs. S. to verbalize concerns about walking. Talking promotes anxiety reduction and enables patient to begin problem solving. My listening showed respect for and interest in her as a person, gave attention, promoted trust in nurse-patient relationship.	Explanation of pool therapy and therapist's help in P.T. seemed to help her figure out for herself that she should walk OK. Mrs. S. came to conclusion after our conversation that she would wait to see progress before assuming she would have trouble walking.

current nursing literature, as well as an ability to use the literature of related disciplines, the natural and behavioral sciences and humanities, will be a necessary part of your continued independent study as you practice nursing.

Evaluation is the step often overlooked or given minimal attention. Yet it is the basis for reassessment and improvement of care and should be included in your written analysis. You may be able to incorporate some of the process recording in your evaluation. Your reassessment is then based on a more complete data base and can be done with a number of interrelated facts, some of which, if missing, would change considerably your approach to the improvement of the patient's care. For example, you may see that the outcome of the bath you've given is increased relaxation for the patient, including a restful nap before lunch, but fail to evaluate the feeling of dependence and loss of self-actualization expressed by the patient verbally and nonverbally. His rehabilitation may then be seriously impaired through inadequate evaluation.

THE NURSE-PATIENT RELATIONSHIP
IN THE NURSING PROCESS

Nursing is based on a concern, direct and indirect, for individuals, families, communities, and all with whom you work.

Defining nursing as a *process* implies that it is an *experience* or a series of happenings shared by the nurse and an individual or group of persons in need of some assistance in dealing with health problems. There is a dynamic quality to these happenings as they constantly change in structure and intensity. As each individual person creates an impact on the other, change occurs. To be able to bring about change in a thoughtful, purposeful manner is a nursing activity [39]. Establishing a helpful relationship is one of the unique functions separating nursing from other health services.

Differences between a Social and a Helpful Relationship

The nurse-patient relationship is a helpful, purposeful interaction between an authority in health care, the nurse, and a person or group with health care needs. Through this relationship the nursing process is put to use, and it must be differentiated from mere association. Social contact with another individual, verbal or nonverbal, may exert some influence upon one of the participants, and needs may be met. But inconsistency, nonpredictability, or partial fulfillment of expectations on the part of one or all concerned often result. A nurse-patient relationship is established *when patient needs are met consistently and unconditionally*.

A working nurse-patient relationship is by definition good, helpful, therapeutic. There is no such thing as a poor nurse-patient relationship; there are only poor or unsatisfactory experiences that prevent establishing the relationship. Interactions moving toward a relationship occur whenever direct patient care, health teaching, listening, or counseling are done, or when patients' activities are being directed or modified in some way.

The following types of interactions are *not* helpful to the patient because needs are met inconsistently or conditionally:

1. Automatic, in which there is no meaning to either person.
2. Impersonally helpful, in which a service is expertly given but no personal interest or empathy is displayed.
3. Involuntary, in which "carrying out orders" is done as a duty, often the result of the nurse's perception of work as just a job to be done.
4. Inconsistent (that which is conditional in nature)—assisting the patient only when his situation is interesting or when it fulfills the nurse's own needs [39].

The nurse-patient relationship is one in which the patient's real complaint is uncovered. The focus is on the patient's needs rather than on your own. The patient is not a social buddy. There is a giving of self in an objective way to the patient and family, yet you do not identify with (feel the same as), pity, or reject the one seeking help. Neither do you feel you are the only person who can help the patient. You utilize the resources that a team can offer whenever it is beneficial to the patient or family.

The Effect of Feelings upon the Relationship

Only through mutual striving for self-awareness and appreciation of the other person's reactions can a nurse-patient relationship grow to maturity. Knowing that each person has needs to be met gives meaning to this relationship. You must expect both positive and negative feelings in yourself and in the patient, and must realize that both can be expressed either overtly or covertly.

The patient's positive feelings may be those relating to a sincere desire to cooperate in his own care and may include a polite manner toward others. The feelings may be a result of his educational, religious, or cultural background, or a combination of these factors. In any event, you are in a position to capitalize on such positive feelings in order to establish rapport and a sense of trust as a foundation for the nurse-patient relationship. Additionally, make every effort to learn the patient's negative feelings: insecurity; distrust of unfamiliar persons, routines, and treatments; or helplessness or hostility because of a lack of control over his own responses—all may be present.

Unfortunately, when either positive or negative overt feelings dominate a patient's behavior, he may be labeled "good" or "bad" by the staff. The "good" patient is the one who never complains, who accepts his illness no matter how distressing or painful it may be, and who receives the care given him without question. The characteristics of the "bad" patient are usually described by staff as demanding, complaining, and displeasing physically and conversationally. He is seen as not helping himself, unappreciative, and uncooperative. Nurses often become upset or judgmental with the intransigent patient as well. He is the one who does not understand the rules in the same way that you do; he interferes with the established routine. Yet, his interference may be an expression of the very self-determination necessary for his rehabilitation[23]. Often the behavior of the person from a different culture, social class, or ethnic group is misinterpreted. When the person's behavior does not match your expectations, do not label it. Rather, try to understand why the behavior might be different.

The positive feelings you may have toward the patient are strongly bound to your commitment to nursing as a way of life. They cannot develop if you are merely doing a job, because the negative feelings we all possess can overpower the positive and interfere with the nurse-patient relationship. Negative feelings, which may at times be expressed in your reactions to patients, will provoke inappropriate behavior. Talking out your negative feelings with the staff is better than unloading them on the patient.

The Effect of Behavior upon the Relationship

To develop an awareness of the feelings you take with you to the patient, examine your behavior to determine whether it is modified for some people in a helping way and for others in a manner that hinders your effectiveness. Modification of your behavior with, or approach to, different persons is a valuable tool. Surely you would behave differently toward the child than toward the aged person. But behaving differently because a person is rich or poor, black or white, quiet or boisterous, grateful or ungrateful, in agreement or disagreement with your value system may prevent you from meeting his needs.

Remembering that all behavior has meaning will help you to sharpen and improve those qualities you possess that produce a positive response in others. When inappropriate reactions do occur, analyze them in terms of what preceded them and of what happened after the incident. Search for clues to establish the meaning of feelings. Using the process recording format, you might record the event by writing the conversation and the nonverbal responses of both you and patient for closer analysis. Discussing the incident with objective persons may help, perhaps in team conference. Become familiar with your own coping mechanisms; seek to understand their relative value and the ways in which you use them in your approach to patient care. Take sufficient care of your personal needs outside the nursing setting so you can give your best professional care to the patient.

Although the relationship with a patient is a reciprocal experience, the responsibility for establishing it and for making appropriate changes in it rests with you, not with the patient. The relationship is based on each person's perceiving the other as a unique individual without stereotyping. Help the patient *not* to see you as the command officer or the "angel in white," and avoid seeing him as a "gallbladder" or a room number.

You may unconsciously exhibit a middle-class tea-and-cookie niceness combined with Puritan morality that insists on uncompromising obedience on the part of nursing student, nurse, patient, and family alike. You may represent a punitive social system, and the person may sense your moral indignation toward health problems that some regard as stemming from "indiscretions": alcoholism, drug addiction, unwed motherhood, obesity, venereal disease, or even diabetes uncontrolled because of dietary carelessness. Superimposed on this may be the ethic of cleanliness in which you loom as a threat to the other, judging him in terms of how clean he is, internally as well as externally.

Hospital administration sometimes contribute to stereotyping by commending the nurse as "good" if she gets the beds and baths finished, the pills passed, the treatments done. Since these things are tangible they do not require time for involvement with patients' reactions, behavior, or qualitative responses of nurse to patient or patient to nurse [18]. Tasks must be done and are vital to patient care, but overemphasis on tasks leaves little time for exploring the meaning of the person's health status and health goals.

Carrying out the patient's planned regimen for health maintenance or restoration will be accomplished more easily because of the nurse-patient relationship, as it will naturally foster the tangible as well as the intangible aspects of your care. Above all, keep expectations mutual and remember that the major characteristic of the nurse-patient relationship is that *the nursing needs of the individual or family are met in an emotional climate of warmth, support, and mutual trust* [39].

Guidelines for the Nurse-Patient Relationship

If you regard your behavior as an influence on the patient's behavior, you will be in a better position to advise specific approaches for bringing about change. You will want to develop the following:

1. *Empathetic understanding*, in which you respond to the person's deeper feelings as well as to his superficial ones.
2. *Positive regard*, through which concern is expressed for experiences, feelings, and potentials, especially important during an illness that erodes self-worth and esteem.
3. *Genuineness,* in which you use communication verbally and nonverbally in a constructive manner to open further areas of inquiry.
4. *Explicitness of expression*, in which your responses permit discussion and full expression in concrete terms about the person's concerns.
5. *Self-exploration*, through which you encourage the patient to be completely himself in his relationship with you.

Working with these dimensions in patient care and evaluating your level of achieving them will help you provide open and honest experiences for your patients—experiences patients must have to be both healthy and free [3].

Phases of the Nurse-Patient Relationship

Unless the encounter is brief, the feelings between you and the patient and his family and the work jointly done evolve through a sequence of phases. The phases are not sharply demarcated, and they vary in duration. They can be compared to human developmental stages because of the degree of dependency-independency and feelings of trust involved: the orientation phase is comparable to infancy, identification to childhood, the working phase to adolescence, and termination to adulthood[5, 17, 36].

The Initial or Orientation Phase of the relationship begins when you first meet the person or family. You might carry out intervention measures shortly thereafter, as you function in the role of technical expert, counselor, teacher, referral person, or substitute mother. However, your main tasks during this phase are to become oriented to the patient's expectations, health needs, and goals through assessment while simultaneously orienting him to your role and health care goals and his role in the health care system. You formulate a tentative care plan. Establishing rapport and showing acceptance are vital for assessing and orienting the other person. Be aware of how you are affecting him and how he is affecting you. During this period, the person clarifies for himself his health status and its meaning to him through your exploration of the many factors affecting him.

The Second Phase, Called the Identification Phase, marks the time when the patient has become better acquainted with you, places his trust in your decisions and actions, works closely with you, follows your suggestions, and at times imitates your behavior. He sees you as "his nurse." You continue the nursing process, actively guiding him but also providing opportunities for his participation in self-care. You accept his dependency without fostering it excessively.

The Third or Working Phase is the time when the patient is becoming more independent, actively using all services and resources offered by the health team. He becomes more assertive and no longer relies so heavily on you. By now he is usually regaining physical and emotional health—optimal function—so his behavior begins to change as he becomes more involved in decision making about certain aspects of his situation. Although he seems more independent and even self-centered, you can now work as equal partners in meeting his health goals. He is preparing for convalescence and discharge from your services.

The Last Phase, Termination, is marked by the patient becoming as fully independent as possible, leaving the health care system to return to the community. Together you plan the management of his health situation after discharge, especially if he will require any special life-style modifications, such as in exercise, hygiene, or diet. This is a time of separation, and both you and he must work through feelings about separation—sometimes past as well as present separations. Mutual attachment develops between you and someone you take care of for a long time, and either one or both of you may feel uncertain about the person's ability to manage without you. Together you need to talk about feelings regarding separation and your confidence in his ability to be independent and remain healthy. Avoid increasing his dependency on you at this time to meet your needs. When he leaves the health care system, both you and he should not feel regret about the termination. On the other hand, if there is need for follow-up visits after discharge, your interest and concern in the patient extend to this on-going care.

Without the nurse-patient relationship, the patient's needs are not met and the nursing process is not in force. Mechanical tasks become an end in themselves, and the patient is not helped to prevent or adapt to his illness.

THE CHANGING ROLE OF THE NURSE

Health care demands over the last several decades have created a situation not only in the United States but also in the world community that requires a complete revision of present health care delivery systems. In the United States, infant mortality is still above what it should be in any country with such rich resources. Death rates for specific diseases, such as cardiovascular, are higher than elsewhere. Health facilities are often built where they are not needed, while rural communities suffer a lack of health care. Moreover, the system is concerned with sickness rather than health.

The fragmentation of care, lack of an organized health delivery system, and a lack of responsiveness to social needs, all discussed in Chapter 2, are reflected in the consumer of health care who is now demanding a new look at the system. He is beginning to demand a voice in planning and policy making. Such changes call for a new relationship between the consumer and health care professionals[21].

A brief review of nursing history will help you understand the present situation and project future trends. You will be part of the force making changes.

Historical Background

Four schools of thought have influenced directions in nursing, the evolution of nursing education, and the effect of education on nursing practice.

From 1900 until the 1950s, the *service* school of thought proposed that nurses be prepared for a service function to doctor and patient. Because of great demands for nurses' services and because of the numbers of nurses serving in the armed forces, various levels of nurses evolved, such as aides, orderlies, licensed practical nurses, hospital diploma nurses, and baccalaureate nurses. Hospital diploma nurses made up the largest number during this period and hence were responsible for integrating these large numbers of ancillary personnel into the system of health care delivery. These nurses had no specific preparation for this administrative role; thus the *administrative* school emerged. The nurses were prepared for management of care and for supervising and coordinating others who gave direct care, rather than for directly giving care themselves.

The *academic* school of thought grew out of the recommendations of the 1948 Brown report in which liberal education for the nurse was stressed[4]. Nursing students seeking academic programs could major only in nursing administration, supervision, or teaching. With the exception of psychiatric nursing, there was no financial support for clinical specialties. Likewise, in 1964, the Department of Health, Education, and Welfare (HEW) sponsored the Nurse Training Act, which provided support for the training of nursing teachers, supervisors, and administrators but offered no support for nurses wishing to seek advanced preparation in clinical areas. Prestige and promotions for nurses were limited to the administrative or academic routes.

The fourth movement, the *clinical* school, grew out of the rebellion against the system that forced nurses away from the patient. *The clinical nurse specialist* developed first, *a nurse with advanced training at the master's level (usually two years in a clinical specialty) who gives expert nursing care to acutely or chronically ill patients or who has responsibility for health maintenance of well clients.* In 1967, a small amount of private foundation support, and later some federal support, were made available to a few experimental programs to prepare clinical nursing practitioners[1].

The direction of nursing is now back to the bedside and into the home and community. Emphasis is on clinical (direct care) activities rather than other duties.

The Nursing Process and the Extended Nursing Role

The development of a physician-extender-type nurse is one approach to returning the nurse to the patient. The family nurse practitioner (PRIMEX),* pediatric nurse practitioner, school nurse, nurse-midwife, and nurse clinician in industry are some examples of the extended role of the nurse. It will take years, possibly 10 to 15, to show any significant increase in the number of medical physicians available, even if medical education is heavily subsidized. Thus a realistic solution to the shortage of physicians and the increasing need for reorganized and refocused health care is extending the nurse's role to provide primary care. In such a capacity, the nurse can perform some of the functions that physicians perform now. Examples of primary-care functions of nurses are discussed in Chapter 2.

Preparation for the nurse of the future is being incorporated into curricula

---

*A term originated by the faculty of the School of Nursing, University of Washington, Seattle, to reflect emphasis on primary care and preventive services.

so that the basic elements of primary care are familiar to new generations of nurses. Continuing education is being stressed to provide nurses educated in conventional ways an opportunity to learn new skills and concepts. Recertification is being examined as a means of documenting new or changed skills among practicing nurses. Physicians and nurses are collaborating to achieve more effective understanding of one another, to redefine the complementary functions of medicine and nursing, and to work out practical applications of new relationships. Analysis is going on in a variety of settings to assess the impact of the extended role on the health care delivery system. These and other measures to improve the availability and effectiveness of health care for the American people were recommended in the 1971 report prepared for the secretary of HEW by the Committee to Study Extended Roles for Nurses[38].

The Nursing Process and the Expanded Nursing Role

Another approach to returning the nurse to the patient is through the expanded role. The future of nursing in the face of a complete revision and updating of the American health care delivery system depends on a compatible fusion of nursing process and redefined role. Nursing is asserting itself as a profession and claiming the right to function independently of the medical profession in giving primary care.

To insure that *process* remains the essence of your nursing care in the expanded role, you can incorporate the following components into your nursing practice:

1. *Separation of clinical from nonclinical activities.* Activities for assisting in the prevention, reversal, or arresting of maladaptive states in patients are clinical and demand your attention. All other activities should be surrendered to persons who do not have your professional education. Clinical activities demand the methods and theory of science.
2. *Constancy of assignments.* The same patient-nurse-physician teams should be established for primary or hospital care. The same nurse can be assigned to the same patients or families daily and thus can be responsible for all their clinical needs. Each nurse then has more knowledge concerning those patients. The quality of care becomes more visible to the person, and he can more readily cooperate in his own care planning. Accountability can be monitored too, and a strong colleague relationship can be built among physician, nurse, patient, and family.
3. *Decentralization of authority and shared power.* Decisions need to be made where the need is ("on-the-spot") if the nursing process is to function in making each person accountable for his actions. Authority must accompany responsibility if accountability is to have meaning. Shared power means that whoever has competence may intervene. Nurses and physicians with similar competence must work toward sharing clinical

activities. At times the nurse will be solely responsible for the patient/family.

4. *Increased flexibility of time with patients.* Innovations in time scheduling will be yours to make as a member of the new generation of nurses. One professional goal is the allocation of nursing time based on the clinical demands of the unit rather than on the traditional three-shift system. Lengthening work days and shortening work weeks may be one way to provide more flexible structuring of time[9].

Individual persons are always responsible for change—persons willing to suggest, to offer alternatives, and to volunteer assistance with new ideas. Use your professional education with its problem-solving approach in working with others in making the nursing process an exciting reality.

Problem Solving versus Research in the Nursing Process

In nursing you will do problem solving and research; both use the scientific method discussed in this chapter. Although problem solving and research are frequently thought of as synonymous, a fundamental difference in purpose exists between them.

The purpose of problem solving is to solve an immediate problem in a particular setting. The solution is not necessarily new knowledge and cannot be generalized to a larger population. Consequently the precision of study is not so exacting, and statistical analyses are seldom done.

The purpose of research is to reveal new knowledge. All elements of the scientific method are precisely followed. The results of a research study cannot be expected to produce information to solve a specific problem.

Knowledge obtained through research may contribute to solution of an immediate problem, and problem solving may reveal new knowledge applicable beyond the immediate situation. But the basic difference remains. Problem solving as a health teaching method is discussed in the next chapter.

Research in Nursing

Historically, nursing research is scarce. Research has been considered the exclusive domain of academicians, nurse-scientists, doctoral candidates—or worse, researchers from other disciplines who have found nurses a rich source of data for study in the behavioral sciences. Study of the nursing profession by behavioral scientists has resulted in certain benefits. Many pertinent facts have emerged from these studies that have given insight to nurses concerning their responses to patients and to each other. However, nursing cannot justify its worth as a separate discipline unless clinical research is performed by its own practitioners. Nurses engaged in direct patient care are best qualified to do nursing research.

Nursing research begins with a *discrepancy, a perceived difference be-*

tween two states of affairs, or an uncomfortable feeling about the status quo. A difference is felt between what is occurring now and things as they could, ought, should, or might be. A gap might exist between what is known and what needs to be known to take action. Or there might be a discrepancy between sets of facts [11].

Your curiosity and your belief in the worth of your practice should guide your interest in nursing research. In the course of your work, if you note that certain situations or sets of circumstances bring about specific patient responses, collecting this data can, over a period of time, result in increased knowledge for nursing. More importantly, it may result in improved care for the patient, family, and community. Epidemiology, a research method, is the topic of Chapter 6.

REFERENCES

1. Abdellah, Faye G., "Extending and Expanding the Scope of Nursing Practice Through the Health Care Team." Paper presented at Conference of the Western Council for Higher Education in Nursing, San Francisco, October 1972.

2. ____, et al., *Patient-Centered Approaches to Nursing.* New York: The Macmillian Company, 1960.

3. Aiken, Linda, and James L. Aiken, "A Systematic Approach to the Evaluation of Interpersonal Relationships," *American Journal of Nursing*, 73: No. 5 (1973), 863-67.

4. Brown, Esther Lucille, *The Future of Nursing.* New York: Russell Sage Foundation, 1948.

5. Burgess, Ann, and Aaron Lazare, *Psychiatric Nursing in the Hospital and Community.* Englewood Cliffs, N.J.: Prentice-Hall, Inc., 1973.

6. Byrne, Marjorie L., and Lida F. Thompson, *Key Concepts for the Study and Practice of Nursing.* St. Louis: The C. V. Mosby Company, 1972.

7. Carlson, Sylvia, "A Practical Approach to the Nursing Process," *American Journal of Nursing*, 72: No. 9 (1972), 1589-91.

8. Chambers, Wilda, "Nursing Diagnosis," *American Journal of Nursing*, 62: No. 1 (1962), 102-4.

9. Christman, Luther, "Process or Role? Outcomes for Nursing," *Utah Nurse*, Winter (1971-1972), pp. 23-25.

10. Ciuca, Rudy L., "Over the Years With the Nursing Care Plan," *Nursing Outlook*, 20: No. 11 (1972), 706-11.

11. Diers, Donna, "This I Believe...About Nursing Research," *Nursing Outlook*, 18: No. 11 (1970), 50-54.

12. Geitgey, Doris A., "Self-Pacing; A Guide to Nursing Care," *Nursing Outlook*, 17: No. 8 (1969). 48-49.

13. George, Madelon, Kazuyoshi Ide, and Clara E. Vamberry, "The Comprehensive Health Team: A Conceptual Model," *Journal of Nursing Administration*, 1: No. 2 (1971), 9-13.

14. Hale, S., and J. Richardson, "Terminating the Nurse-Patient Relationship," *American Journal of Nursing*, 63: No. 9 (1963), 116-19.

15. Harris, Barbara L., "Who Needs Written Nursing Care Plans Anyway?" *American Journal of Nursing*, 70: No. 10 (1970), 2136-38.

16. Henderson, Virginia, *Nature of Nursing*. New York: The Macmillan Company, 1966.

17. Hofling, Charles, Madeleine Leininger, and Elizabeth Bregg, *Basic Psychiatric Concepts in Nursing* (2nd ed.). Philadelphia: J. B. Lippincott Company, 1967.

18. Ingles, Thelma, "Understanding the Nurse-Patient Relationship," in *Issues in Nursing*, eds. Bonnie Bullough and Vern Bullough. New York: Springer Publishing Company, Inc., 1966.

19. Kalkman, Marion, *Psychiatric Nursing* (3rd ed.). New York: McGraw-Hill Book Company, The Blakiston Division, 1967.

20. King, Imogene M., *Towards a Theory for Nursing*. New York: John Wiley & Sons, Inc., 1971.

21. Kramer, Marlene, "The Consumer's Influence on Health Care," *Nursing Outlook*, 20: No. 9 (1972), 574-78.

22. Levine, Myra, "Adaptation and Assessment: A Rationale for Nursing Intervention," *American Journal of Nursing*, 66: No. 11 (1966), 2450-53.

23. _____, "The Intransigent Patient," *American Journal of Nursing*, 70: No. 10 (1970), 2106-11.

24. Lewis, Edith P., "Accountability: How, for What, and to Whom?" *Nursing Outlook*, 20: No. 5 (1972), 315.

25. Lewis, Lucille, "This I Believe...About the Nursing Process: Key to Care," *Nursing Outlook*, 16: No. 5 (1968), 26-29.

26. Maslow, A. H., *Motivation and Personality*. New York: Harper & Row, Publishers, 1954.

27. Mayers, Marlene, *A Systematic Approach to the Nursing Care Plan*. New York: Appleton-Century-Crofts, 1972.

28. McCain, R. Faye, "Nursing by Assessment—Not Intuition," *American Journal of Nursing*, 65: No. 4 (1965), 82-84.

29. McCarthy, Rosemary T., "A Practice Theory of Nursing Care," *Nursing Research*, 21: No. 5 (1972), 406-10.

30. McPhetridge, L. Mae, "Nursing History: One Means to Personalize Care," *American Journal of Nursing*, 68: No. 1 (1968), 68-75.

31. Murray, Ruth, and Judith Zentner, *Nursing Assessment and Health Promotion through the Life Span*. Englewood Cliffs, N.J.: Prentice-Hall, Inc., 1975.

32. Orlando, Ida J., *The Discipline and Teaching of Nursing Process*. New York: G. P. Putnam's Sons, 1972.

33. ____, *The Dynamic Nurse-Patient Relationship*. New York: G. P. Putnam's Sons, 1961.

34. Palisin, Helen E., "Nursing Care Plans Are a Snare and a Delusion," *American Journal of Nursing*, 71: No. 1 (1971), 63-66.

35. Pardee, Geraldine, D. Hoshaw, C. Huber, and B. Larson, "Patient Care Evaluation Is Every Nurse's Job," *American Journal of Nursing*, 71: No. 10 (1971), 1958-60.

36. Peplau, Hildegard, *Interpersonal Relations in Nursing*. New York: G. P. Putnam's Sons, 1952.

37. Pierce, Lillian M., "Usefulness of a Systems Approach for Problem Conceptualization and Investigation," *Nursing Research*, 21: No. 5 (1972), 509-13.

38. Report to the Secretary of Health, Education, and Welfare from the Committee to Study Extended Roles for Nurses, "Extending the Scope of Nursing Practice," *American Journal of Nursing*, 71: No. 12 (1971), 2346-51.

39. Travelbee, Joyce, *Interpersonal Aspects of Nursing*. Philadelphia: F. A. Davis Company, 1967.

40. Wiedenbach, Ernestine, *Clinical Nursing: A Helping Art*. New York: Springer Publishing Company, Inc., 1964.

41. ____, "The Helping Art of Nursing," *American Journal of Nursing*, 63: No. 11 (1963), 54-57.

CHAPTER 5

Health Teaching: A Basic Nursing Intervention

Study of this chapter will enable you to:

1 Discuss why teaching is a major nursing responsibility.

2 Differentiate the traditional and simple definitions of *teaching, learning,* and *education* from the nontraditional and complex.

3 Describe changing educational trends, with an emphasis on the future.

4 Identify the varied opportunities for teaching health promotion.

5 List the fundamentals of teaching.

6 Explore the many facets of creativity and learn how to apply them in teaching-learning.

7 Discuss and translate into practical examples various teaching-learning theories.

8 Compare methods of teaching, including various individual and group approaches, and predict when each might be appropriate.

9 Discuss the significance of home and agency teaching.

10 Sharpen your ability to identify significant teaching-learning opportunities through analysis of a case study.

11 Teach patients, families, and coworkers in the nursing setting when appropriate.

When you entered nursing you may not have understood that to nurse is to teach. Teaching provides one of the major ways to help another adapt.

If you search out teaching-learning literature, you may find it uninteresting. Why? Suppose that a teacher has successfully created a process in which active, vibrant people have gained new insight. They are excited, perhaps transformed in their attitudes. When the teacher attempts to describe this process he is suddenly imprisoned in words. He has to design terms to differentiate his process from another process. Thus you are confronted with such words as *altercasting, self-actualization, behavior modification, proactive learning, interpersonal interaction, role playing,* and *operant conditioning,* all of which sound lifeless and boring.

This chapter does not attempt to review the many teaching-learning theories. Rather it presents various theories and methods which seem applicable to nursing and which you can begin to use.

This writer has not attempted to emulate educational jargon, but she is also imprisoned in words. You must take the words and phrases and apply them to people, yourself included, making the ideas alive and active. Only then will you experience the teaching-learning process.

DEFINITIONS

Learning is the acquiring of knowledge or skill; teaching is providing another with knowledge and insight [10] . These definitions are deceptively simple. Popular magazines, textbooks, library shelves are full of theories and explanations about how these processes take place. Yet no one can say learning *will always* take place under certain conditions or teaching *will never* take place under certain conditions. In spite of myriads of information, people with their unique minds and personalities are always modifying the existing theories.

In actuality, teaching and learning cannot be separated, for while a person is teaching he is also learning, or at least he should be. Perhaps the substandard use of *learn,* as in the sentence, "I'm going to learn you something," has more accuracy than people have thought. Both of these terms connote a lifelong process, an internalization (learning) of thoughts, attitudes, facts, and a consequent externalization (teaching) of those thoughts, attitudes, and facts. Teaching and learning can be conscious and formal, as in the announced situation, "Today we are going to learn about the digestive system." Or they can be unconscious and informal, as when a mother frowns and says with a certain tonal emphasis, "What is *that* smell?" The listening and watching child combines a certain smell with a negative mental attitude.

One word which connotes a chilly, stiff learning process is *pedagogy*. Originally the word meant teaching children, but today it refers generally to teaching. Unfortunately, most knowledge about learning is taken from studies of children and animals, and most knowledge about teaching comes from teaching children who were in compulsory attendance. Thus many times adults are taught as though they were children. To combat this erring process, Knowles has coined a new word, **andragogy**: *helping adults learn* [16]. Consequently he turns from traditional pedagogical methods. His ideas will be more thoroughly considered later in this chapter, for they are significant to use in patient teaching.

The word *education* has traditionally meant a process that transmits the culture. But the word originally came from a Latin word meaning "to draw out." Although we are more familiar with education as a cramming full of facts and information, the other side of the definition is to draw out the mysterious hidden qualities within a person. The amount of education a person has gained · and retained has long been measured by IQ (intelligent quotient) tests. But many qualities cannot be measured this way. The IQ test cannot measure how much creative imagination a person has, how much ambition, perseverance, or willingness to cooperate [25]. And these qualities are significant, though often not considered or given priority. Thus a balanced definition of *education* is the *continuing process of using immeasurable inner resources to gain external information.*

EDUCATION: HISTORICAL PERSPECTIVE

Toffler says that the educational system is dying—a startling thought. He traces the stages of education in America [37]. In stage 1, history was important. People looked to the past for knowledge, guidance, and strength. Teaching came primarily through family, religious institutions, and apprenticeships. The teacher and learner were spread throughout the community.

Industrialism and the mechanical age ushered in stage 2. New skills were required and the educational system took on a factory appearance. Assembly-line students were taught by specifically trained teachers in a central location. One writer relives such an educational experience as he passes his former elementary school. He is sick with his old fear of the factorylike structure with its castle facade. Perhaps his experience is extreme, but he doesn't associate school with learning, only with the necessity to get ahead, to compete with classmates, to make a good impression on the grim teachers who gathered the little robots (students) into the human factory to shovel food (knowledge) into the body [14].

Toffler insists that in our present stage 3, the new technological era, where more sophisticated machines perform more frequently, where communication systems connect most world points, and where environments are ever-changing, we need a superindustrial education. He calls for teachers and learners who can adapt to change, who plan for future change, and who understand the impetus toward the future. No longer can a person use the skills of his father for the rest of his life. In fact, he may not even be able to use what he was recently taught in school. Teaching and learning must again take place in various settings within the community, but with much greater speed then in stage 1. Education must be a lifelong process, not a phase of experience finished in 21 years.

Skills are then needed in three areas: learning, relating, and choosing. People must learn how to learn. With such rapidly changing information, they must know the process of discarding obsolete data in order to take on new. They must learn to relate under new conditions. Mobility has caused less stable friendships. People now cope with more loneliness and less reliance on groups of people. With so many choices available for the person, some goals and priorities must be set. Along with data, people must acquire behavioral skills or "life know-how."

Teachers, including yourself as nurse-teacher, must themselves adapt to the present age, examine their teaching methods and goals, provide people with information about what the future will hold for them, and help people anticipate these conditions. Teaching can no longer present all facts, all history. The probabilities of the future must be considered.

THE NURSE AS TEACHER-LEARNER

As a staff nurse or unemployed nurse, you may be more of a teacher than someone actually called a "teacher." A history instructor may teach high-school students from 9:00 A.M. to 3:00 P.M. five days a week. But you can spend nearly every waking moment in teaching health promotion. You teach through example: through health precautions and personal hygiene.

If you have a family, either children of your own or brothers, sisters, and parents, you constantly do health teaching. You may lock the medicine and caustic material in a cabinet, explaining the dire results of taking too much internally. You may notice early diabetic symptoms in your father and direct him to an internist for tests. You may quickly take the proper first-aid action when your sister fractures a bone. You will additionally be a teaching guide to your neighbors and friends.

Teaching those near you takes on unprecedented magnitude when you analyze the barrage of so-called health information directed at us daily through communications/advertising media: natural or organic foods are superior to processed foods; certain vitamins and minerals will provide pep and sexual vigor; certain exercises will promote breast development. Or again, certain procedures will grow hair on a bald male head or remove hair from a female face; a particular cream will slow down the aging process; a certain diet will cause drastic weight reduction; certain medications will wake you up, put you to sleep, or remove all your aches in moments.

Obviously, Americans are concerned with staying slim and appropriately masculine or feminine, with looking young and retaining their vigor. They have a fear about their own and their loved ones' health. You can supply sound information on the essentials of good nutrition, exercise, and rest while pointing out that people must accept periods of strain, fatigue, lesser energy, and the aging process. You won't always teach with words alone. Your standards of cleanliness—for example, how frequently you wash your hands—will be imitated by your children and observed by your patients.

You will teach no matter what professional position you hold. The staff nurse can teach while giving a bath. The nurse in the doctor's office or clinic can do spot teaching while preparing a patient for examination. The public health or visiting nurse can teach while working with specific situations in the home. The industrial nurse can teach while taking down worker information. Of course, the nurse is also a teacher while instructing students, but teaching is more basic than a professional job.

In trying to help each individual reach his maximum health potential you must consider the total person. His culture, social class, religion, environment, definition of health and illness, developmental stage, whether or not he is in a crisis, and what kind of communication he responds to will affect his understanding and your consequent teaching. Thus, this entire text and *Nursing Assessment and Health Promotion through the Life Span* together provide a foundation from which you may glean teaching and learning concepts [22].

You might ask yourself: What does the person want to learn? How can he best be taught? Can I help him project a positive image of what he will be in the future? For example, can I help the diabetic think of himself as slim, healthy, and enjoying the proper foods rather than as a deprived person who will moan and reminisce about his delicious sugary desserts? Can I help him understand that he must continue to learn about his disease and possible new treatments as medical research probes now-unknown possibilities? More importantly, can I be a stabilizer in the midst of change? Can I improve my skills in the three crucial areas of learning, relating, and choosing?

FUNDAMENTALS OF TEACHING

Although no set rules can be laid down as absolute standards for effective teaching, the following suggestions are recommended:

1. Be trustworthy and consistent.
2. Have self-esteem and enthusiasm. Generate a sense that what you are teaching will benefit the learner.
3. Don't discuss your personal problems with a patient.
4. Think through your teaching image. What do patients learn from your cleanliness (or lack of it), dress, posture, tone of voice, gestures, and yawns?

5. Know your teaching area. Organize and present your material so that patients feel you know what you are doing.
6. Review and evaluate your teaching methods for effectiveness.
7. Utilize available teaching methods, resources, various emotional climates, and referral systems when appropriate.
8. Record your teaching experience and share these notes with other staff members (or teachers from other disciplines) who may instruct the patient.
9. Be realistic about teaching and learning. Accept good days and bad days. Sometimes you will be elated, sometimes depressed about results.
10. Respect the patient as more important than a procedure, a potential disease process, or a research project.
11. If you ask the patient to do something, explain why.
12. Distinguish between lack of intelligence and misunderstandings caused by cultural, ethnic, or religious differences, and do not equate intelligence level with educational level.
13. Strive for learning from inner motivation through recognition of need, not from outward pressure.
14. Practice sensing the moment of learning. A sense of appropriate timing is essential in teaching.
15. If you write instructions, write legibly.
16. Plan for interruption.
17. Don't overwhelm with technicalities.
18. Give reinforcement regarding progress.
19. Accept errors in the learning process without harsh judgment but with correct information.
20. Don't allow your racial bias to control your attitude about another's ability to learn.
21. Don't reinforce destructive thinking. When a patient says, "My mother died of this disease," don't reply, "It's a real killer. My two aunts died from it too."

CREATIVITY

Assume that your best teaching device is you. You may be open to new knowledge, and you may agree with the fundamentals of teaching but not always know how to implement them. Thus you will benefit from the following investigation of creativity and its application to teaching and learning.

What is *creativity*? The word has been used freely. It has been defined as a process, a product, a personality, and an environmental condition. *Creativity is the ability to sense gaps or problems with known information, forming ideas or hypotheses about what should be done, testing and modifying those ideas, communicating those ideas, and taking appropriate action in a unique way* [39].

From this process you will obtain ideas or carry out activities that are new, unique, and useful to you, even though they may not be new, unique, or useful to other people.

An appropriate question might be, "How do you sense gaps and problems?" Without this essential tension in thinking, the rest of the process will not follow. One answer is to improve your observation. People can look at a slowly changing object for years and not notice the change, as the exterminator proves who points to a foundation beam largely devoured by termites. The astonished homeowner says, "I've gone by here every day for a year but didn't notice the change." Or less dramatic, can you describe in detail from memory the tree outside your kitchen window?

These are two examples (or at least one, if you can describe that tree in detail) of lack of sight perception. Other senses that need sharpening are sound, touch, sensation of movement, taste, and smell. Re-create in your mind the following sensations: the voice of your mother or father when you were little and being reprimanded, the feel of the hair on your pet dog, the sensation of your body as you hiked the last 100 feet of the mountain last summer, the taste of lemon juice, the smell of cooking broccoli. Practicing this kind of observation exercise of your sensory memory will improve your teaching because you will have a broader sensitivity base from which to sense gaps and problems.

Observing emotional reactions is also significant as you work with patients. Can you re-create the emotion of despair you felt when, after working hard and counting on a certain achievement, you failed the test, were disqualified in the race, or didn't get the job or school position you wished? How did you feel when you lost the love and understanding of someone you were counting on? You really can't walk a mile in the patient's shoes, but your helpful understanding of his emotions, through understanding your own, can increase the value of your teaching.

Lowenfeld lists this quality of sensitivity in observation among his criteria for creativity, along with fluency of ideas, flexibility, originality, and the ability to redefine or rearrange, analyze, synthesize, and coherently organize problems[17]. You might display fluency of ideas as you think of the various ways you could apply a bandage, form recipes, or adjust meals in a particular situation. You might show flexibility as you quickly incorporate changing circumstances into a situation. For instance, a procedure doesn't work because a previously unknown factor has been introduced. Instead of saying, "It won't work," you take the factor into account and get desirable results.

Originality is variously defined. Some say there are no new ideas and therefore no true originality. Others say that every time you associate or combine two or more ideas that you already have and come up with a new perspective, you have been original.

The rest of Lowenfeld's criteria work into a systematic process. You redefine a disease process with new research results or you rearrange a procedure with the new knowledge that the patient is left-handed instead of right-handed.

You analyze, or take apart, the significant factors involved in an unwed mother's situation. You synthesize, or put the parts back together, when you help a senior citizen create a new way of life. You exhibit coherence or organization when you arrange all the aspects of any teaching plan to form a unified working unit.

Creativity, then, conjures up visions of curiosity, imagination, discovery, innovation, and invention, and is a number of abilities rather than a single characteristic. The creative person can see many relationships among elements, relationships that baffle the conformer, the person who does only what is expected and does not ruffle the sytem. The creative person isn't always accepted by the traditional teacher because he has to be dealt with uniquely; he can't be treated in the ordinary way. Can you tolerate creativity in your patients? Will you help them learn through exploring, manipulating, questioning, experimenting, testing, and modifying rather than by accepting your word as final authority?

Torrance contends that smothering creativity is an American phenomenon[39]. He points out that adults often repress fantasies, hold back learning, and overemphasize sex roles in children. Creativity will emerge if family life and childrearing are organized so that every child has the opportunity to reach his potential[35]. By the time a child enters school, the foundation for creative development has been laid. Schools will then influence further development.

During their children's elementary years, Americans tend to stress conformity to the peer group, use punitive discipline, orient their children to success, equate divergency with abnormality or delinquency, and make a sharp distinction between work and play. In their high-school years, American youth are frequently pressured into striving for popularity, achieving high grades, getting work done on time, and making conventional occupational choices. In college (as well as high school) American students are sometimes forced to overemphasize the acquisition of categorized knowledge, memorization of facts, and standard testing. Thus, covering subject matter rather than studying in depth, and separating knowledge into arbitrary categories rather than seeing the interrelationships can often be the result. You may recognize this pattern in your own experience. One adult writes that as a child he was fascinated with the circus[4]. He spent every possible moment absorbing the aura of its life. Pressure to conform, however, pushed him into the conventional education route and he eventually acquired a Ph.D. in geography and a responsible college faculty position. Still, even with a family of four children to support, he would fantasize and dream about the circus. He is unique because with his family's approval, he quit his job and joined a circus, an unusual turn of events in American culture.

As you teach patients, some basic suggestions may be useful to foster creative learning:

1. Allow opportunity for creative behavior, such as providing for independent learning through the study of appropriate literature or asking questions that require more than recall.

2. Develop your own skills in creative learning according to methods described later in the chapter.
3. Reward creative achievements by respecting unusual solutions and by not threatening with immediate evaluation before an idea is completely tested.
4. Develop a constructive, rather than critical, attitude toward information gleaned.
5. Establish creative relationships, especially with children. Permit one thing to lead to another and embark on the unknown; yet provide adequate guidance.
6. Provide for continuity of creative development in solution finding [39].

Creativity is *not* synonymous with *permissiveness* or *chaos*. You are the resource, the organizer. Often you will be authoritative. You will say, "Sugar elimination will modify your diabetic condition. Omitting egg yolk will help lower your cholesterol. Chewing sugarless gum will cut down on dental caries. Adequate exercise will strengthen those muscles." But how you then help the patient work with those facts in his own situation will reveal either your authoritarian or your creative teaching manner.

SOME IDEAS TO CONSIDER

In addition to developing a creative teaching manner, you may want to ponder the following ideas concerning the nature of teaching and learning that have often been overlooked. The following ideas originated in various disciplines: psychoanalysis, adult education, language and communication studies, anthropology, and nursing.

Significant Learning

Carl Rogers defines *significant learning* as learning that makes a difference—that affects all parts of a person and influences his behavior, course of action, attitude, and personality [29]. Rogers substantiates his claim that such learning does take place by citing his experience with psychotherapy. He assumes that it can also take place in an educational setting under certain ideal conditions: (1) The person must clearly perceive the problems and issues that he wishes to resolve. (2) You, the nurse-teacher, must be openly aware of the attitudes you hold and accept your own real feelings. (3) You must accept the person as he is and understand his feelings. (4) Resources (such as literature about health promotion, crutches, cookbooks, yourself) should be given if they are useful to the patient and not an imposition. (5) Evaluation should be conceived as knowing the patient is adequately prepared to solve his problem if he so desires, but leaving him free to choose whether he wishes to put forth the required effort.

Two college students, both taking an education course and writing papers on learning theories, were overheard in the following conversation:

Did you get your term paper on learning written?

Yes, I'm almost done. I've found one article that expresses exactly what I believe. I'll try to work it in with all the hairy material the prof expects.

(Significant learning?)

Pedagogy versus Andragogy

The saying from the Talmud, "Much have I learned from my teachers, even more from my classmates, but most of all from my students," has special significance in Knowles's theory of adult education. As a person matures, according to Knowles, he (1) moves from dependency to a self-directing position; (2) accumulates experiences that become an increasing resource for learning; (3) moves in the direction of learning that harmonizes with his current developmental tasks; and (4) makes the transition from subject-centered, postponed applications characteristic of children's education to problem-centered, immediate applications of knowledge [16].

As a nurse-teacher you may be working with a variety of age groups. Some will be self-directing adults. You can apply these crucial assumptions as you teach adult patients and their family members if you let them to some extent help plan and conduct their own learning programs. Build on and make use of their life experiences to gain greater learning, and be sure learning is appropriate to their developmental tasks. (For example, don't try to get the 40-year-old heart patient to plan his retirement if he still has realistic aspirations for becoming a company vice-president.) Teach what is significant to their particular life problems, not what you think is a good subject. You may need to help them in the organization of material, in refocusing thinking, in reassurance by pointing out what they already know, in giving authoritative answers when needed, and in helping those who do not learn well alone.

Likewise, you must adjust to the children and youth you teach, to their dependency needs, their lack of experience, their developmental tasks, and their lack of sophistication in problem solving. Children lack the seasoned habits of adults and may respond more quickly to a change in pattern. You have a special responsibility to children as a teacher of health promotion because eating, exercise, and health practices become routinized early in life. The child who comes to you may have had little health teaching at home or in school. A recent questionnaire filled out by 910 early elementary classroom teachers (kindergarten through third grade) revealed generally low nutritional-knowledge scores[27]. Obviously, such teachers are not teaching good nutritional habits to their pupils.

The child may be inspired to learn through playing games, reading appropriate books or cartoons, or using puppets. Simple drawings, with explanations in appropriate-age-level language, may help explain a body part, a procedure, or what a medicine will do in the body.

Language: Prohibitor in Teaching-Learning

Language, our primary tool for education, can open up new worlds to people or leave them in a state of confusion. Nonverbal behavior is also significant. Communication developed first through the physical movements of people or objects; then through drawings, which represented objects or needs of people; next through giving spoken names to important ideas, concepts, and objects; and finally through establishing written signs to correspond to these names[9].

We sometimes forget that written signs have no physical resemblance to their referents. Two people must have a mutual understanding about the meaning of a word, or communication does not occur. We also do not have distinct and separate signs for each observed occurrence. Thus, although dwellings can be generally subdivided into houses, apartments, condominiums, and mobile homes, even these words cannot give a unique description of your dwelling. Because we cannot keep producing exact sounds for all different experiences, we have words that have many different meanings—such as *fast*, which can mean a speed, a dye that remains in place, or a certain type of friend. *High* can mean a physical elevation, a degree of alcohol or drug intoxication, a musical pitch, or a kind of religious ceremony; it can mean "grave" or "serious" (as in *high treason*), or "expensive" or "costly." *Reading* a skin test is not the same as *reading* an essay. Furthermore, the mind seems to decode messages in relationship to its own background situation, prejudices, and moods. For example, a person can hear and repeat exactly what you have said, without believing a word of it.

Given such possibilities of faulty language communication, even if technical language is adjusted to the patient's level and even if explanations are logically coherent and complete, the patient should have additional understandable experiences about the new concepts he will learn. His comprehension must not be evaluated totally on the basis of his language or reading response. Because motion pictures, television images, photographic slides, and pictures look like their referent, and the first two also sound like their referent, these and other (audio)visual aids should be strongly considered as adjuncts to verbal explanations.

Culture: Prohibitor in Teaching-Learning

The preceding ideas on adult education may work well in American majority culture, but may fail miserably in a culture where authority is unquestioned and where concepts of self-help and audience participation are not valued. For instance, in a strict patriarchal system, if a married woman is a patient, you should teach the husband what must be done.

Cultural and subcultural expectations have a powerful effect on behavior—yours, the patient's, and the family's. Accepting what the group believes to be true on the main issues of life is beneficial to all members of society. When one is relieved of the need to make choices, peace of mind and security are found. Thus health education to change habits is likely to fail unless social pressures to maintain the old customs are overcome. At the same time, the new proposed behavior cannot cause too much insecurity, uncertainty, or mental stress.

People conform to the expectations of prestigious members of society, and prestige may have nothing to do with money. Thus important persons need to be consulted and be given an opportunity to maintain their prestige by having a significant part in the changing of health habits. Programs are accepted only to the extent that local representatives—priests, teachers, grandparents, shop stewards, doctors— take part in planning and conducting them.

Ritualistic customs or behaviors are usually tied to elementary functions of of life—menstruation, feeding, gestation, defecation. Sometimes the ritual is harmful to health, but attempts to change it may cause resistance because time has sanctified the custom. Examples are female circumcision, defecation in open places, and food taboos for pregnant women.

Every culture accepts and absorbs new ideas provided they do not conflict with its own fundamental tenets. All new ideas are at first judged according to existing customs and beliefs and then gradually accepted if there is sufficient likeness to what already exists.

Consider the following suggestions in promoting health education and changes in health practices in any culture:

1. Get intimately detailed knowledge of beliefs, attitudes, knowledge, and behavior of the cultural group and evaluate their psychological and social functions. Try to share the feeling of the culture. Avoid being culture-bound: do not automatically reject concepts and patterns different from personal ones.

2. Identify numerous subcultures, as programs based on premises valid for one group may not be successful with another group.

3. Determine leadership patterns within a community or group. Define the decision makers in the family and larger social institutions, the status of various groups within the community, as well as the status of the health worker in comparison to these groups.

4. Remember that every culture is layered: each has certain characteristics that are manifest and others that are latent—certain components that comprise the stated ideal pattern of behavior but that are seldom practiced. Consider and study both levels. Least visible are the values that give direction and meaning to life.

5. Don't make direct attacks on the fundamental beliefs of the group; instead, patiently and gradually change ideas by appealing to the group's desire for health and normality. Avoid abrupt change. Use *linkage ideas, ideas consistent with both public health and the cultural belief system.* If no common ground exists, you should add on your idea to the cultural ideas[11].

6. Consider unanticipated consequences of the health education program and estimate how permanent the introduced changes are expected to be. Con-

sider the untoward consequences of the program. Positive results from your teaching in one situation may be considered negative in another situation.

7. Beware of the aspiration gap. Expectations of better living or health conditions, once aroused, are likely to rise more rapidly than improvements in the actual life situation. Supplying help and hope runs the risk of intensifying rather than satisfying felt needs, as rising aspirations outrace material gain, causing discontent and disillusionment. Programs of preventive health measures are the most difficult to establish because of the low value on health, the lack of understanding of cause and effect or the reasons for preventive measures, and the existence in local cultures of competitive preventive measures[6].

For the results of a detailed project that tested the survival power of medical ideas across a language-translation barrier, see Hanson and Saunders[11]. Chapter 10 deals extensively with the significance of culture in health promotion.

Other Prohibitors in Teaching-Learning

A nursing student, somewhat dissatisfied with her nursing education, used analogy to make a point. She compared some of her nursing instructors to delicate flowers who wilted as teachers. She declared that when she taught, she would be like a dandelion—tough, common, almost indestructible, and with functional component parts[3].

The idea is commendable, but a caution is needed. Although armed with the best of theory and methods and with respect for the patient, you will at times fail to impart positive health habits through teaching knowledge based on scientific information.

You will be dealing in health education with many myths and forms of unconscious resistance. Some people try to undermine their own health as a means of attracting attention or avoiding a hated job. Others, out of desire to belong, will hold on to a false diet theory. Some believe the whole body is a mobile dirt factory with a constant need for cleaning. Even health educators, although highly trained formally, are subject to these devices and beliefs. You may need to teach other teachers.

Occasionally situations arise where significant learning simply can't occur. Maybe you remind the patient of her employer whom she detests. Or if you are a black female heterosexual health teacher working with a white male homosexual patient, you may not succeed in teaching him because of prejudice.

In a hospital setting, the question of who shall teach, and when, may be impossible to answer. Health professionals cannot decide who should teach about diagnosis, nurse or physician. And if both, how? Aiming primarily for efficiency runs counter to allowing teaching time. The physician suddenly writes the discharge order. No teaching time is available.

Teaching can be harmful if goals are unaccepted, inappropriate, misunderstood, or not broken down into manageable steps. If teaching materials are not appropriate, if teaching is not thorough, or if evaluation is not adequate, the patient may be confused, lose his self-confidence, and be unable to adapt to his health problem[26].

Obviously the hardest look you take must be at yourself. Communication is often easiest with a person of one's own class or status group because you both share similar premises. But what happens when basic premises are dissimilar? Sometimes you fail.

Failure need not be permanently defeating. Sometimes it furthers the maturing process. Thus you should evaluate and revise working principles from your varied experiences in an attempt to produce better results (and to realize when you can't). This is analogous to the step of evaluation in the nursing process.

METHODS OF TEACHING

Techniques of Teaching

Methods or techniques of teaching are nearly as varied as people. A given technique can be effective in one setting and totally inappropriate in another. The key is in planning the technique for the specific situation.

Basically, a climate for teaching-learning must be set. All involved must want teaching and learning to occur and anticipate an improved self-image as a result of learning. Time must be set aside for in-service teaching preparation and for patient teaching. General team or individual goals must be set. Teaching guidelines and audiovisual materials must be available. The actual setting for the teaching-learning must be conducive. For example, learning is difficult in an overcrowded, poorly ventilated room where people are looking at each others' backs or are uncomfortably seated.

Your responsibility is to know your patient and his situation. You might write individual teaching guides on your patients that include such items as: (1) the nature of the person's disease, including the person's normal functions, pathological changes, and results of the changes; (2) hospitalization and nursing care measures, such as diagnostic procedures, treatments, medications, fluids, diet, and rehabilitation; (3) discharge and home care, including diet, fluids, medications, activity, dressings, rest, general hygiene, prophylaxis, special equipment, and suggestions for improvisations; (4) community agencies and resources; and (5) helpful bibliography[38]. Obviously age, mental and emotional attitudes, family status, and other factors affecting the patient's learning should also be included in this guide. With this on-going information you can construct a design for teaching, made up of various appropriate techniques.

Using the nursing care plan with teaching as an integral part is discussed in Chapter 4. Just as a work of art calls for unity, continuity, and a certain sense of pace and movement, so does teaching. These guides or plans provide the basis for such a design.

Although there are certain techniques that generally work better than others, in certain situations, there are no definite rules. *A teaching method represents a way of thinking.* You must choose a method that you can effectively use and that patients can benefit from.

Table 5-1 depicts some techniques for producing desired behavioral outcomes[16]. You can use your creativity to adapt these methods to your specific situations.

TABLE 5-1

Some Techniques for Producing Desired Behavioral Outcomes

RATIONALE	TEACHING METHODS
If you wish to:	*Use:*
impart *generalizations* about experience.	lecture, symposium, reading, audiovisual aids, a book- or pamphlet-based discussion.
apply information to experience through insight and *understanding.*	feedback devices, problem-solving discussions, laboratory experimentation, group participation, case problems.
build *skills.*	role playing, drill, coaching, demonstration, and return demonstration.
create new *attitudes.* (Attitudes are learned through repeated reinforcement of a response to a stimulus. If a response different from the original one is given and reinforced over a period of time, a change in attitude occurs, evidenced by a change in behavior in a particular set of circumstances [21]. Eventually the attitude may become a value.)	reverse role playing, experience-sharing discussion, counseling-consultation, environmental support, games designed to produce certain attitudes, and nonverbal exercises which draw out certain attitudes through gestures, posture, and facial expression.
change *values* through the rearrangement of the priority of beliefs.	speakers who have adjusted satisfactorily to a certain condition now facing the patient, biographical or autobiographical reading, drama, philosophical or direct-value-placement discussion with provision for reflection.
promote new *interests.*	field trips, audiovisual aids, reading, creative experiences.

Individual and Group Teaching

Some techniques are best suited for teaching on an individual basis, while other methods should be used for large groups or several subgroups.

Individual Teaching can be provided through programmed learning, reading material, audiovisual aids, and one-to-one instruction. *Programmed learning provides material in carefully planned sequential steps that leads the person to a mastery of the subject.* The material is presented through program instruction books or a *teaching machine, a simple manually operated machine or a complex computer.* One frame of information is presented at a time. The learner then tests his grasp of the information in the frame by writing his response to a question, usually a multiple-choice type. The book or machine then gives the correct response. If the learner's response was incorrect, the program then presents (or, in the case of a book, directs him to turn to) a repetition of the information or a more detailed explanation, depending on the program and his response. The advantages of this method include logical presentation, active learner participation, immediate disclosure of correct response, reinforcement of material, and individual pacing[7].

Another method of giving individual instruction is by providing factual material. The health organizations discussed later in this chapter provide preventive health-teaching literature as part of their programs. Evaluating the benefits gained from these materials is difficult because people who receive the material often do not respond to the organization's request for feedback, even when given a stamped answer form. One study tried to determine the effectiveness of breast self-examination by seeking the reactions of 383 women one year after they received teaching kits with filmstrip, teaching notes, and commentary; only 41 percent responded. Women in the upper half of the social scale reacted more favorably: 48 percent of them had established an examination pattern (though not necessarily monthly, as the material suggested)[12]. The tendency of upper-class persons to read better and to respond more readily to scientific health teaching than lower-class persons seems evident here.

Other factual reading materials include autobiographies of persons with certain disease processes and "how-to" books by persons who have experienced certain health problems directly or indirectly and want to pass along suggestions to others. Fiction can also provide valuable insights into physical and mental illness.

With the constant introduction of more sophisticated audiovisual equipment into the teaching-learning area, you can get and adapt these devices to individual learning. A recorder and cassettes explaining preventive measures, disease processes, or specific instructions can be loaned to the patient. He can stop the cassette at any point and replay necessary portions until he is satisfied with his learning. Closed-circuit television or videotape setups allow the person to hear and view material. You can be involved in producing teaching cassettes and television or videotape programs.

These methods of individual instruction are only individual to a certain point. Only when the patient can check his learning with a resource person, ask further questions as necessary, and have help in making personal applications, will learning become significant. That process involves you. The person doesn't learn from a machine alone.

Group Teaching can meet the person's need to achieve status or security through being a group member. Patient groups provide a channel through which feelings and needs can be expressed and met, especially if the patients have similar problems, such as a colostomy or diabetes. Thus you can use the group process to enhance health teaching or for therapy to aid coping with problems. You may also have an opportunity to work with a group that has formed to accomplish some specific goal, such as losing weight, promoting research to find a cure for cancer, or providing guidance to parents with mentally retarded children. In some cases information is not enough. Social support is also necessary, especially when engaging in a lesser-valued activity—like not eating sugar when society says that dessert is the best part of the meal. One study of hospitalized diabetics, some taught individually and some taught in a group by a nurse specialist, showed that the latter demonstrated as much or more knowledge and skill in urine testing as the former[23].

In another study 25 experimental patients participated in a small group session the night before surgery. They discussed their concerns and fears and learned what to expect and how to aid in their convalescence. A randomly selected matched control group of 25 patients who underwent similar surgery but who received only routine care were compared, after surgery, with the first group. Results showed that extra preparation increased patient participation, decreased tension and anxiety, and led to more rapid postoperative recoveries[31].

One minister who had visited hundreds of patients on the night before surgery said, "Fear of the unknown is what I continually find. I don't necessarily mean about the outcome of the surgery, although that is involved. I mean they don't even know about the recovery room process. Instead of giving spiritual help, I find myself telling them many details which the nursing staff should have taught. With these important details at their command, I can see their anxiety lessen." Small group sessions could reduce those fears.

Not only should the rather complicated procedures such as surgery and its accompanying routines be explained. Positive results have also been obtained with minor procedures. For example, one group was told what sensations to expect and then had blood-pressure cuffs placed on their arms and the pressure pumped up to 250 mm Hg. Another group was told only of the procedure—that is, "Your blood pressure will be taken." The conclusion was that accurate expectations about sensations do reduce stress, but that patients should be told only about sensations usually experienced, not those rarely experienced[13]. Excessively detailed explanations can raise, rather than lower, anxiety.

If you work with a group, you will have to initially set a working social climate. People don't automatically start revealing their problems and supporting and helping each other. You must use some introduction technique that focuses on the individual, his personality strengths and resources, rather than on his disease or problem. (He already knows why he is there.) Each person can introduce himself if the group is small. If the group is large (25 or more), you can break it up into subgroups of 5 each and allow each of these subgroups at least 20 minutes to plan a presentation utilizing one of the following creative techniques. In *the inquiring reporter*, one person in each group (or subgroup) is chosen to compose a feature story about the personalities and resources of his group members. He then presents the story to the total group in 3 minutes. In *the living newspaper*, each group picks a type of newspaper feature—a news story, column, book review, or editorial, for example—and presents a 3-minute group description through that format. In *the television variety program*, each group has a 3-minute segment to present its members through interview, skit, song, or comedy. These methods produce immediate ego-involvement, create an atmosphere conducive to participative learning and sharing of problems and resources, and start the spirit of creative inquiry [15]. You can think of other introductory techniques for your particular group situation.

Whatever your reasons for teaching the group, you must assess needs and interests, define your purposes and objectives, and construct a design. As you teach, you can rely on many approaches to accomplish your purpose.

A sample of group approaches that you could use follows:

1. *Support groups.* The total group breaks up into subgroups of three or four people. The purpose is for subgroup members to support one another. If one person misses a session or doesn't understand a procedure, the other members of his subgroup are responsible for getting the missing information to him. Each has a feeling of being active and of being responsible to one another, and each can clarify his own understanding as he teaches someone else.

2. The *whip group.* This is a variation of the support group, in which one person in each subgroup is designated to interpret the concepts being taught. Misunderstandings can be caught early, as periodic times are designated for interpretation and discussion.

3. *Directive note taking.* The entire group listens to a lecture for 2 or 3 minutes. Then all stop and write notes on what was said. The teacher checks sample summaries to see how well the ideas are getting across. This procedure is repeated until the end of the session.

Problem Solving

Another approach to teaching-learning is the problem solving technique, useful with either individuals or groups, and which is essentially the creative process discussed earlier in this chapter. Parnes outlines a seven-step creative problem-solving process that can be written out to clarify thinking [26]. He starts with *confronting "the mess,"* acknowledging the predicament and the resultant dissatisfied

feelings. Creative efficiency is increased if people understand the psychological process by which they operate. Thus the emotional and irrational factors in peoples' thinking are more urgent than the intellectual and rational[39].
People are free to go on more effectively after acknowledging this first step.

The second step is *clarifying the "fuzzy problem,"* writing a factual rather than an emotional explanation of the situation by answering such questions as who? what? when? where? why? and how? The third step is *fact finding*, writing information the patient would like to have related to the situation described. The fourth step is *problem finding*, listing all the creative-type questions or challenges suggested by the preceding two steps, such as: "How might I...?" and "In what ways might I...?" The fifth step is *idea finding*, or deferred judgment, selecting the most likely ways of solution finding. The sixth step is *solution finding*, in which the best approaches are evaluated; and the seventh step is *acceptance finding*, or adoption of solution. These steps are merely guides to be adapted to personal and group characteristics *(see Figure 5-1)*.

Some persons are capable of going through these seven steps relying only on their insight. Others can work through the steps themselves, but will need you to present the plan to them. And still others will be so engulfed in "the mess" that they will need your careful guidance to move them toward a solution.

Other Approaches

Appropriate visual aids should be used with whatever method is used. Letting people work with their hands as well as their minds is often effective. Groups may make a collage from magazine pictures—for example, foods acceptable to a diabetic versus unacceptable foods; good hygiene versus poor hygiene; elements of health versus elements of illness. Patients are also eager to get *handouts,* appropriate visual or written materials that they can keep. Ideally they will use this material and even pass it on to a relative or friend. You must know each patient's reading ability (or lack of it) and select materials accordingly. Not being able to read is a source of embarassment to patients. Go over the handout with the person; do not just hand it to him.

Teaching client-rights utilizes a direct approach with either individual persons or groups. Although persons may have vast resources within themselves, they sometimes do not use them because they have been taught to respect the doctor: "Do not question his judgment. He is too busy to explain." While you and the patient should respect the doctor, he should also respect you and the patient. While we question the plumber about the new parts he is putting in our sink, ask their cost, and refuse to pay if the work is ineffective, we often don't question the doctor about medications we take, their cost, or his service fee. And we pay whether we are satisfied or not.

One study questioned 60 patients in a teaching hospital about the drugs they were taking, and concluded that: (1) patients have little information about

FIGURE 5-1

Seven-Step, Creative Problem-Solving Process

	(Monologue of a 55-year-old woman who has just learned, after routine bloodwork in a clinic, that she appears to be a borderline diabetic. She leaves without getting an adequate explanation.)
1. Acknowledging *the mess* (emotional aspects).	1. I can't possibly change my ways. I love desserts. I can't cook without sugar. My husband and friends won't accept me. I'll never go to another party. I can't stand to have diabetes.
2. Identifying the *fuzzy problem* (known facts).	2. Yes, I have been awfully thirsty lately. And that cut on my foot healed so slowly. I have been too tired to carry on my usual work.
3. Looking for *additional helpful facts*.	3. Maybe there is a diet I *can* follow. Maybe I can find a cookbook which will teach me to cook without sugar. Maybe I will have more energy and be a better companion to my husband if I look into the management of diabetes.
4. Asking *creative questions* to help deal with steps 2 and 3.	4. Where can I get this cookbook? Where can I get more literature on diabetes? How can I test my urine myself? Who can help me?
5. Selecting *tentative solutions*.	5. Let's see, I could call Jane's family doctor. I think she said he works with diabetics. Or maybe I can find a doctor who specializes in diabetes. I can look in the phone book to see if a diabetic association exists. I can talk to Mrs. Jones; she has had diabetes for 10 years and seems to handle herself well.
6. Evaluating tentative solutions and selecting a *solution*.	6. Well, I think I better find a specialist. If I have diabetes, I want to get all the facts. I'll also call Mrs. Jones; she can probably give me lots of hints from her everyday life.
7. Accepting the findings through *adopting a plan* of action.	7. I'm glad I found out while I'm borderline. Lots worse things could happen. I will follow the regimen. It should help me live longer.

the medications they are taking; (2) younger patients know more about their drugs than older ones; and (3) patients who would like more information do not ask[18]. Another study confirmed that patients want specific information about their condition[8].

Table 5-2, based on suggestions from a medical physician, indicates how patients can get specific information[24].

Evaluation

Evaluation—judging how effective teaching has been—is essential to stimulating growth and improvement in teaching, which is of no value if it does not lead to improved practice. Evaluation is difficult because patients cannot always be followed long enough to see the results of teaching, and human behavior is so complicated that true changes are hard to measure.

TABLE 5-2
Teaching Guide for Client's Rights

FIVE DOs	FIVE DON'Ts
1. When you call the nurse or secretary for an appointment, state your request or problem so she can schedule appropriate appointment time.	1. Unless an emergency arises, don't take up extra, unplanned-for time. For example, don't say, "Oh, while I'm here for my ear infection, why don't you do my complete physical."
2. Organize thoughts about your present health status or illness and write them down so you can present pertinent facts to the doctor. These will aid him in giving a thorough examination or in making a diagnosis.	2. Don't lie to yourself or to the doctor. Don't let fear cause you to ignore a situation which may need immediate but minimal treatment.
3. Cooperate during the physical exam and allow the doctor to be complete. Don't tell him to skip certain procedures.	3. Don't tell the doctor to give you pills. Don't feel cheated if you don't get medication; many illnesses are minor and self-limiting. Your own observance of a health-promotion regimen may be all you need.
4. Ask your doctor about proper diet, work load, exercise, and rest to help you maintain maximum health. Ask about realistic limitations. If ill, ask your doctor questions about cost of treatment, medication, diagnosis, causes of condition, chances for recovery, or whatever you want to know related to situation. If you have more questions after you leave, write them down and call back for answers. If hospitalized, continue to ask questions about drugs and on-going treatment.	4. Don't ask for unnecessary hospitalization for X-rays or tests because the insurance will pay or because grandma is burdensome. Talk with your doctor about alternate plans which will promote long-range health for everyone involved.
5. Follow instructions after health promotion plan is established. After time, effort, and money are spent, you are the only loser if you refuse to follow suggestions or directions.	5. Don't leave the doctor's office dissatisfied. At least express and explain your feelings. The doctor needs to understand your point of view. Maybe a change can be made or perhaps you need additional information to understand a suggestion or decision.

Evaluation can be informal or formal. Informal judgments are made constantly. A patient makes compliments or complains. You react to these judgments. You observe how well a patient dresses a wound, irrigates a catheter, or cooks a meal. You may write evaluation notes on his learning ability. By questioning yourself about his understanding, you mentally evaluate a situation and decide whether his behavior has improved or worsened, thus adding to your evaluation material. You might even ask patients to evaluate their learning and your teaching, using a rating scale or checklist.

Every person connected with a teaching-learning program should be involved in evaluating it. Depending on the specific situation and program, these people might include the participants (patients and teachers); the program director and staff, who can see the program as a whole; the directing committee, who establish objectives and policy; and outside experts, who can be totally objective. Community representatives can supply valuable evaluative information when the teaching is aimed at serving the general public [16].

HOME TEACHING

So often there is no continuity in teaching from health care agency to home. Ideally all teaching should include the patient's family and its particular circumstances in the plan, but in a setting other than the home the true circumstances often cannot be discerned. When a mother takes a child back to the clinic for the third time with pneumonia, the doctor and nurses may reprimand her for not taking better care of her child. She may be too proud to say she can only afford to keep one room partially warm, that she doesn't have enough quilts, and that their diet consists mostly of rice.

Sometimes lower-class persons give up before they ever get started on a health-promotion plan because they know they cannot afford the fancy equipment or the expensive nutritional supplements recommended by the hospital staff.

The nurse who goes into the home can, in one-half hour, make observations that could never be made under any other circumstances, and certainly not in a hospital room. When you enter the home, you see, smell, hear, and feel how the people think and live. Peeling plaster, unpainted walls, holes in the floors, spilled old food underfoot, the smell of urine, piles of dirty clothes, oppressive heat or pervasive cold all give information regarding health (or lack of it). A row of shined shoes, a picture of Jesus or a nun, a certain painting, photos of children and relatives, framed certificates, rows of books or of store-bought medicine also give valuable information. These are extensions of the personalities. From these observations you can begin realistic health teaching as part of your nursing intervention.

One visiting nurse said her goal was to teach health promotion under existing conditions, to make patients both comfortable and as healthy as possible in their own circumstance. She said that if a patient needed a diet change for heart disease or diabetes, she would ask him to keep a record of everything he ate for three days. Then she would plan an adequate diet around that information. She felt it was futile to drastically change the existing plan, to take away all his favorite foods and add new ones that he didn't like or didn't want to try [44].

Five Families

The following synthesis takes place in the mind of a visiting nurse as she spends part of her day in the inner city, doing health teaching along with other care.*

*One of your authors collated the following from the cases of two visiting nurses. The names are fictitious.

Of the five families depicted, four of them, all on welfare, have the **matrifocal family structure**: *there is no male living permanently in the home.* The matrifocal family structure requires a different teaching approach from that taken with the middle-class families with an adult male present. Yet unless you are in the home, you might not realize the necessity for this.

Use the following narrative as a guide to focus on what types of information you can glean and what teaching you can do in the home as opposed to an agency setting.

I awaken the Green family at 8:00 A.M. on an August morning. They generally sleep from 1 or 2 o'clock in the morning, after it cools off a little, until 10 or 11, when it starts to get hot again. While I bathe and tube-feed 10-year-old Kevin, who has Dawson's syndrome, I carry on a constant dialogue with him (although he can't talk) and his mother. I assure Mrs. Green that she is an adequate mother and is giving adequate care when she tells me that the doctor seems surprised that she can make astute observations about her son's condition. "After all," she says, "I am the mother, and I have raised several other children." I give her information on what medicine to use for the bedsore and how to apply it, tell her what vitamin supplement has the same ingredients for less money, and tell her not to take the feeding tube out even though she thinks Kevin can swallow again. I see her worn look from the round-the-clock care and I tell her I'll send a home aide in for two hours tomorrow so she can go out to get her hair cut and set. The patient follows me with his eyes and I am not fooled by his lack of words. I give him gentle instructions and he co-operates.

I next stop at Mrs. Allen's home. She is an "agency hopper" and has been offered countless opporunities to help her four-year-old, Sarah, who has cerebral palsy. She doesn't want to let me in because her child has soaked the bed and she doesn't have any clean diapers in the house. I am finally admitted. I ask where Sarah's eye glasses are. They are lost. When Mrs. Allen finds them, I realize they have been squeezed out of shape. I suggest a guard. Mrs. Allen says a guard doesn't work, but I explain how it work. I ask if Mrs. Allen has been down to pick up Sarah's braces and walker. She hasn't. Although she is getting all equipment free, she complains that she doesn't have time to make these trips. I point out that both for Sarah's health and so the mother will have less of a burden when Sarah is older, she should follow through with the use of this equipment, which is designed to help Sarah function at optimum level.

My next visit is to Kathy, a teenager who has given birth to twins. She is back home with her mother in a crowded flat. I am visiting her to see how she cares for the infants. I know that I cannot insist on a separate room for the infants because eight people must sleep in two rooms. I have, however, recommended a space for the infants' items—a space which is kept clean and is off-limits to the rest of the family. I have purposely *not* recommended a fancy, expensive sterilizer, but rather a simple sterilizer which can be used on the gas stove and which can serve as a cooking pot when its original purpose is served. I am happy to see the pride this young girl is taking in providing the best care she can for the children. She asks questions about what cereal and juice will be most likely to agree with her six-week-old infants. I outline a simple nutritional plan. She gives me a photo of the twins as I leave.

My next case is a new one. A physician has asked me to make the initial assessment of a mother, Mrs. Wheeler, who has seven young children and who thinks her youngest might be mentally retarded. I ask many questions and the children all volunteer answers. I watch the youngest carefully. I use my growth-and-development education. I sense a gap. The mother is talking like a Ph.D. graduate but is living in culturally deprived conditions. I will need to think more before I make any recommendations.

My final case is Mrs. Lawton, a terminal cancer patient. She took care of herself until she was in too much pain to do simple chores, after which her sister took over. But her sister, without a full night's sleep in three weeks, called the American Cancer Society, who recommended a visiting nurse. Initially, I have given and left instructions for giving daily mouth care, as the patient's mouth is caked with residue. I have ordered perineal pads from the cancer society (free) so that the sister will have less sheet washing, and have told the sister that Mrs. Lawton is eligible for Social Security as both of them were unaware of this opportunity. I have suggested a medicine schedule for optimum pain relief, have recommended more and certain kinds of fluids after evaluating Mrs. Lawton's diet, and have made a clinic appointment for her. The sister, lacking private transportation, called one ambulance service that charges $40 to take the patient either to or from the hospital. I have recommended a service for $20 and explain that the American Cancer Society will pay for $15 of that. The sister is grateful for the information and demonstrates her ability to follow through on these and numerous other suggestions.

Not everyone wants or needs a nurse in the home, but a lack of follow-up in home health teaching exists. A routine phone call to patients who have been seen in other circumstances can determine if a home visit would be helpful.

AGENCY TEACHING

Effective teaching often involves making a pertinent referral. After you understand the health status of the person and of his family and his home situation, you can refer the person to the agency that can give him the most help. In fact, you should not attempt to provide services in areas where you are not fully trained, especially if expert service is simply a matter of proper referral.

Survey your local community for health-teaching agencies. You should know which services you can expect from these agencies. Larger cities sometimes have community-service directories that give this information. Keep abreast of newly added programs. Don't overlook church and club groups that sponsor or help with health education.

Chapter 2 outlines some basic types of health agencies. Table 5-3 presents some specific service and educational agencies. These services are not inclusive, and vary with location. The table does, however, point out the vast resources available.

CURRENT CHALLENGES

Teaching-learning is important at any stage of the wellness-illness continuum, but recently more emphasis is given to teaching health promotion and early prevention. You now have a brigade of definitions, theories, methods, and agencies to assist you in teaching. But before you can teach effectively you must have a wellness orientation rather than a pathological orientation. Health educators should shift their emphasis from pathology that has never been experienced to things the person has done and enjoyed and will be unable to continue to do if health behavior is not implemented[34].

Not only should you teach health promotion and prevention measures to lay people. You may need to direct your teaching toward those health educators who continue to focus on only the curative process. You may also establish courses to teach schoolteachers, firemen, policemen, ambulance attendants, or health-agency workers—those who are in a direct position to aid in illness or injury prevention and control.

Health Behavior

Health behavior is any activity, undertaken by a person who believes himself to be well, to avoid an illness. The person might undertake certain measures to promote and maintain wellness or to detect aberrations in their early or covert states[40].

Practicing health behavior or teaching health behavior is not dramatic. One nurse said that teaching proper diet, weight control, the need for rest and sleep, the importance of exercise, cleanliness, periodic health examinations, and immunizations is so humdrum. Yet these areas of teaching can eliminate much time, effort, and money spent on teaching in later disease stages as well as eliminate suffering for the person.

Providing you have a wellness orientation, you still must deal with the

TABLE 5-3
Agencies to Utilize in Health Teaching

AGENCY	SERVICES
American Cancer Society	Provides a service director who will guide family of cancer patient to community resources. Sponsors rehabilitation programs. Gives financial, equipment, and service aid. Prints literature on different types of cancer, and preventive and early diagnostic measures. Advocates nonsmoking and avoiding overexposure to sun; monthly breast self-examination; regular mouth, proctoscopy, and total health checkups; yearly cervical "Pap" test.
American Dental Association	Refers patients to dentists. Intervenes between patient and dentist if patient has complaint about treatment. Prints educational material in cartoon form for children and pamphlet form for adults on proper brushing, nutrition, and importance of periodic cleaning by dentist or hygienist. Defines eight areas of specialization in dentistry.
American Diabetes Association	Teaches about all phases of diabetes from detection through treatment. Prints magazines, newsletters, visual aids. Sponsors speakers' bureaus and camps for diabetic children. Provides test kits for detection, nutritionists for proper meal planning, cookbook for home use, scales for food weighing, identification bracelets.
American Heart Association	Supports research. Prints books, pamphlets, and visual aids to teach prevention and care measures. Offers nutritionist services and a cookbook, speakers' bureau, screening projects (EKG and blood glucose level test) at certain industrial centers. Incorporates a course (in at least one city) on the prevention and treatment of heart disease into the college curriculum of future elementary-school teachers.
The Arthritis Foundation	Prints extensive literature on different types of arthritis, those affected, Social Security benefits for arthritics, medication, diet, approved exercises, quackery, homemaker hints, home care programs. Supports and finances research.
Visiting Nurse Association	Provides home care and services through registered nurses; home health aids; physical, occupational, and speech therapists; social service workers; nutritionists.

patient where he is—culturally, socially, and developmentally. The average layman does not place health in the same level as does the health worker. The layman generally takes health action only when he believes that he is susceptible to a health threat that could have serious effects on his life, when he knows what actions to take to reduce the health threat, and when the health threat is greater than the action threat[30].

Consider the following case study in terms of information from Chapters 1 through 8 on wellness orientation and behavior, nursing process, adaptation, crisis, teaching-learning attitudes and techniques, and referral systems. Project how topics in Unit II, such as culture, social class, family, and developmental study of the young adult [22] will be useful in full assessment and intervention.

Case Study

Mr. H. R. is a well-educated 38-year-old middle-class, white male living in a major metropolitan area where sophisticated medical facilities abound. Because of a lifetime of allergies and a Bilroth II surgery two years ago for a bleeding duodenal ulcer that left only one-third of his stomach remaining, Mr. H. R. is conscientious about his health habits. When he went to his allergist for his annual checkup, two abnormalities were found: an irregular prostate nodule and hyper-lipoproteinemia Type IV. After a trip to a urologist that disclosed that his prostate nodule was not alarming and a second trip to his allergist for another blood test, Mr. H. R. had spent $108 and had a confirmed diagnosis of hyperlipoproteinemia Type IV.

The allergist hurriedly explained the diagnosis: "Fat in the blood, not too serious, could cause diabetes or atherosclerosis in ten years, a familial tendency, better tell your brothers; they might have it too. Call my secretary in two days for an appointment with a dietician." End of conversation.

Mr. H. R. went home and told his wife. He explained the situation as best he could. The word itself, *hyperlipoproteinemia*, had a horrendous sound. He couldn't pronounce it, only guess at the syllables. The wife, also well-educated, called the allergist to get more details. His secretary said the doctor was too busy to talk then but would call back. He did, and gave the same fast explanation. He added, for "consolation": "Another type is worse. The diet won't be bad."

Two days later Mrs. H. R. called the secretary and was told to go to the dietician's office in a certain large city hospital any day that week and the diet plan would be ready. Mrs. H. R. waited several days to allow adequate time. Then with her three-year-old child she drove to the hospital, spent 45 minutes finding a one-way street that would lead her to the proper parking lot, and walked at least a mile hunting for proper elevators. She asked directions several times, as no signs were available, and finally found a small cluttered office labeled "Dietician."

Mrs. H. R. announced herself and her intention to the three people sitting at desks in the office, and one person said, "The dietician isn't here right now." There was no indication that anyone expected Mrs. H. R., no offer for her to wait in a certain place, and no explanation of when the dietician would return.

Mrs. H. R. and her child walked through the halls until the dietician returned in one-half hour. The dietician didn't recognize the situation. Finally, after searching, she found a small note, under numerous large papers, listing Mr. H. R.'s name, doctor, and type diet needed. No offer was made to get chairs for Mrs. H. R. and her child. While the dietician searched for a book with the proper diet, Mrs. H. R. found chairs.

The dietician said, "Have you been on this diet before?" "No," said Mrs. H. R., not understanding that the dietician thought the diet was for her and not her husband.

The dietician asked, "Did the doctor explain this condition and diet to you?"

"Not very well. I'd appreciate a more detailed explanation."

The dietician quickly responded. "Oh, you'll have to ask your doctor. I'll have to work this diet out now. It calls for 2500 calories. Do you eat *that much*?"

"Oh, no, it's for my husband," said Mrs. H. R. The dietician seemed relieved. After she had worked out the portions allowed per meal, the dietician said, "This is a low-animal-fat and low-carbohydrate diet. You'll have to weigh the meat." She then started reading the portions for each meal.

Mrs. H. R. had to stop her to ask, "Why low-carbohydrate when the problem is high fat?"

"Carbohydrate pushes up the fat," answered the dietician. "We don't know why."

Mrs. H. R. stopped her again, "How will I weigh the meat? On a scale?"

"Yes," said the dietician.

Mrs. H. R. had visions of standing on a bathroom scale and holding 6 ounces of meat. She knew it wouldn't register properly. "Well, what kind of a scale?" she asked.

"Oh, there are special meat scales which you can buy at drugstores," said the dietician, and she rummaged through several drawers and brought one out to show Mrs. H. R. She then resumed the explanation. "Now, the important thing is to cut out animal fat. Only certain lean meats are acceptable; also, no butter, no milk except skim, only three eggs a week; no sweets, especially ice cream."

Mrs. H. R. was in a state of emotional shock. Her husband, born and raised on a big dairy farm in Wisconsin, was a meat, butter, egg, and whole-milk advocate. "One luxury we will have, no matter what our finances," he had told her 13 years ago when they were first married, "is butter." She thought of the two eggs and bacon he ate ritually every morning, how he would shudder as he looked at the slightly blue cast of the skim milk, and how ice cream in the freezer as a must for bedtime snacks would be no more.

The dietician was saying, "Do you understand?"

"I understand all too well," replied Mrs. H. R.

The dietician took that as a sign to end the session, never sensing that Mrs. H. R. didn't understand all the aspects of the diet, but understood something quite different—the emotional aspect. Therefore, there was no attempt to work out a sample diet. The dietician, a city raised woman originally from Hawaii, had no knowledge of the German farm heritage she was dealing with.

The dietician said she didn't work with this type of diet much and seemed glad to be done. It was late Friday afternoon and of course she was anxious to be done working for the weekend, Mrs. H. R. thought.

Before she left, and as she picked up old diet menus and pencils that her child had been playing with, Mrs. H. R. said, "Oh, what about my husband's food allergies? Did you account for them?"

The dietician looked blankly. "No, I didn't know about them. But just omit any foods on the diet that he's allergic to."

Mrs. H. R. decided not to mention certain food restrictions from the surgery. She knew the dietician wouldn't know about that either.

So after a mile walk back to the car and a six-mile ride home in rush-hour traffic, Mrs. H. R. arrived home to present her husband with his new eating regimen. Obviously the presentation was poor, and Mr. H. R. was too depressed with the initial ideas to discuss any more that evening.

Fortunately, because Mr. H. R. was young and had a strong desire to live healthfully, had long-range plans for his professional future, and wanted to share a long life with his wife and children, he determined to follow the recommended program.

Because his wife had some health education, they were able, when refreshed the next day, to sit down and comprehend the diet booklet. Mrs. H. R. took the initiative in planning menus and buying the suggested food for a prompt beginning. She was able to integrate the new menus with allergy and postsurgery restrictions and took notes on unanswered questions so that she could call the dietician and ask for specific information.

Several days later Mrs. H. R. called the dietician about essential information that had been omitted. She asked what comprises one measurement of certain acceptable fats, what category (fat, carbohydrate, or protein) the bedtime snack should be taken from, and what sugar substitute was recommended. The dietician had only partial answers. Mrs. H. R. then called the allergist, whose response was, "I've never seen the diet. I don't know what you mean, but I'll find out."

He did call back with answers, but Mrs. H. R., her confidence in the health team shaken, decided she had to find someone with more definite answers. She contacted two nurse friends, one of whom got her literature on the disease and menu plans from the American Heart Association. The other nurse friend told her that research was being done on the disease in another local hospital. Mrs. H. R. called the research group and asked for the name of a private physician specializing in lipid metabolism. She contacted the doctor, and he said he would get Mr. H. R.'s records from the allergist and would check his lipids again in two months. (The allergist was acquainted with the lipid specialist, but had not thought to recommend him.)

Mr. H. R., having read that diabetes often accompanies his condition, asked the lipid specialist if a glucose-tolerance test should be done, as suggested in the literature. The specialist said, "By all means. It should have been done originally."

The bill from the specialist for the initial visit and tests was $55. The triglycerides, the portion of the fat not dissolving properly, were still not at a normal level. The specialist examined the diet and said that the carbohydrate intake recommended by the dietician was too high. He rearranged the diet.

Mr. H. R.'s diet, calling for lean meat, eliminated many "stretch" or cheaper foods such as hot dogs, hamburger, and bologna. Sweets were all but eliminated. He had to eat large quantities of nuts and olives to prevent weight loss. The family food budget increased about $10 to $15 per week, since Mrs. H. R. put the entire family on the diet. (The children may also have the disease, although it usually cannot be diagnosed until after 30.)

In another two months the lipids were checked again. The diet had worked: the triglycerides were normal. A half-year had elapsed since the allergist detected Mr. H. R.'s condition; nearly $200 had been spent for medical expenses, and the family food budget had increased considerably.

This is only one case, but it has implications for many others. How many people can be expected to practice health behavior if they are impersonally shuttled from specialist to specialist with no continuity? How can they practice health behavior if they are overwhelmed with medical terminology hurled at them in various fragments? If they do not have the money to pay for special treatment, foods, or other required items, what course can they take?

A worthwhile exercise would be to construct an optimum teaching-learning situation for Mr. H. R. and his family. Then translate that program into terms appropriate for a welfare patient, and for a newly rich patient, using information from this chapter and Chapter 12. You have a current challenge.

REFERENCES

1. American Cancer Society, St. Louis, public service literature.
2. American Dental Association, St. Louis, public service literature.
3. Bayer, Mary, "The Red Dandelion," *Nursing Outlook*, 21: No. 1 (1973), 32.
4. Boas, Charles William, "The Circus," *Guideposts,* July 1973, pp. 16-19.
5. Carlson, Carolyn, *Behavioral Concepts and Nursing Intervention*. Philadelphia: J. B. Lippincott Company, 1970, pp. 269-79.

6. Cassel, John, "The Social and Cultural Implications of Food and Food Habits," Paper presented at the Joint Session of Dental Health, Food and Nutrition, Public Health Education, and Public Health Nursing Sections of the American Public Health Association, 84th Annual Meeting, Atlantic City, N.J., 1956.

7. Cleino, Bettie, "Teaching Machines and Programmed Learning," *Journal of Nursing Education*, 3: No. 1 (1964), 13-15.

8. Dodge, Joan, "What Patients Should Be Told: Patients' and Nurses' Beliefs," *American Journal of Nursing*, 72: No. 10 (1972), 1852-54.

9. Gardner, C. Hugh, "Educators' Failure at Communication," *Intellect*, 100: No. 2350 (1973), 486-88.

10. Guralnik, David, ed., *Webster's New World Dictionary of the American Language* (2nd college ed.). New York: The World Publishing Company, 1972.

11. Hanson, Robert, and Lyle Saunders, *Nurse-Patient Communication: A Manual for Public Health Nurses in Northern New Mexico*. Washington, D.C.: United States Department of Health, Education, and Welfare, 1964, pp. 121-62.

12. Hobbs, Patricia, "Evaluation of a Teaching Programme of Breast Self Examination," *International Journal of Health Education*, 14: (1971), 189-95.

13. Johnson, Jean E., "Effects of Structuring Patients' Expectations on Their Reactions to Threatening Events," *Nursing Research*, 21: No. 6 (1972), 499-503.

14. Kazin, Alfred, "The Human Factory," in *A Walker in the City*. New York: Harcourt, Brace and World, Inc., 1951.

15. Knowles, Malcolm S., "Teaching-Learning Teams in Adult Education," in *The Changing College Classroom*, eds. P. Runkel, R. Harrison, and M. Runkel. San Francisco: Jossey-Bass Inc., Publishers, 1969, p. 257.

16. _____, *The Modern Practice of Adult Education*. New York: Association Press, 1970, pp. 37, 39-40, 225, 271, 294.

17. Lowenfeld, Viktor, "Creativity: Education's Stepchild," in *A Source Book for Creative Thinking*, eds. Sidney J. Parnes and Harold F. Harding. New York: Charles Scribner's Sons, 1962, pp. 9-17.

18. Marks, Janet, and Margaret Clarke, "The Hospital Patient and His Knowledge of the Drugs He Is Receiving," *International Nursing Review*, 19: No. 1 (1972), 39-51.

19. Matheney, Ruth, B. Nolan, A. Ehrkart, and G. Griffin, *Fundamentals of Patient Centered Nursing* (2nd ed.). St. Louis: The C. V. Mosby Company, 1968, pp. 141-46.

20. Morgan, Fred, *Here and Now*. New York: Harcourt, Brace & World, Inc., 1968.

21. Moss, Fay, "The Effect of a Nursing Intervention on Pain Relief," *ANA Regional Clinical Conference*. New York: Appleton-Century-Crofts, 1967, pp. 247-54.

22. Murray, Ruth, and Judith Zentner, *Nursing Assessment and Health Promotion through the Life Span*. Englewood Cliffs, N.J.: Prentice-Hall, Inc., 1975.

23. Nickerson, Donna, "Teaching the Hospitalized Diabetic," *American Journal of Nursing*, 72: No. 6 (1972), 935-38.

24. Nolan, William, "Rules to Make You a Better Patient," *Today's Health*, 51: No. 4 (1973), 41-42, 66-67.

25. Pardue, Austin, "Don't Be Frightened by Failure," *Guideposts*, May 1973, p. 26.

26. Parnes, Sidney J., *Creative Behavior Workbook*. New York: Charles Scribner's Sons, 1967.

27. Peterson, Mary E., and Constance Kies, "Nutrition, Knowledge, and Attitudes of Early Elementary Teachers," *Journal of Nursing Education*, 11: No. 4 (1972), 11-15.

28. Redman, Barbara, *The Process of Patient Teaching in Nursing* (2nd ed.). St. Louis: The C. V. Mosby Company, 1972, pp. 150, 153.

29. Rogers, Carl, *On Becoming A Person*. Boston: Houghton Mifflin Company, 1961, pp. 279-94.

30. Rosenstock, Irvin M., "What Research in Motivation Suggests for Public Health," *American Journal of Public Health*, 50: No.3 (1960), 295-302.

31. Schmitt, Florence E., and Powhatan J. Wooldridge, "Psychological Preparation of Surgical Patients," *Nursing Research*, 22: No. 2 (1973), 108-15.

32. Schweer, Jean E., "Teaching Students to Teach Health Care to Others," *Nursing Clinics of North America*, 6: No. 4 (1971), 682-84.

33. Smith, B. Othanel, *Teachers for the Real World*. Washington D.C.: The American Association of Colleges For Teacher Education, 1969, pp. 7-8.

34. Suchman, Edward, "Preventive Health Behavior: A Model for Research on Community Health Campaigns," *Journal of Health and Social Behavior*, 8: No. 3 (1967), 197-209.

35. Sutterly, Cook, and Gloria Donnelly, *Perspectives in Human Development*. Philadelphia: J. B. Lippincott Company, 1973, pp. 181-85.

36. The Arthritis Foundation, St. Louis, public service literature.

37. Toffler, Alvin, *Future Shock*. New York: Random House, 1970, pp. 342-67.

38. Tollefsrud, Valborg, "We're for Educating Our Patients," *American Journal of Nursing*, 56: No. 8 (1956), 1009-10.

39. Torrance, Ellis Paul, *Creativity*. Washington D.C.: National Educational Association of the United States, 1963.

40. Wu, Ruth, *Behavior and Illness*. Englewood Cliffs, N.J.: Prentice-Hall, Inc., 1973, p. 112.

Personal Interviews

41. Bringewatt, Mark, student of Malcolm Knowles, May 17, 1973.

42. Byrne, John, and Mary McElfresh, director and educational director, respectively, St. Louis Visiting Nurse Association, July 6, 1973.

43. Goldberg, Mrs. Virginia, program director, St. Louis Heart Association, June 29, 1973.

44. Morris, Virginia, and Verna Andrews, registered nurses, St. Louis Visiting Nurse Association, July 12, 1973.

45. Sellars, Ernest, director, St. Louis Diabetes Association, July 2, 1973.

46. Zentner, Reid, cooperative work training coordinator, Alton, Illinois, public school system, May 5, 1973.

CHAPTER 6

Concepts
of Epidemiology

Study of this chapter will enable you to:

1 Define *epidemiology, agent, host,* and *environment.*

2 List types of agents and describe the interaction of agent, host, and environment.

3 List and discuss the key concepts applicable to the epidemiological method.

4 Compare the epidemiological method with the nursing process.

5 Define and discuss the types of epidemiological studies—descriptive, analytic, and experimental.

6 Discuss the application of epidemiology to nursing.

7 Do an epidemiological study with an instructor's supervision.

Before proposing health practices you must know the health status of a certain population. Health and illness patterns can vary considerably among groups in a pluralistic society. You and all other health workers therefore require an understanding of epidemiology and its relevance to health care. Emphasis in this chapter will not be on statistical incidence of disease but rather on the use of the scientific method for data collection and planning of health care.

EVOLUTION AND DEFINITION

Historically the emphasis of epidemiology was on investigating an *epidemic, the unusually frequent, widespread occurrence of a disease; and included tracing a disease source, controlling its spread, and initiating measures to prevent recurrences* [5]. From studying such diseases as cholera, plague, smallpox, yellow fever, and typhus, several significant contributions materialized. Microorganisms were discovered as causative agents of disease, immunology developed, and new knowledge regarding the transmission of disease was acquired [7].

Today epidemiology is concerned with much more than epidemics. The scientific method used to study contagious disease now pervades every aspect of the nursing process and extends to every area of nursing. *Epidemiology now includes the study of the incidence, distribution, and dynamics of health states, noninfectious and infectious disease, disability, and mortality within groups of people.* The premise is that deviations from health are the result of the imbalance among agent, host, and environment. Therefore, problems of normal aging, chronic and degenerative diseases, congenital defects, accidental injuries, mental illness, nutritional disorders, and social pathology are also current subjects of epidemiological investigation. The ultimate goal of epidemiology is the prevention of disease and disability.

Key Concepts

There are two key epidemiological concepts. The first is that people are studied in groups. In order to identify the factors that are essential or contributory to a particular disease or threat to health, comparisons of those afflicted with those not afflicted must be made. Thus, after the appropriate population or group is selected, all persons are subject to investigation [5].

The second key concept is that the natural history of disease must be observed. Factors in the initiation of the disease, the possible course from beginning to cure or death, and environmental or genetic factors modifying the course are all examined. Through the study of the balance and change among agent, host, and environment, epidemiologists analyze their data to describe the *incidence or frequency of occurrence,* the distribution, and the cause of disease [19].

INTERACTION OF AGENT, HOST, AND ENVIRONMENT

The Agent

The nature of the interaction among agent, host, and environmental factors determines the relative health or disease status of a population. *An agent is an element, a substance, or a force, either animate or inanimate, that initiates or perpetuates a disease under proper environmental conditions or following contact with a susceptible host.* Causative agents may be biological, chemical, nutrient, physical, mechanical, or psychological in nature.

Biological agents are living parasites of man. These include insects, worms, protozoa, fungi, bacteria, rickettsiae, and viruses. Malaria is considered to be the most important global parasitic disease, both in terms of *morbidity, number of people with the disease, and mortality, number of deaths caused by the disease.*

Chemical agents may be *exogenous substances, those arising outside the body* and creating harmful change in tissue, such as dusts, gases, vapors, and fumes. Or they may be *endogenous substances, those arising within the body*, usually normal products of metabolic activity that when produced in excess cause disease. Examples of the latter are gout, which results from excess uric acid production because of disturbed purine metabolism, and peptic ulcers, caused by excessive gastric secretion.

Nutrient agents, also chemical in nature, are distinguished by an over-abundance or lack of one or more basic dietary elements—fats, carbohydrates, protein, vitamins, minerals, or water. *Physical agents consist of several kinds of atmospheric abnormalities*, such as extreme temperature, intense sound, and excessive radiation. *Mechanical agents produce undue force or friction on the body,* resulting in crushing wounds, sprains, dislocations, or fractures. Some mechanical forces may be accidental or peculiar to certain jobs, such as the trauma to the hands from motor-driven drills used in demolition work[3].

Although some do not consider psychological factors to be true agents, stress sometimes causes headaches, nausea, vomiting, diarrhea, peptic ulcers, hypertension, and a number of other conditions. Some diseases may have multiple causative agents. Therefore, agent categories should be carefully reviewed when analyzing any disease process or health threat.

The Host

The host is a person or organism capable of being infected or affected by an agent. Many factors affect a human host's relative susceptibility or resistance to a disease agent, including age, sex, race, cultural habits, customs of living, nutritional status, occupation, and income. Other factors include normal body-defense mechanisms, heredity, and general constitutional makeup. Chapter 1 discusses these characteristics[5].

The Environment

The *environment*, capable of preventing, suppressing, or contributing to disease, accidents, or death, is *all the external conditions and influences affecting the life and development of an organism*. Chapter 1 discusses specific environmental variables.

Clark has proposed an analogy using the principle of the lever and fulcrum (see Figure 6-1). Health equilibrium is dependent on the weights at each end of the lever and on the position of the fulcrum. Environmental factors are the fulcrum, and agent and host factors are the opposing balances. When the system is in balance, health prevails. When any force changes and the balance is altered, the likelihood of disease or other threats to health increases[3].

EPIDEMIOLOGICAL METHODS

An epidemiological team, using the entire community as its laboratory, may include doctors, nurses, laboratory experts, microbiologists, geneticists, sanitary engineers, anthropologists, and statisticians. They may study a self-limited problem, such as an outbreak of food poisoning; a short-term problem, such as a schoolchild's infectious hepatitis; or a long-range problem, such as hypertension.

Scientific Approach

Epidemiological investigations adhere to the basic principles and procedures of the scientific method discussed in Chapter 4. Once a problem is identified, steps in the scientific method are employed. Data are produced from pertinent and accurate observations; measurements are then analyzed, employing various statistical methods; conclusions are drawn; and practical application is made. The exact starting point in any investigation depends on the type and extent of the problem, the interest and experience of the investigators, and the ultimate objectives[3, 7].

Case Studies

A classic example of an epidemiological study that utilized an orderly fashion of investigation (although not the exact scientific method) is the "Broad Street Pump problem," conducted more than 100 years ago by John Snow. A clinical investigator now considered a pioneer in the field of epidemiology, Snow showed continued interest in cholera and explained its mode of spread, even though the living causative agent had not yet been discovered[17].

An epidemic outbreak of cholera occurred in the Broad Street area of London, with some 500 fatalities. Snow carefully defined the problem and examined the existing information relating to deaths from cholera. His hypothesis was that cholera results from an invasion of a morbid poison that enters the

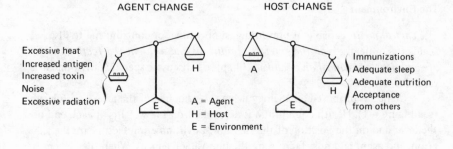

AGENT CHANGE   HOST CHANGE

Excessive heat
Increased antigen
Increased toxin
Noise
Excessive radiation

H   A

A = Agent
H = Host
E = Environment

Immunizations
Adequate sleep
Adequate nutrition
Acceptance
from others

EQUILIBRIUM OF AGENT, HOST, ENVIRONMENT

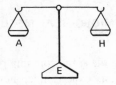

A   H

E

Environmental change in favor of the
agent, increasing susceptibility of host

Environmental change in favor of the
host, decreasing agent potential

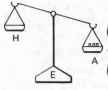

Poor aseptic measures
Crowding
Air pollution
Water pollution
Food contamination

Family harmony
Adequate shelter
Eradication of rats
Sunshine

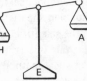

FIGURE 6-1
Interaction of Agent, Host, and Environment

alimentary tract, multiplies, and is excreted and so spread to others. He tested
his hypothesis many times and in different ways. He examined the water from
the well used by a number of the townspeople, the Broad Street Pump. Initially,
he observed a minimal amount of impurities and retested it several times. He
found variations in the amounts of impurities but concluded that at the beginning of the outbreak the water had been more impure. Snow then visited the
families of dead cholera victims. The majority of them lived near the pump or
had drunk water from the pump shortly before their death. His study indicated
that there had been no outbreak or increase of cholera in the area except among
persons drinking water from the Broad Street Pump. Snow made a report of his

findings, and the handle of the pump was removed the following day. All of this work was accomplished in one week.

When Snow observed still more deaths reported during the following weeks, he began to collect additional data. Although some of those infected reportedly had not drunk water from the Broad Street Pump, Snow felt they had unknowingly taken some, since proprietors in the area had utilized the water for mixing drinks, preparing food, and a variety of other uses. He also discovered that although a workhouse, brewery, and manufacturing plant were located near the pump, only men working in the plant were among the casualties. He learned that the workhouse and brewery utilized water from wells located on their premises, which were apparently not contaminated, while the manufacturing plant had utilized the Broad Street Pump.

All the reports of cholera in this study originated with water from a contaminated well or pump. Snow carefully analyzed his data about cholera and developed a complete list of recommendations to prevent its transmission. This study shows how the basic principles of scientific problem solving were utilized even before the discovery of the causative agent.

You may be wondering if it is feasible for persons other than members of an epidemiological team—or an individual practicing nurse—to do such a study. It is indeed. A nursing student conducted a small study while taking an epidemiology course. She used the scientific method to study conditions of refrigerators in a nurses' residence. Steps of the study included: (1) describing the quantity of food stored and cleanliness of selected refrigerators; (2) examining the possible relationship between poor conditions and the refrigerator's potential for harboring disease organisms; and (3) noting the possibility of a relationship between poor refrigerator conditions and incidence of gastrointestinal illnesses in the student users[18].

The investigator gave consideration to all potential agent, host, and environmental factors relating to the refrigerators and the users. The concepts of disciplines such as public health, nutrition, and microbiology were involved. The results showed a possible relationship between gastrointestinal disturbances in certain nursing students and their consumption of food stored under poor refrigerator conditions. Therefore, even a small study (in this case resulting from an assignment to develop problem-solving skills) can uncover a very practical epidemiological problem. Further investigation would provide more conclusive results. More importantly, further illness from these conditions could be avoided.

Types of Investigations

Epidemiological investigations may be either descriptive, analytical, or experimental.

Descriptive epidemiology focuses on describing the occurrence and distribution of disease or health states. Questions about who is affected and where and when are answered so that health care workers can be alerted to outbreaks of disease and can be provided with historical information about disease during a specific time[6].

Descriptive information lends itself to formation of hypotheses—for example, the association between a season and disease, age and disease, or place and disease. Hypotheses can then be tested to discover the causes and mechanics of disease in analytical or experimental studies.

Analytical investigations explore the possible association between a cause or contributing factor and disease. These studies may be conducted *by beginning with a disease* (such as cancer) *and looking backward at its possible causes, called a retrospective* or *case-history study*. Or they may be conducted by *beginning with exposure to a suspect factor*, such as nicotine and tar content in cigarettes, and *looking forward to possible results, a prospective* or *cohort study*. The goal in both types of studies is to learn if exposure to factor *x* increases the risk of development of a specific disease[5, 12].

Associations that have been discovered by analytic studies are often very suggestive of a causal relation, but they never prove that a causal relation exists. Only experimental investigations provide the scientific proof.

Experimental investigations provide a test of an association by introducing an experimental condition (for example, a therapeutic drug) *in a test group but not in a comparable control group, and observing the effect over a period of time*. These studies are best conducted under "double-blind" conditions, in which neither the observer nor the subjects know which subjects belong to the test and which to the control group. Using this procedure insures objectivity and allows for more accurate estimation of the experimental agent's effect[7].

Application

In order for epidemiology to serve its full purpose, it must be applicable to ordinary circumstances of community life. In the United States, epidemiologists serve the people mainly through affiliation with national, state, or local governments. A few function internationally, while yet others work for private agencies or corporations[5].

At the national level, epidemiological practice is concentrated in two programs within the United States Public Health Service. One program, the National Communicable Disease Center, is located in Atlanta, Georgia. The other program is primarily concerned with noncommunicable disease and is located at the National Institutes of Health in Bethesda, Maryland.

At the state and local levels, epidemiological practice is related to disease and accident surveillance, detective work, disease and accident control, and prevention activities. Surveillance, utilizing some formal system of data collection, tabulation, and evaluation, is the primary concern. Usually this basic surveillance information is available at the local level of government. Sources of data may come from schools, physicians, laboratories, concerned individuals, hospitals, community health nurses, and a variety of other sources. Epidemiologists may study the data for time variations in occurrence, distribution, or related health threats.

For example, you may notice that there are more automobile accidents on a certain street in the winter; that incidence of tuberculosis has declined over a certain period; or that the incidence of mild gastroenteritis and mild hearing loss has increased during the summer. You may then use the data in a variety of ways: report it to a state health department, make referrals to other agencies, plan health programs, provide information for legislative action, or investigate a communicable disease.

The term denoting investigation of an outbreak that has been identified through surveillance is *detective work*. As in a police investigation, suspense is involved, clues are needed, suspects are questioned, facts are analyzed, and results are obtained. Ideally, the villain is found. The epidemiologists then focus on prevention or minimization of recurrences through control and prevention activities[5]. Examples of control activities include mass immunization against rubella, venereal disease clinics, and education about risk factors associated with certain diseases or accidents. Epidemiologists must validate the need for everyday control activities, determining that the community needs the program.

Epidemiologists have many opportunities to stimulate innovative ideas to benefit the health of people. For example, epidemiological data in a mental health center revealed a high rate of failure for teenage marriages. All of the failing teenage marriages had two facts in common: (1) the marriage occurred because of pregnancy, and (2) there were at least two children involved. At the time of failure, the partners were completely fed up with marriage and children. The treatment team was concerned not only about the many pairs of teenagers who were trying marriage and parenthood before they were ready but also about the children involved. Hoping to meet community needs, the team surveyed the local annual incidence of such marriages, the incidence of failure, what happened to the families after failure, and the apparent differences between marriages which failed and those that did not. They then shared the results with family doctors and ministers[9].

Family doctors confirm pregnancy, deliver babies, supply medical care to these families, and are "in" at both the beginning and end of marriage. The doctor, through counseling and marriage education, could help in preventing some marriage failures and unplanned babies. Because clergymen perform most teenage marriage ceremonies, often after the marriages have been arranged by parents to solve the problem of pregnancy, clergymen could also be crucial in prevention. They could help work out plans that might correct rather than compound the mistakes. One Catholic priest in the area concluded that he would perform no more pregnancy-propelled teenage marriages because they were not holding[9].

In implementing this study or any program utilizing epidemiological data, the local community must be involved: clergy, welfare caseworkers, lawyers, school administrators and counselors, nurses, doctors, parents, and civic groups. Innovation does not occur without a receptive attitude.

ROLE OF THE NURSE IN EPIDEMIOLOGY

You can use epidemiological concepts regardless of the practice setting, for you will be observing and influencing a primary agent-host-environment triad: the patient or family (host); the hospital, home, or community setting (environment); and the agent, whatever it is—known or unknown[21].

You may be a formal member of an epidemiological investigation, identifying the need for and participating in the design of the study as well as collecting data. For example, in a school you might observe that there has been an increase in the number of accidents over a two-month period and feel an investigation is warranted. You may initially work alone, examining some sociological characteristics of the children in relation to causes or influencing factors associated with accidents, before alerting other team members.

Because health records are often used for data collection, you must do a thorough assessment of the people receiving care and record the information accurately. You may use records to identify and observe health trends in the people being served. In a community agency setting, you may observe that the same people with high-risk characteristics, such as teenagers or low-income groups, are missing prenatal appointments every week. You should then conduct an informal investigation to identify and possibly eliminate or modify barriers preventing such people from keeping their clinic appointments.

You may also support epidemiological investigations. Some studies, such as nutrition studies, are conducted over extended periods of time. Because of the relationship you can develop with the family, you may become the liaison who interprets the study to the people and gives them explanations, support, or encouragement while participating in the study. You may offer comprehensive nursing care as a bonus for participation in a study[6].

Application of general health-promotion measures, including education about health, is part of epidemiology. In a school setting you help provide a suitable atmosphere and instill positive health education at an early age. In a hospital setting, you have daily opportunities to help restore people to health and then assist them to learn how to maintain it. You may help prevent and control disease. For example, you may conduct screening programs or immunization clinics during which you explain the need for the program and provide the necessary followup care. You may identify and implement control measures, perhaps as a member of the hospital infection committee. You may set up and explain isolation to a patient, prepare a patient to enter a tuberculosis hospital, or send a child home from school because of suspected ringworm.

Be aware of epidemiological investigations in the literature. Results of existing studies may provide clues for investigations in your nursing practice, or they may identify nursing needs of specific population groups. Many nurses employ epidemiological methods every day in their practice, but are not aware of the professional terminology. If you have not previously understood the day-to-day relevance of epidemiology, perhaps you can begin to actively utilize this approach in providing patient and family care.

REFERENCES

1. Beland, Irene L., *Clinical Nursing: Pathophysiological and Psychosocial Approaches* (2nd ed.). London: The Macmillan Company, 1970.
2. Burton, Lloyd E., and Hugh H. Smith, *Public Health and Community Medicine*. Baltimore: The Williams & Wilkins Company, 1970.
3. Clark, E. Gurney, "The Epidemiologic Approach and Contributions to Preventive Medicine," in *Preventive Medicine for the Doctor in His Community* (3rd ed.), eds. Hugh Rodman Leavell and E. Gurney Clark. New York: McGraw-Hill Book Company, 1965, pp. 39-123.
4. Corrigan, Marjorie, and Lucille Corrigan, *Epidemiology in Nursing*. Washington, D.C.: The Catholic University of America Press, 1966.
5. Fox, John P., Carrie E. Hall, and Lila Elveback, *Epidemiology: Man and Disease*. London: The Macmillan Company, 1970.
6. Freeman, Ruth B., *Community Health Nursing*. Philadelphia: W. B. Saunders Company, 1970.
7. Goerke, Lenor, and Ernest Stebbins, *Mustard's Introduction to Public Health* (5th ed). New York: Macmillan and Company, 1968.
8. Kallins, Ethel L., *Textbook of Public Health Nursing*. St. Louis: The C. V. Mosby Company, 1967.
9. Kiesler, Frank, "Programming for Prevention," in *Community Mental Health: Social Action and Reaction*, eds. Bruce Denner and Richard Price. New York: Holt, Rinehart & Winston, Inc., 1973, pp. 101-11.
10. Lester, Mary R., "Every Nurse an Epidemiologist," *American Journal of Nursing*, 57: No. 11 (1957), 1434-35.
11. Levengood, Robert, Paul Lowinger, and Kenneth Schooff, "Heroin Addiction in the Suburbs: An Epidemiologic Study," *American Journal of Public Health*, 63: No. 3 (1973), 209-13.
12. McMahon, Brian, and Thomas Pugh, *Epidemiology: Principles and Methods* (2nd ed). Boston: Little, Brown & Company, 1970.
13. Nordsiek, Frederic, "An Epidemiological Approach to Obesity," *American Journal of Public Health*, 54: No. 10 (1964), 1689-98.
14. Parrish, Henry, Gerald Wiechmann, Janet Weil, and Carole Carr, "Epi-

demiological Approach to Preventing School Accidents," *Journal of School Health*, 37: No. 5 (1967), 236-40.

15. Paul, John R., *Clinical Epidemiology*. Chicago: The University of Chicago Press, 1966.

16. Roueche, Berton, *Curiosities of Medicine*. Boston: Little, Brown & Company, 1970.

17. ____, *Eleven Blue Men*. New York: Berkley Publishing Company, 1953.

18. Sheetz, Anne, "An Investigation of Residence Refrigerators," *Nursing Outlook*, 14: No. 9 (1966), 54-57.

19. Van Peenan, Huber J., *Essentials of Pathology*. Chicago: Year Book Medical Publishers, Inc., 1966.

20. Winslow, C., W. Smillie, J. Doull, and J. Gordon, *The History of American Epidemiology*. St. Louis: The C. V. Mosby Company, 1952.

21. Zeis, Dolores, *Epidemiology as a Contribution to Nursing Practice*. A Report to the Workshop, Epidemiology for Nurses, St. Louis, June 1 and 2, 1970. St. Louis: St. Louis University and Metropolitan College in cooperation with United States Department of Health, Education, and Welfare, Public Health Service, 1970.

CHAPTER 7

Application
of Adaptation Theory
to Nursing

Study of this chapter will help you to:

1 Define *adaptation, adjustment,* and key concepts related to adaptation.

2 Discuss the application of adaptation theory and related concepts to nursing.

3 Discuss examples of physiological processes that are adaptive.

4 Differentiate between stress and anxiety and describe physiological, emotional, and behavioral reactions to psychological stress.

5 Discuss examples of and factors influencing cultural and social adaptation.

6 Identify adaptive behaviors used in family interaction.

7 List examples of situations or behaviors that interfere with adaptation.

8 Discuss nursing measures that will assist the person or family to adapt to or cope with internal or external changes (physical, emotional, social, cultural).

9 Identify various body rhythms and give examples of body rhythms that maintain adaptation.

10 Analyze effects upon patient care when body rhythms are considered in medical and nursing practice.

11 Discuss nursing measures to assist the person's maintenance of normal biological rhythms during illness.

12 Relate mobility to physical, emotional, and social adaptation.

13 Define *immobility* and describe the dimensions of immobility.

14 Discuss the physiological effects of immobility upon the various functional areas of the body and related nursing measures to enhance or restore adaptive processes.

15 Describe the effects of emotional or behavioral immobility and nursing measures that enhance or restore psychological adaptation.

16 Work with a patient to maintain or restore physiological and emotional adaptation.

A concept that lends itself readily to the science and art of nursing is **adaptation**. *Through this process man, either individually or in groups, constructively copes with conditions imposed internally or externally in order to meet his needs.* These new, different, or threatening conditions—stimuli, forces, stressors, pathologies—may be entirely beyond man's control or may result from his freedom to choose alternatives. The term **adjustment** *refers to minor changes in customary behavior to more effectively meet life's problems.*

Adaptation and life are synonymous; each involves the whole organism. Adaptation permits forward movement by reducing or negating the effects of discord, deviance, or adverse forces accompanying change. No adaptation is permanent or static, because change is constant. Change or adaptation should be accomplished without excess physical illness, loss of long-range goals or values, psychological disintegration, or disruption of the person's overall social functioning.

The definition of *health* and its related concepts outlined in the first chapter of this book introduced you to the concept of adaptation. Although adaptation as a concept is not emphasized in other chapters, its implications permeate the book. An appropriate teaching method promotes adaptation. Epidemiological discovery of or controlling of disease patterns aids adaptation in a person or group. Behavior in the phases of crisis is the person's way of adapting. Environmental, cultural, religious, social-class, and family influences are integral factors in adaptation. In each developmental era the person undergoes adaptive changes[35]. This chapter will explore the application of adaptation to nursing practice.

ADAPTIVE PROCESSES

Although adaptive processes may appear to be strictly physiological, they affect the whole person. Thus the key concepts discussed here regarding these processes in general should be considered in relation to psychological, sociocultural, and family adaptation as well. Nursing implications are related throughout.

Homeokinesis

Homeokinesis refers to the ability of the organism to preserve its integrity through change and the element of motion that is characteristic of physiological adaptation. Dynamic, self-regulating processes work to maintain or to restore the internal environment to normal. This involves *negative feedback, wherein a deviation in one direction results in a reaction in the opposite direction*. The classic example of this is the maintenance of a relatively constant environment in the home by means of a control device, a thermostat.

The Body as an Open System

Physiological adaptation may be considered by viewing the body as a complex open system in which a dynamic balance is maintained with the surrounding environment. Each of the interrelated subsystems (organs, tissues) of the body is an open system made up of additional subsystems (cells). Levels of organization within and among systems include the cellular, structural, organ-system, and physiological-process aspects[48]. For example, the regulation of body temperature involves skin, respiratory, circulatory, and neurological structures. Variations in the degree of adaptation also may occur. Changes in function of one body part mediate change elsewhere. Examples include the carotid sinus reflex that slows the heart rate, thereby reducing blood pressure through decreased vasoconstriction, and eye adaptation to light and dark through pupil dilation and changes in the rods and cones. Increased production of antibodies occurs in response to the presence of foreign protein in the form of a bacterium. And decreased oxygen tension at higher altitudes increases blood hemoglobin content[26].

Basic adaptive responses are known sufficiently to permit prediction of outcomes, and these relate directly to many aspects of nursing care. For example, detection of *hyperpyrexia*, an *increased body temperature*, in the patient will permit you to plan for his increased perspiration, resultant dehydration, increased cardiac and respiratory rates, increased surface heat loss, and eventual decreased metabolism leading to a decreased heat production[31]. Plans for fluid replacement, rest, conservation of body heat, and monitoring of vital signs will be some of the basic components of the febrile patient's care plan. Special skin care will promote adaptation of the integumental system, preventing skin breakdown caused by deprivation of moisture and nutrition to the skin during hyperpyrexia.

Progressive segregation, in which the open system divides into a hierarchy with subsystems, causes progressive "mechanization" or a fixed arrangement. This imposes restraints on the free interplay of the subsystems and limits their potential function[30]. An example of this is the difficulty encountered when a person tries to void in a supine position. The "mechanized" positions are sitting or standing.

Maintaining a Steady State

Man's functioning as an integrated behavioral unit can be viewed on a continuum: at times he is operating as a stable integrated unit with consistent, orderly behaviors and at other times he is an unstable, ineffective, nonintegrated unit in coping with stimuli. (This process can be related to the agent-host-environment interaction explained in Chapter 6.)

In the *stable or steady state there is optimal energy balance between utilization and conservation.* Any disturbance in a system stimulates return to a steady state or *equifinality, a characteristic or original state that the organism strives by nature to assume through self-regulatory processes*[30].

All people have a potential for energy imbalance and inappropriate energy allocation. One of the best ways to assess imbalance is to note inconsistency between behaviors: the person says one thing and does another. For example, the apparently calm, friendly patient may actually be feeling great anxiety, undergoing great energy utilization, and experiencing covert behavioral and physiological instability. Illness is also likely to cause energy imbalance, which indicates that the body's responses are inadequate to its special needs. Illness may be regarded as a life process that is regulating or striving toward normalcy following a disturbance to the system. Recovery is an adaptive response to maintain the body's integrity, a reestablishment of equifinality, the steady or stable state. Chronic disease or disability represents an altered state between usable energy and the steady state. When all man's regulatory processes are properly functioning, he is in a steady adaptive state. He can then deal most effectively with whatever situations he meets.

Freedom within the steady state refers to the wide choice of activities and environments available to the organism for survival. For example, man can survive by eating a wide variety of foods. Yet stability may be best achieved by limiting the variety of foods. The creation of microenvironments, such as the centrally heated and air-conditioned home, is a means of attaining stability. But to remain ideally comfortable, man must then forever after stay in his home, avoiding out-of-door activities—an unlikely possibility.

The Adaptation Syndrome

Stress is a physical and emotional state always present in the person, intensified when environmental change or threat occurs internally or externally to which he must respond. The manifestations of stress are both overt and covert[9, 44].

The person's survival depends upon constant mediation between environmental demands and adaptive capacities. Various self-regulatory mechanisms are in constant operation, adjusting the body to a changing number and nature of internal and external stressors, agents, or factors causing intensification of the stress state. Stressors (stress agents) include cold, heat, radiation, infectious organisms, disease processes, mechanical trauma, fever, pain, imagined events, and intense emotional involvement. A moderate amount of stress, when regulatory mechanisms act within limits and few symptoms are observable, is constructive. The exaggerated stress state is recognized when stressors are excessive or intense, limits of the steady state are exceeded, and the person cannot cope with the stressors' demands.

Responses to stress are both local and general.The *Local Adaptation Syndrome*, typified by the inflammatory response, *is the method used to wall off and control effects of physical stressors locally*. When the stressor cannot be handled locally, *the whole body responds to protect itself and insure survival in the best way possible through the General Adaptation Syndrome*. The general body response augments bodily functions that protect the organism from injury, psychological and physical, and suppresses those functions nonessential to life. The General Adaptation Syndrome is characterized by Alarm and Resistance stages and, when body resistance is not maintained, an end stage, Exhaustion [44, 45].

The General Adaptation Syndrome

The *Alarm Stage* is an *instantaneous, short-term, life-preserving, and total sympathetic-nervous-system response* when the person consciously or unconsciously perceives a stressor and feels helpless, insecure, or biologically uncomfortable. This stage is typified by a "fight-or-flight" reaction[44]. Epinephrine is released from the adrenal medulla and at the adrenergic nerve endings and is transported to the target areas. Generally the person is prepared to act; he is more alert and able to adapt.

Physiologically, the following responses occur when the sympathetic nervous system is stimulated:

1. Cardiovascular rate and output are increased, making more blood available, so that the pulse increases in rate and strength of beat; palpitations or arrhythmias may occur; and blood pressure rises.
2. Blood supply is shunted to the brain, heart, and skeletal muscles rather than to the periphery, causing the skin to be pale, ashen, and cool to touch.
3. Respiratory rate and depth are increased to assure adequate oxygenation.
4. Salt and water are retained by the kidneys to bolster blood volume, contributing to a fuller blood pressure and reduced urinary output.
5. Metabolism is increased up to 150 percent, providing immediate energy

and producing more heat. Thus body temperature may rise, perspiration ensues, and mild dehydration follows. (Dry lips and mouth are not uncommon.) If metabolism remains high for some time, insomnia and then fatigue occur.

6. Hyperglycemia results from glycolysis in the liver to meet energy demands after initial hypoglycemia.
7. Muscle tonus is increased so that activities may be better coordinated; however, the person may be more rigid or have tremors. Tense musculature, especially of the trapezius muscle in the neck-shoulder area, causing headache, is not unusual.
8. Pupils dilate so that maximum light can be used in viewing a situation. Vision is initially sharp.
9. Sodium chloride in the extracellular fluid is reduced, while potassium levels are increased.
10. Less essential functions such as digestion and excretion are diminished and sphincters tighten. The person may be unable to void or void only small amounts while feeling a strong urge, feel anorexic, or become constipated and distended with flatus[9, 21, 44, 45].

To complicate assessment, there are times when *parts* of the parasympathetic division of the autonomic nervous system are inadvertently stimulated during a stressful state because of proximity of sympathetic and parasympathetic nerve fibers[9, 21, 44]. With intensification of stress, opposite behaviors to the above are then observed:

1. Cardiovascular output may diminish, causing a slow, thready pulse and a drop in blood pressure.
2. Blood supply does not remain shunted to vital organs but returns to the periphery, causing flushed, hot skin and feelings of faintness.
3. Respirations may become difficult because of constricted bronchi. If considerable carbon dioxide has been exhaled earlier with deep respirations, hyperventilation with accompanying tremors, syncope, and dizziness may occur.
4. The elevated body metabolism uses much energy; body reserves of glycogen may be depleted and the person feels nauseated and hungry when hypoglycemia occurs.
5. Muscle tonus may relax, so that incoordination results. Increased blood flow through the muscles affects alertness and cognition and may cause syncope.
6. Pupil dilation may become fixed, causing blurred vision; or constriction may occur, reducing acuity.
7. Sphincters have diminished tone and gastrointestinal secretion and propulsion increase, so that the person has involuntary urination or defecation or urinary frequency and diarrhea[9, 21, 44, 45].

The **Stage of Resistance** *is the body's way of adapting, through an adreno-cortical response to the disequilibrium caused by the stressors of life* [44] . Because of the adrenocortical response, increased use of body resources, endurance and strength, antibody production, hormonal secretion, blood sugar levels, and blood volume result to sustain the body's fight for preservation. Body response eventually returns to normal.

Stress is additive. The repeated exposure to stress, even when the stressors are of widely differing kinds, including people and their feelings, ultimately takes a toll on the individual. Ordinarily the body sooner or later copes adequately with stress—even cumulative stress—and the excessive or undirected energy produced as a response. The **Stage of Exhaustion** *occurs when the person is unable to continue to adapt to internal and external environmental demands.* Physical or psychic disease or death results because the body can no longer compensate for or correct homeostatic imbalances. Manifestations of this stage are similar to those of the Alarm Stage except that all reactions first intensify and then diminish in response and show no ability to return to an effective level of function. Frequent or prolonged General Adaptation Syndrome response triggers disease through adrenocortical hypertrophy, thymolymphatic atrophy, elevated blood glucose, ulceration of the gastrointestinal tract, reduced tone and fibrosis of tissues, and vasoconstriction [44] .

Health care workers are concerned with promoting the resistance stage and preventing or reversing the exhaustion stage, whether through drugs, bedrest, medical treatments, crisis intervention, psychotherapy, or social action. Ideally, you should identify potential stressors that the person might encounter and determine how to alter the stressors or best support the person's adaptive mechanisms and resources physically, emotionally, and socially, since the person will respond as an entity to the stressors.

PHYSIOLOGICAL ADAPTATION

The processes of homeokinesis, maintenance of a steady state, and the General Adaptation Syndrome just described all affect physiological adaptation.

Adaptation to the Environment

Adaptation enables living organisms to respond to changes in their environment in such a manner that injury or disease is prevented or damage repaired. Adaptation assists man to function within a normal range. The following two experiments demonstrate man's adaptation in response to environment [49] .

In one study, sweat production increased in men encased in ventilated suits for two hours each day for several days. The men were warmed to a uniform oral temperature on each testing occasion, but they consistently perspired more profusely on successive days. This change was a result of increased adrenal medulla production of epinephrine and norepinephrine resulting from the stressor heat[49]

In another study, the circulating number of erythrocytes in men taken to high altitudes increased because of lower atmospheric oxygen. On successive days, erythrocyte production in the bone marrow was increased, carrying more oxygen to the tissues. This resulted from release of erythropoietin from the kidneys because of low oxygen tension in the kidneys[49].

Oxygen-Carbon Dioxide Exchange

Normal physiological processes of the body are also examples of adaptation. For example, oxygen is essential for man's survival. *Respiration is the transport of oxygen from atmosphere to the cells, subsequent utilization, and transport of carbon dioxide from the cells to the atmosphere*[2, 3].

All cells need oxygen for metabolic functions, but some react to a lack of oxygen with more devastating results than others. The cells of the cerebral cortex, myocardium, and kidney tubules do not adapt to a lack of oxygen and are highly susceptible to anoxia.

Varying situations in the body alter and change the normal oxygen needs. Metabolic requirements change as a person grows older. Changes in activity demand more or less oxygen; for example, during sleep or at rest less oxygen is needed than for exercise or strenuous work. Nutritional status is significant, since oxygen combines with a carbohydrate, fat, or protein to produce energy. The rate of chemical reaction in the cells during metabolism depends upon the concentration of oxygen in the extracellular fluids[2, 3].

Respiration is divided into various phases[2, 3]. Each has an ability to adapt to the body's changing needs.

Phase 1 is ventilation, the transportation of air from atmosphere to alveoli through inspiration and the return of air from alveoli to atmosphere by expiration. This particular function is measured through the respiratory rate, which indicates respiratory integrity and oxygen need. The rate of ventilation, an adaptive mechanism, is directly proportional to the need for oxygen or need to eliminate carbon dioxide.

Phase 2 involves diffusion of oxygen and carbon dioxide across the alveolar and capillary membranes. Normal adaptive mechanisms within the lung shunt the passage of gases, at varying times, for the purpose of maintaining a constant homeostatic level.

Phase 3 involves transportation of oxygen and carbon dioxide within the blood stream by hemoglobin. Adaptive mechanisms involving the blood buffer system maintain an equilibrium in this area.

Phase 4 involves oxidation-reduction reactions in the cells. Adaptation occurs as membrane permeability and transport of gas alter in response to metabolic changes.

Phase 5 involves the chemical and neurological regulation of respiration. Regulatory mechanisms adapt to alterations as necessary. For example, a high blood carbon dioxide stimulates the respiratory center through chemical changes in the blood, so that the person breathes faster, thereby reducing carbon dioxide. The opposite occurs with low blood carbon dioxide.

Certain protective biological mechanisms of the respiratory tract minimize the harmful effects of inspired air. These mechanisms, which allow the individual to adapt to environmental changes, can be classified as either functions of the system or integrated processes. The functional mechanisms include the cilia, which cleanse the inhaled air, and the length of the passageways, which gives moisture and warmth to the air mix before entry into the lung. The integrated mechanical and neurological processes are the sneeze and the cough. Within the lung itself are certain capabilities to deal with microorganisms; this process of adaptation includes healing, fibrous tissue changes, and local or systemic pathophysiological changes.

You have a vital role in prevention of respiratory problems, which are often avoidable. As a citizen and nurse, you must fight legally and personally the problem of air pollution. Generally, health measures to maintain a sound state of physical fitness are important in keeping up physical defenses that combat disease. For example, persons with allergies to airborne substances should be desensitized.

Body Defenses to Disease

The human body is equipped with various internal and external mechanisms that are adaptive: They help to reduce injury and prevent invasion by pathogenic microorganisms, thus promoting and maintaining a healthy status. When these mechanisms fail, various disease states result: neoplastic, infectious, viral, toxic, or traumatic.

External Defenses. Some of the principal external defenses of the body are the skin, mucous membranes and their secretions, the skull, and reflex movements. The first line of defense is the unbroken *skin* and *mucous membranes* that protect the deeper tissues from mechanical and chemical injury and provide a barrier against the penetration of bacteria. The skin and mucous membranes are constantly in contact with microorganisms. Certain microorganisms that are regularly present on these coverings constitute their normal flora of resident bacteria. When the person's resistance is lowered by injury to the tissues or by a disease process that reduces general resistance, these resident microorganisms, as well as pathogenic microorganisms, flourish[23]. Pathogenic microorganisms may gain entry through any portal of entry: broken skin or mucous membranes, the respiratory or gastrointestinal tracts, the vagina, or blood vessels, especially the veins. Microorganisms are spread through direct contact, droplet infection (organisms that are sneezed or coughed), food and water, insect and animal bites, or contaminated equipment, such as in intravenous or intramuscular administration of medications.

Reproduction of resident skin flora and the growth of pathogenic microorganisms are minimized by lack of sufficient moisture and the presence of specific antibacterial and antifungal organic acids. A surface film on the skin, which consists of secretions from sebaceous glands and sudoriferous (sweat) glands and of products of *cornification* (the process whereby the epidermis hardens), provides an acid environment and has antibacterial and antifungal properties. These properties enable the film to act as an antiseptic, to neutralize acid and alkali substances, and to interfere with the absorption of toxic agents[17]. Since some soaps are highly alkaline, their excessive use should be avoided to prevent the removal of this protective surface film.

The epidermis, which is partially composed of a layer of dead cells, serves as another defense mechanism. As the cells of the epidermis die, their protein material undergoes a change. The new protein form is called *keratin*, a tough, fibrous protein that causes the epidermis to become highly resistant to environmental elements, including bacteria, fungi, parasites, and most injurious chemicals[20]. If this layer of skin (also called the horny layer) is broken, physical and chemical agents can enter the body[22]. Therefore, protect yourself and the patient from scratches, cuts, and any breaks in the continuity of the skin.

Mucous membranes line cavities or passageways of the body that communicate to the exterior. These membranes secrete a fluid, *mucus*, which consists of several mucopolysaccharides, inorganic salts, water, and epithelial cells. The membranes and mucus serve to decrease bacterial invasion and lessen the severity of chemical or mechanical trauma[21].

The surface of the stomach is lined with mucus-secreting cells, while the deeper mucosa tissue contains gastric and pyloric glands[21]. The pyloric glands secrete a thin mucus, and the surface mucous cells secrete a viscid, alkaline mucus. Together these secretions coat the stomach mucosa and help prevent injury of the underlying tissues from such factors as digestive enzymes, hydrochloric acid, and abrasive foods. The parietal cells of the gastric glands secrete a solution that contains hydrochloric acid. This acid environment acts as a barrier to destroy most pathogens that enter the digestive tract. However, the acid environment of the stomach can be diminished temporarily by such foods as milk and eggs; thus the protective action of the acidity is decreased[17]. Remember this when planning or instructing patients in diets that must contain large quantities of milk, milk products, and eggs.

Some mucous membranes in the digestive tract secrete substances that have bacteriostatic properties. For example, the mucous membranes in the intestines secrete certain enzymes capable of destroying pathogens[24].

The genitourinary tract is also lined with mucous membranes. Pathogens entering the vagina are usually destroyed by the acid secretions produced by the cells lining this area. Frequent vaginal irrigations, or douches, will lower the acidity in the vagina and therefore lessen the protective function of the mucous membranes there[24].

A ciliated mucous membrane lines the respiratory tract. The external nares are surrounded by fine hairs that block pathogens from entering the nose; pathogens that do enter are trapped by mucus secreted by the cells lining the nasal passageways. Inhaled bacteria escaping these two defense mechanisms are usually blocked by *cilia* (hairlike projections), whose wavelike motions move the pathogens toward the pharynx, where they are swallowed or expectorated.

The eye is protected by several defense mechanisms. The skull provides a *bony orbit* that protects the eyeball (as well as the brain and vital centers) from mechanical injury. The *eyelids*, which are lined with a conjunctival membrane, serve as protective coverings for the eyeball. *Eyelashes*, lining the free edges of the lids, act to prevent foreign bodies from entering the eye. Tears or *lacrimal fluid*, secreted by the lacrimal glands, have a lavage action which serves to wash foreign bodies out of the eye and to dilute irritant materials. Excessive tear formation occurs any time a foreign particle or other irritant gets on or near the eye. The lacrimal fluid also contains an enzyme, *lysozyme*, which functions to destroy bacteria[20].

Some *reflex* or *involuntary acts* assist the body to rid itself of pathogens. Sneezing and coughing eliminate pathogens from the respiratory tract, while vomiting and diarrhea help to eliminate them from the gastrointestinal tract. The reflex of blinking renews the tear film over the cornea and prevents the entrance of foreign material. Reflex muscular movement, such as removing the hand from a hot stove or foot from a sharp object, prevents injury.

Internal Defenses. The primary internal defenses include the reticuloendothelial system, leukocytes, the inflammatory process, and the immune response. The reticuloendothelial system and the leukocytes (white blood cells) combat any infectious agent that tries to invade the body. They function in two different ways to prevent disease: (1) destruction of invading pathogens by a process called *phagocytosis*, and (2) formation of *antibodies* against the pathogens[21].

Phagocytosis, an important mechanism in the prevention of disease, is performed by phagocytes, special cells capable of ingesting and digesting bacteria and dead tissues. In order to promote phagocytosis, *opsonins* (globulin molecules) combine with the bacteria and dead tissues and increase their cohesiveness with the phagocytes. Some pathogens may survive and multiply in the phagocytes, rather than be destroyed, and are transported in the bloodstream from one part of the body to another. Some phagocytes—for example, the stationary macrophages—are capable of forming immune bodies against foreign agents.

Phagocytic cells are classified according to size as macrophages and microphages. *Macrophages* are either stationary or mobile. The stationary cells, *tissue histocytes,* are permanently located in the interstitial tissues of the *reticuloendothelial system, which is composed of connective-tissue cells widely scattered throughout many vascular and lymph channels,* including the bone marrow, spleen, liver, and lymph nodes. The reticuloendothelial system serves as the primary line of defense after bacteria have invaded the body. The mobile macrophagic cells are *lymphocytes* and *monocytes,* which are formed in the lymph nodes.

Microphages are smaller and more numerous than the macrophages, and the phagocytic power per cell is greatly reduced. The microphagic cells are *granulocytes,* which are formed in the bone narrow. After their formation, the granulocytes are transported throughout the body via the blood. Jointly, *the granulocytes, lymphocytes, and monocytes are referred to as **leukocytes,*** mobile units of the body's defense system[2, 21].

Both the reticuloendothelial system and leukocytes serve an important function in the inflammatory reaction. *When body tissue is injured by trauma or invaded by bacteria, a local reaction called **inflammation*** occurs. Since inflammation is one of the most common body responses to injury, knowledge of the inflammatory mechanism provides a basis for understanding many infectious and noninfectious diseases.

First, there is an accelerated blood flow to the site because of a dilatation of the adjacent capillaries. This process increases the amount of oxygen and nutrients in the area and produces *redness* and *heat* at the site. An accompanying increase in the permeability of the capillaries causes white blood cells and serum to escape into the surrounding tissues. The accumulated fluid (blood cells and serum) causes area *swelling,* and pressure on the nerve endings produces *pain.* Together, the pain and swelling produce *limitation of movement.* Thus the cardinal signs of inflammation are redness, heat, swelling, and limitation of movement. Pain as a subjective symptom results[24].

With the increased number of localized white blood cells during the inflammatory reaction, phagocytosis occurs. The phagocytes engulf and destroy the pathogens. Dead phagocytes, pathogens, tissue cells, and tissue fluid accumulate. This accumulation is known as *pus.* The dead pathogens and tissue cells are eventually carried away by the leukocytes via the blood and lymph. Those in the bloodstream are carried to the spleen, liver, and bone marrow, where the phagocytic cells (macrophages) engulf and digest them. Those in the lymph stream are filtered out by the lymph nodes and ingested by phagocytic cells[24].

The third major internal defense mechanism of the body is its immune response to bacteria or injury. Hawker suggests that humoral immunity depends on the formation of antibodies which react with and neutralize the infective properties of invading pathogens. Organic substances capable of inducing antibody formation are called *antigens*. Antibodies are formed principally by plasma cells, which develop from small lymphocytes under stimulation by antigens. The plasma cells are scattered throughout the reticuloendothelial system. Once the antibodies are formed, they are contained in serum globulins, especially the gamma globulins[23].

The immune response is divided into two classifications, active and passive; each can be either induced naturally or artificially.

Natural active immunity occurs when the host's body produces antibodies following the invasion of pathogens. During the course of the disease, the antibody titre increases. Depending on the identity of the causative agent, the titre remains elevated for months or even years after the symptoms of the disease have disappeared. Eventually the titre will fall; however, if the host is exposed to the same pathogen, rapid antibody production occurs[23]. Natural active immunity can be acquired from subclinical forms of disease and from repeated contacts with pathogens not virulent enough to produce disease[6]. Chickenpox, mumps, and smallpox usually confer permanent immunity after recovery from a single attack.

Artificial active immunity occurs after an individual is inoculated with a specific antigen that stimulates the production of antibodies. The two main agents used for these inoculations are vaccines and toxoids. *Vaccines* are prepared from microorganisms that are living, attenuated, dead, or inactivated. Living vaccines are usually prepared with organisms of lower virulence; attenuated or weakened strains are used in the Bacillus-Calmette-Guerin (BCG) vaccine for tuberculosis. The vaccines for whooping cough and typhoid fever are prepared from dead bacteria, and the vaccines for measles and influenza are prepared from inactivated viruses. A vaccine can be prepared from a strain that does not produce disease in humans but that compares with the antigenicity of human strains—for example, the use of cowpox vaccines for smallpox vaccinations.

Toxoids are prepared from attenuated forms of toxins (poisonous chemical substances produced by certain bacteria). When introduced into the body, attenuated toxins stimulate the production of antitoxins. Toxoids are used to immunize the host to such diseases as diphtheria, scarlet fever, and tetanus[6].

Passive immunity occurs when the person receives resistance to a disease by receiving antibodies from an external source. In *natural passive immunity, antibodies pass from mother to the fetus by way of placental transmission.* This immunity is temporary, lasting only days to months. In the case of measles, the newborn is protected for approximately six months[4]. Bowen reports that transmission of antibodies from mother to baby by colostrum and milk secreted by the mammary glands is almost negligible, contrary to previously held ideas[6]. *Artificial passive immunity occurs when immune bodies or antibodies for specific diseases are obtained from other human beings or animals and injected into a person who has been exposed to the same disease and who needs antibodies to prevent the establishment of the disease.* These antibodies provide temporary immunity, allowing the person time to produce his own antibodies. Tetanus antitoxin and gamma globulins for hepatitis and German measles provide this form of protection [6].

Transfer of pathogenic microbes can be prevented and controlled through proper personal hygiene habits. Covering the mouth and nose when coughing or sneezing, disposal of contaminated tissues, and control of dust and particulate matter minimize spread of airborne droplet infection. Thorough handwashing, use of individual equipment, and disinfection and sterilization of equipment prevent direct spread of microorganisms through touching of contaminated areas of articles. Foods and liquids require careful handling by few people so they do not become sources of infection.

Immunizations and various *medications* (such as antibiotics) also aid man's natural defenses by producing a desired effect on a particular body system. *Biological rhythms* are also increasingly understood as essential to adaptation. A later section of this chapter discusses this subject in detail.

Motion is synonymous with life and adaptation. When either the internal or the overall mobility of the person is interfered with, adaptation is inadequate. The hazards of immobility and nursing measures for dealing with them are discussed in detail further on in this chapter.

PSYCHOLOGICAL ADAPTATION

Whether life offers psychological threat involving loss and suffering or the challenge of goal attainment, adaptational tasks will be necessary for psychological growth. The term *coping* is sometimes used to refer to *the psychological way by which man deals with life's demands and goals* [29].

Key Concepts

Psychological adaptation refers to behavioral adequacy in attaining appropriate human relationships. Adaptation is achieved through the personality structure called the *ego, that part of the person concerned with the processes of judgment, thinking, memory, perception, discrimination, motor activity in response to perception, understanding, association, communication, control over behavior, and use of adaptive or defensive behaviors* [9, 14]. The ego refers to what we commonly think of as the conscious self.

*Failure to satisfy basic innate or acquired needs or to reconcile conflicting value systems constitutes **psychological stress**.* Stressors may exist in the real world or only be perceived as real by the person; both may come from either the external or internal environment of man. Each person's individual perception of events determines his reaction; this accounts for the wide variety of possible responses to a given situation [9, 14, 15].

Adaptive behavior helps the person to adjust to or cope with certain circumstances, while *defensive behavior causes the person to alienate himself from certain circumstances or to avoid life's demands and goals.* Patterns for both these behaviors originate in the early formative years of childhood, when anxiety and discomfort with people are first experienced, and are learned without much awareness on our part. By adulthood these patterns are usually fixed, unconscious, and automatic. Current experiences sometimes reactivate feelings and behavior associated with long-forgotten experiences and bring forth responses similar to ones that were originally adaptive but may now be inappropriate, useless, or incapacitating. Thus what was once adaptive behavior becomes defensive.

Generally, defensive behavior is an exaggerated response to experience perceived or anticipated as a threat to one's self or to a situation inconsistent with one's existing self-image[9, 14]. A certain behavioral response is used too frequently or for too long. The experience is temporarily rendered harmless by being distorted or denied to awareness. For example, if a normally active person sprains an ankle, he may insist on continuing his routine activities, denying the implications of the sprained ankle. Such behavior is defensive. To admit the necessity of staying off the sprained ankle is adaptive, since healing is fostered through rest of the part.

Adaptive behavior is maximum when the person is feeling a sense of discovery, a purposeful changing of self, or creativity. The adapting person is not necessarily happy, content, or a conformist. But he is living constructively and in as much harmony with his culture and others around him as possible to allow for a balanced satisfaction of needs[9, 14].

The processes or functions of the ego help the person to delay gratification, presume a sense of reality, and feel a sense of mastery or achievement in the world. The ego also mediates among inner demands, needs, impulses, and drives (the *id*) and the internalized prohibitions and rules of society, parents, and outer reality (the *superego*). As the ego becomes stronger in its role as mediator between inner demands and outer reality, more efficient and complex mechanisms are developed for adaptive behavior. Thus the person can adapt emotionally to his surroundings, physical or social.

The well-organized, adapting ego can recognize anxiety (feelings) as a signal in a situation and can cope with this situation and feelings. Mechanisms of adjustment are not used too frequently, too intensely, for too long a duration, or too rigidly. The underdeveloped, maladaptive ego has either no organized behavioral mechanisms for response to anxiety or uses the same defensive mechanisms rigidly in every situation, to an excessive degree, for too long a duration. Such a person is vulnerable to small amounts of anxiety and cannot adapt to his feelings. Mental illness occurs in such persons[14, 15].

The human psyche is highly versatile in arranging or using adaptive behaviors. Such versatility is fortunate, since the anxious, uncomfortable person thus has many resources to draw upon and can use a combination of behaviors. But people generally use only certain mechanisms that work best for them, thus establishing styles of adjustment by which others can predict their behavior.

172 | Application of Adaptation Theory to Nursing

Nevertheless, a common core of needs, drives, patterns of responses, and other psychological phenomena can be identified. Understanding the similarities and general patterns of behavior promote an understanding of man's psychological adaptive potential.

Behavioral patterning, using a cluster of behaviors that have a common goal and are used with predictability and regularity when a person is faced with a similar stimulus or need, is an adaptive process that minimizes the amount of energy needed to cope with changing surroundings and promotes stability or a steady state[9]. Behaviors previously successful are repeated, usually without thinking, so that the myriad of daily routine activities are done automatically. *Nursing Assessment and Health Promotion through the Life Span* explores some of the normal behavioral patterns in each life era[35]. The person does not substitute new behaviors unless they seem advantageous; and the substitution depends upon the source and intensity of stimuli and upon a comparison of the satisfaction provided by the established behavior pattern with the predicted satisfaction to be gained by changing behaviors. People vary in the ease with which they can change or adapt.

The interruption during illness of these patterns, whether related to eating, bedtime, work, socialization, or hygiene, constitutes a crisis. You will assess behavioral patterns and help the person cope or adapt to the changed internal environment (illness) and the changed external environment (health care system). Chapters 3, 4, 5, and 8 discuss the ways in which you can assist.

The body usually maintains or regains internal constancy through automatic regulatory mechanisms without conscious effort. Man's relationships with others, however, are dependent upon his behavior, whether consciously or unconsciously motivated. Therefore, the person is usually more concerned about others and the external environment than his body, unless the malfunctioning body part interferes with daily activity. For example, an illness is of secondary concern to the person who is about to experience a business loss or feels he has great occupational obligations.

One study gathered the life histories of three groups of individuals: (1) expatriate anti-Communist Chinese students in New York, (2) American workers who were frequently ill, and (3) American workers who were usually healthy. Results indicated that the healthiest persons were those whose life situations satisfied their particular needs and goals, however they might differ from the population in general. The interviews revealed that clusters of illness tended to occur during significantly stressful periods when the person was striving to adapt to what he perceived to be threatening environmental demands[47]. A longitudinal study of discharged Navy men revealed the same relationship between stress-evoking life situations and clusters of illness[38].

Although *stress* and *anxiety* are terms used interchangeably, they are not the same. *Anxiety is the psychological response to excessive unchanneled energy resulting from the stress reaction; it is a vague, diffuse feeling of dread, uneasi-*

ness, or general discomfort resulting from perception of a threat to the self, real or imagined [9, 14].

Anxiety is the response to feeling helpless, isolated, alienated from others, insecure, an object rather than a unique, worthwhile person. Anxiety, like stress, is subjective and indirectly observable. Severe anxiety immobilizes the person. But using the energy generated from the stress state (as explained in the discussion of the Adaptation Syndrome), to create a plan of action or goal mobilizes or motivates the person under stress.

The energy aroused by the stress state, manifested in feelings of anxiety, can be dissipated or reduced in intensity by walking, talking, crying, or other physical and social activity. However, frequently the ill person has limited ways of working off tension.

Certain variables alter the stress state and resultant anxiety: the physical and mental status of the person and his age, temperament, and health status; the kind, nature, or number of stressors; the duration of exposure; and past experiences and reactions to similar stress.

Manifestations of Anxiety

People use a variety of behaviors to cope with anxiety or to attempt to change a stressful situation. Redistribution of energy is often not consciously recognized; thus a person may be unaware of his behavioral shifts, although others notice them. Certain behavioral changes may be the best the person can do at the time, although to an objective observer they seem inadequate. You must be observant of the following responses that may indicate psychological stress:

1. Overt behavior or personality changes, including an increase in the number or variety of activities undertaken; disorganized, persistent use of a single pattern; and inefficient, regressive behavior.
2. Inappropriate, exaggerated emotional reactions to usual environmental conditions.
3. Disturbed consciousness and memory.
4. Disturbed thought processes, including decreased problem-solving abilities; inability to comprehend, use, or follow directions; delusions; phobias; unfounded suspicions.
5. Perceptual disturbances, including illusions or hallucinations involving any of the five senses.
6. Somatic (physical) symptoms or altered physiological status.
7. Overuse of unconscious mechanisms, such as rationalization, denial, isolation, displacement, fantasy.
8. Inability to carry out usual, appropriate social behaviors.

The General Adaptation Syndrome described earlier can be modified to assess psychological adaptation. In the *Alarm Stage*, the person has an increased ability to perceive data, comprehend relationships, and do problem solving. He feels mildly anxious but can cope with the situation. Should the feelings of alarm persist, the degree of anxiety heightens and other types of psychic behavior may be evoked that are less adaptive: irritability, anger, demanding, denial, withdrawal, crying, hypersensitivity to noise and confusion, hallucinations, loquaciousness, silence, and eventual panic if the stimuli are overwhelming. Exposure to intense psychological stimuli can cause death.

During the *Resistance Stage*, psychological adaptive mechanisms include the behaviors typical of moderate anxiety. The person has a narrowed perceptual field but the ability to focus on a delineated subject or situation, while shutting out irrelevant distractions. He can comprehend relationships; has a strong feeling of persistence; shows stereotyped, rigid behavior; but does problem solving to directly attack a problem. Various ego adaptive mechanisms may be used, though not excessively—for example, sublimation, reaction formation, rationalization, selective inattention, displacement, or overcompensation. The Resistance Stage involves some deliberative change of behavior as the person gets in control of himself, others, or the inanimate environment.

Should the person's attempts at coping with the feelings involved in a situation be unsuccessful, the *Stage of Exhaustion* would be manifested by physical or mental illness (neurosis, psychosis). Now the person gives up coping attempts or uses inappropriate or ineffective behavior. Without help, the person might indeed become chronically ill or even die.

Intervention for the person passing through these stages is crisis intervention, discussed in Chapter 8; relevant techniques of therapeutic communication are discussed in Chapter 3.

Five-Phase Analysis. Another way of assessing psychological adaptation is by identifying five phases of behavior. *Phase I* deals with man's identity and values. Man's identity is in an on-going state of evolution as he thinks, perceives, and experiences emotion in his interaction with others, although he has basically one conception of himself that exists at all times. Many values make up this self-identity and are essential to biological integrity and to a satisfying and secure existence. In this phase man is adaptive.

Phase II recognizes that there are potential stressors threatening the values of the self-concept. These are anticipatory in nature, dependent upon cognitive (thought) processes, and may be felt when alone or with others. For example, the parent views his child's illness as a threat to his personal values regarding the child's biological integrity, and the child in turn senses the parent's discomfort in addition to his own physiological distress. The child feels anxious and personally threatened as a result.

Psychological stress characterizes the third phase and is the emotional response that activates the fourth or adaptive phase. In *Phase III* you will observe signs of psychological stress or anxiety described earlier, such as impaired thinking, hostility, helplessness, or hopelessness. As the person comes to sense that his goals of security and need-satisfaction are not being met, he tries to re-solve the situation through adaptive maneuvers in order to maintain his sense of self. At this point you will need to validate your observations with the patient and other health team members in order to understand the meaning of the emo-tional experience to the patient. Chapter 4's suggestions for rewriting conversa-tions in order to analyze their meaning are helpful in this regard.

In *Phase IV*, behavior is aimed at resolving the conflict between values held and the stressors impinging upon them. The person's behavior may not involve problem solving or be effective unless he receives help.

The use of cognitive coping styles for the person involves problem solving and learning. The focus here is more on the stressor (the situation or event) than on the emotional response. Part of the learning process may be a restructuring by the individual of the threatened value. You will need to assess the person's feelings accurately and help him toward independence by teaching him more about his reactions and how to cope with his situation. Often the person's powers of observation and attention are altered by anxiety, especially if it per-sists over a prolonged period. Such alterations may result in selective inattention, denial, autistic invention, or hallucinations. Since observation and logical think-ing are crucial to decision making, you must use careful assessment to determine the specific nature of the patient's responses.

Noncognitive measures are used to seek immediate relief from the dis-comfort of the emotional response to the stressor. These are usually in the form of conversion patterns or defense mechanisms. They appear to be automatic. Aggression, withdrawal, or somatization are examples of defensive patterns. Aggression may be in the form of blame, resentment, expressions of anger or frustration, or manipulation. Silence, apathy, or alcoholism may be expressions of withdrawal. *Somatization, the development of physical symptoms*, releases emotional tension and diverts attention to the self rather than to the stressor or emotional response to stress. Noncognitive measures create a myriad of nursing problems, for they alter relationships so vital to the fulfillment of basic needs. Finally, noncognitive measures that worked once may fail to serve as success-fully later and may then lead to the last crisis phase in psychological adaptation.

Individuals do not always reach *Phase V*, the stage of inadequate adapta-tion, total panic, or disintegration of control. Problems may be resolved through problem solving, or noncognitive defensive measures may relieve the discomfort before a crisis occurs.

ANTHROPOLOGICAL ADAPTATION

A culture makes adaptation possible through its ideas, inventions, and customs. Together with physiological adaptive processes, culture is a powerful force. For example, man is able to live in a wide variety of climates because his body has adjusted gradually to permit survival. Man also heats and cools his environment for comfort, controls predators and parasites, and domesticates animals and plants for his needs. Man has constructed a variety of life styles and patterns of social relationships to guarantee his survival and to free himself from the limits of his physical environment. Prescribed cultural norms are the most effective adaptive mechanisms man uses: they affect his physical, social, and mental well-being; aid adaptation to diverse situations, environments, and recurring problems; and teach about other environments to which he may have to adapt. In addition, some adaptive modifications are achieved through genetic, physiological, and constitutional capacities that have been transmitted for generations through natural selection or cultural conditioning. Physical mutation may also promote permanent change in a group if it enables the person to successfully compete and live, promoting adaptation.

Different forms of physical or cultural selection are:

1. Survival of the fittest, in which persons who cannot cope or who have dysfunctional mutant genes are most subject to an inability to reproduce or to early death. This is most intense where resources are scarce or competition is intense.
2. Modification of the environment to help the person with a condition that interferes with optimum health. An example is treatment of diabetes, inherited by a recessive gene, which enables a normal life span and adaptation in other spheres.
3. Cultural changes that strive to make man diversified. Mass uniformity prevents adaptation to changing and diverse environments. For example, persons living in different regions of the same culture often live differently in some respects while adhering to the overall value system.
4. Cultural conditioning or teaching the person how best to survive in his own environment and life situation[12].

Culture allows diversity within a framework of uniformity (customs, traditions). Lately cultural differences are becoming more recognized as factors to be dealt with in nursing practice, especially in the United States with its pluralistic society. Nursing care plans in America, however, often fail to recognize the special care requirements of patients from diverse sociocultural backgrounds and have, instead, a strong reference to Anglo-American values. Lack of diversity in your thoughts and actions prevents your adaptation to the patient as a person as well as your aiding his adaptation to his illness state. Unit II provides information to widen your understanding in this respect.

SOCIAL ADAPTATION

People need other people to become and remain socialized; hence *social adaptation, adjusting the self to a group,* is essential. Sensory-deprivation experiments indicate that a continual flow of changing sensory stimuli is necessary for the person's mental health. The infant needs stimulation through touch from another human being. Withholding caresses and normal human contact or similar emotional deprivation ultimately results directly or indirectly in physical as well as mental deterioration.

As the person develops, he learns to accept symbolic rather than actual touch, until the mere act of verbal recognition serves the purpose. That people recognize one another's presence, and thereby offer the social contact necessary for the preservation of health, is more important than what is said.

Sensory stimulation that keeps certain parts of the brain active appears necessary in order to maintain a normal waking state. This need to be recharged by stimulation, and especially by social contact, may be regarded as one of the biological origins of group formation. The fear of loneliness (or of lack of social stimulation) is one reason why people are willing to resign part of their individual desires in favor of group consensus, while at the same time developing a high proficiency in getting as many satisfactions as possible from socialization.

Through social adaptation man receives spiritual and emotional nourishment. He gets responses to his love and creativity. He can attain power and prestige. Threats to man's ability to perform in these areas produce the everyday stresses than can cause disability and disease[47].

Responses to Social Change

It is impossible to generalize concerning social adaptation, or to define it as social striving or obtaining cultural goals. The individual's response must be objectively considered. For example, persons who are comfortable in a social climate of brotherly love and unworldliness would find it hard to survive or be happy in a competitive world.

As man becomes a more specialized being, his responses to adaptational needs are more varied and his ability to select certain aspects of the environment to which to respond increases. The most evolved responses of social adaptation are those in which the individual or group modifies living habits or the environment, or both, to achieve comfort and pleasure in survival[13].

Man adheres to societal expectations, and social behavior evolves from assuming particular social roles. Behavior toward others is prescribed by *social norms, rules which define and prescribe performance and attitudes for persons in particular social positions.* There is a certain assumed degree of stability about norms, so that each person knows what to expect from others. How norms are lived depends on the person's conception of his role and the adaptive reactions of others, as well as on his own adaptive abilities. If mutual expectations are not met, adaptation to a situation is difficult.

Social change is rampant in today's world. Unsuccessful social adaptation to rapid change can contribute to illness, such as ulcers, heart disease, or arthritis. Illness, in turn, may force more social adaptations on the person[1, 14].

Modern man is increasingly exposed to stresses of a symbolic nature. For this reason his goals and values determine the response of his whole being toward health or disease. As time evolved, values and goals became a way of life to man, and his performance has reflected the worth of his values. In both social and bodily health he has often been more maladapted than not, more sick than well.

Modern Western civilization requires use of traditional adaptations as well as new ones to cope in a changing society. Conflict between the pressures of one's past and pressures newly encountered brings problems for those who change environments, whether the new one be another country, a different work climate, or a new social position. The social and cultural pressures a person feels, his psychological drive, and his innate abilities all influence his interpretation of and response to illness.

The only stable thing in life is change. Man's mind has created social change, on-going and relentless. Reason has aided man in his adaptation but created challenges as well. Power beyond the dreams of the past has built a scientific technology that protects man from the elements and from other destructive forces in the environment, but with this life have come new hazards of injury, death, and changes in the air he breathes and the food he eats.

Illnesses related to modern technology and to man's social relationships are gaining attention. Society requires that people live together without destroying each other; differences in people and ideologies must be tolerated for survival. Adaptations fraught with stress accompany these developments. You will need to view man in the context of his biological tendencies, his learned patterns of response, and the pressures, both tangible and intangible, to which he is exposed. Your assessment of the person must include a search for the forces that arouse, and the mechanisms that regulate, his adaptive efforts[47].

Toffler has confronted us with the concept of "future shock," a force he predicts will insure adaptational breakdown unless man can come to grips with rapid social change[46]. Toffler describes the frequent shifting of families from one place to another, alterations in bureaucratic structures that may speedily engulf the worker in change, and diversity of options and continuing novelty in many life situations. The disposable, transient culture makes it difficult for man to establish roots or pass on culture as a guideline to future generations.

Because of the "future shock syndrome," the risk of illness can be predicted from the amount of change present[46]. If a person is in the equivalent of the Alarm Stage continually, body defenses weaken. Extreme examples of persons caught in rapidly changing environments are the combat soldier, the flood victim, the culturally dislocated traveler. Other examples include the aged who are uprooted and the person who moves from a rural to an urban environment.

The principles of crisis therapy discussed in Chapter 8 will be useful in helping people adapt to social change. You must constantly adjust to new surroundings, or create new ones, in order to remain adaptive. In nursing, you adjust in the work environment to changing patient groups, and the patient adjusts to the sick role and health care system and workers. You can also develop for yourself and teach others about adaptive behaviors to overcome the stress of constantly changing life, since to deny change is occurring is to distort reality. Change will seem easier if you are the one initiating at least part of the change. At times you can purposefully focus on one aspect of a situation; eventually, however, awareness must expand to include the total situation.

Find a place for temporary isolation, a retreat where you can shut out the noise and in which you can maintain the same environment and routine. Equally indispensable is a set of values, be they religious, ethical, or philosophical, that will serve as guiding principles in a variety of situations.

FAMILY ADAPTATION

Adaptive responses in the family, a social unit, represent the means by which it maintains an internal equilibrium so that it can fulfill purposes and tasks, deal with stress and crisis, and allow for growth of individual members. Some capacity for functioning may be sacrificed in order to control conflict and aid work as a unit. But the best-functioning family keeps anxiety and conflict within tolerable limits and maintains a balance between effects of the past and new experiences [32].

Ideally the family achieves equilibrium by talking over problems and finding solutions together. Humor, nonsense, shared work, and leisure all help relieve tension. The family members know that within their confines certain freedoms exist that are not available elsewhere. Yet even the most stable family will briefly utilize the following behaviors to cope with stress, which in turn promotes more stress. However, these mechanisms are not overused in healthy families[32].

Adaptive Mechanisms in Family Life

Family conflict may be avoided or minimized through scapegoating, coalitions, withdrawal of emotional ties, fighting, use of family myths, reaction formation, compromise, or designation of a family healer. Two or more of these mechanisms may be used within the same family. If these mechanisms are used excessively, however, they become defensive and are unlikely to promote resolution of the conflict, so that the same issue will arise repeatedly[32].

Scapegoating or Blaming involves labeling one member as the cause of the family trouble and is expressed in the attitude, "If it weren't for you... ." Or one member may offer himself as a scapegoat to end an argument by saying, "It's all my fault." Such labeling controls the conflict and reduces anxiety, but it prevents communication that can get at the root of the problem. Growth toward resolution of the problem is prohibited.

Coalitions or Alliances may form when some family members side together against other members. Antagonisms and anger result. Eventually the losing party tries to get control.

Withdrawal of Emotional Ties, loosening the family unit, and reducing communication may be used to handle conflict, but then the family becomes rigid and mechanized. Family members are also likely to seek affection outside the family, so that the home becomes a hotel with everyone superficially nice. In some families there is no show of emotion, as this signifies to them loss of control or giving in to unacceptable impulses.

Repetitive Fighting through verbal abuse, physical battles, loud complaints, curses, or accusations may be used to relieve tension and allow some harmony until the next round. The fight may have the same theme each time stress hits the family. The healthy family allows some "blowing up" as release from everyday frustrations, but does not make a major case out of every minor incident or temporary disagreement.

Family Myths or Traditional Beliefs can be used to overcome anxieties and maintain control over others. Such statements include: Children are seen, not heard; We can't survive if you leave home; Talking about feelings will cause loss of love. In the healthy family, members encourage growth and creativity rather than rigid control.

Reaction Formation is seen in a family in which there is superficial harmony or togetherness. Traumatic ideas are repressed and transformed into the opposite behavior. Everybody smiles but nobody loves. No one admits to having any difficulties. Great tension is felt because true feelings are not expressed.

Resignation or Compromise may provide temporary harmony when someone gives up or suppresses his needs for assertion, affection, or emotional expression for the sake of keeping peace. The surface calm eventually explodes when unmet needs can no longer be successfully suppressed.

Designation of One Person as Family Healer or Umpire involves using a "wise one" (most often in the extended family) or a minister, storekeeper, bartender, or druggist to arrange a reconciliation between dissenting parties. Part of the dynamics sometimes underlying the helper role is that the referee gets great satisfaction from finding someone worse off than himself. The healer feels a sense of heightened self-esteem or omnipotence. A variant of the healer role is that of family "protector," where one person takes all the stresses upon himself in order to save other members stress or conflict. One person ends up fighting the battles for everyone else in the family.

You may find yourself in the role of family healer. Help the family to develop harmonious ways of coping and avoid the protector or omnipotent role.

INADEQUATE ADAPTATION

Disturbances in adaptation (nonconstructive behavior) result in illness or various disorders—physically, emotionally, socially. Some behaviors that are adaptive for a time become defensive or inadequate if used for prolonged periods. Illness or sensory distortions may in turn cause or further enhance disturbed adaptation. Inadequate adaptation may occur when there is:

1. Failure to sense change, present or coming; selective focusing on the here-and-now.
2. Adherence to values or beliefs no longer considered valid by the social environment.
3. Undue commitment to unrealistic, immoral, unethical, or inhumane goals.
4. Use of adaptive mechanisms no longer appropriate.
5. Resistance to rational change.
6. Presence of physical disease or disability.
7. Sensory distortion or deprivation.
8. Failure to discriminate because of thought disturbances or organic problems.
9. Severe anxiety feelings.
10. Overspecialization, limiting one's ability to adapt to new and changing circumstances.
11. Focusing on the involved body part or only one aspect of a situation rather than the entire body or situation[34].

Yet *apparently maladaptive behavior should be considered as the best that the person is capable of at that time.* So-called deviant behavior may actually be adaptive and may eventually promote constructive change in or for the person or group. For example, adaptive deviance is seen in the patient who demands control over himself and his treatment, or in the nonconformist nurse who views a situation from a different perspective, acts accordingly, and improves nursing care as a result. Also, inadequate behavior in one person may permit others in a group to function appropriately as a result. For example, when a person is sick his symptoms and problems may inadvertently preserve family equilibrium by drawing attention away from family conflicts. The sick member may be designated the scapegoat or patient, even though other family members are more socially or emotionally ill.

IMPLICATIONS FOR NURSING

Adaptation is a concept that can provide a unifying structure for nursing practice. It can link together the mass of information considered necessary to professional nursing practice. It helps you see how various factors affecting man do not exist in isolation but in a multidimensional whole. It helps you more accurately predict and more effectively help each person adapt to his crisis, illness, or disability.

If you are in a leadership position, teach your coworkers to report signs and symptoms of adaptational failure—such as restlessness, withdrawal, rigidity in behavior, or inability to make a decision—just as they would note a disease symptom. Your knowledge of the patient's *accustomed* adaptive pattern, obtained through a nursing history, will help you formulate a plan of care to meet his special needs. Assess the person's needs, ways of coping, and the predominant stimuli affecting him. If inadequate adaptation is occurring, attempt to modify or manipulate the stimuli to make a positive response possible. Adjusting the physical environment or using methods of purposeful communication are examples of ways to enhance adaptation.

You can use adaptation theory as an independent nurse practitioner. You might be available in a community to promote adaptation where circumstances are making harmful demands—where a disease has broken out or a natural disaster occurred. Or you might do health teaching, diet counseling, support before surgery, discharge planning, and health maintenance among those persons in the community who have health problems in varying degrees.

Whatever the setting in which you practice, your assessments must be based on scientific knowledge combined with an appreciation of the individual's behavioral responses. When your intervention influences adaptation favorably and promotes social well-being, it is *therapeutic*. If you cannot alter the course of adaptation and your best efforts only maintain the status quo or slow up a downhill course, you are acting in a *supportive* role[27].

Adaptation as a concept is applicable to the nurse as well as the patient, for you will have to adapt to a new and different perspective and life style as you involve yourself actively in the profession. You may feel threatened at times by the challenges. An understanding of yourself and your adaptive capacities will help you to keep faith in yourself and your ability to cope, to adapt, to learn, to grow. You will become more comfortable with change and challenge, recognizing that they are part of normal adult living.

So far this chapter has considered the concept of adaptation in its broadest sense. The two sections comprising the rest of the chapter deal with matters crucial to adaptation: the maintenance of biological rhythms, and the hazards of immobility. Related nursing responsibilities are also discussed in each section.

REFERENCES

1. Alexander, Franz, "The Development of Psychosomatic Medicine," in *New Dimensions in Psychosomatic Medicine,* ed. C. W. Wahl. Boston: Little, Brown & Company, 1964.

2. Beland, Irene, *Clinical Nursing: Pathophysiology-Psychosocial Approaches* (2nd ed.). New York: The Macmillan Company, 1971.
3. Bendixen, H. H., *Respiratory Care*. St. Louis: The C. V. Mosby Company, 1968.
4. Benenson, Abram, *Control of Communicable Diseases in Man*. Washington, D.C.: American Public Health Association, Inc., 1970.
5. Bergersen, Betty S., "Adaptation as a Unifying Theory," in *Theoretical Issues in Professional Nursing*, ed. Juanita F. Murphy. New York: Appleton-Century-Crofts, 1971.
6. Bowen, Eleanor, *Biology of Human Behavior*. New York: Appleton-Century-Crofts, 1968.
7. Burd, Shirley F., "A Psychological Approach to Adaptation," in *Theoretical Issues in Professional Nursing*, ed. Juanita F. Murphy. New York: Appleton-Century-Crofts, 1971.
8. Burnes, A. J., and S. J. Roen, "Social Roles and Adaptation to the Community," *Community Mental Health Journal*, 3 (1967), 156.
9. Byrne, M., and L. Thompson, *Key Concepts for the Study and Practice of Nursing*. St. Louis: The C. V. Mosby, Company, 1972.
10. Conroy, R. T. W. L., and J. N. Mills, *Human Circadian Rhythms*. London: J. & A. Churchill, 1970.
11. Coulter, P., and M. J. Brower, "Parallel Experience: An Interview Technique," *American Journal of Nursing*, 68: No. 5 (1968), 1028.
12. Dobzhansky, T., "Man and Natural Selection," in *Man in Adaptation: The Biosocial Background*, ed. Y. A. Cohen. Chicago: Aldine Publishing Company, 1968, pp. 37-48.
13. Dubos, René, *Man Adapting*. New Haven: Yale University Press, 1965.
14. Engel, G., *Psychological Development in Health and Disease*. Philadelphia: W. B. Saunders Company, 1962.
15. Evans, Frances Monet Carter, *Psychosocial Nursing: Theory and Practice in Hospital and Community Mental Health*. New York: The Macmillan Company, 1971.
16. Finch, A., "A System for Learning," *Nursing Outlook*, 19: No. 5 (1971), 332-33.
17. Frobisher, Martin, L. Sommermeyer, and R. Fuerst, *Microbiology in Health and Disease*. Philadelphia: W. B. Saunders Company, 1969.
18. Ganong, William, *Review of Medical Physiology*. Los Altos, Calif.: Lange Medical Publications, 1971.
19. Goode, W. J., *The Family*. Englewood Cliffs, N.J.: Prentice-Hall, Inc., 1964.
20. Grollman, Sigmund, *The Human Body: Its Structure and Physiology*. New York: The Macmillan Company, 1969.
21. Guyton, Arthur, *Basic Human Physiology: Normal Function and Mechanisms of Disease*. Philadelphia: W. B. Saunders Company, 1971.

22. Hadley, B., "Evolution of a Conception of Nursing," *Nursing Research*, 18: No. 5 (1969), 400-4.

23. Hawker, Lillian, and Alan Linton, eds., *Microorganisms: Function, Form, and Environment*. New York: American Elsevier Publishing Company, Inc., 1971.

24. Johnston, Dorothy, *Total Patient Care: Foundations and Practice*. St. Louis: The C. V. Mosby Company, 1968.

25. King, Imogene, *Towards a Theory for Nursing*. New York: John Wiley & Sons, Inc., 1971.

26. Langley, L. L., *Homeostasis*. New York: Reinhold Book Corporation, 1965.

27. Levine, M., "Adaptation and Assessment: A Rationale for Nursing Intervention," *American Journal of Nursing*, 66: No. 11 (1966), 2450-53.

28. Levinson, D. J., "Role, Personality, and Social Structure in the Organizational Setting," *Journal of Abnormal Psychology*, 58 (1959), 170.

29. Lipowski, Z. J., "Physical Illness, the Individual, and the Coping Process," *Psychiatry in Medicine*, 1: No. 4 (1970), 91-102.

30. McKay, Rose, "Theories, Models, and Systems for Nursing," *Nursing Research*, 18: No. 5 (1969), 393-99.

31. McLeod, Dorothy L., "Physiological Model," in *Theoretical Issues in Professional Nursing*, ed. Juanita F. Murphy. New York: Appleton-Century-Crofts, 1971.

32. Messer, Alfred, *The Individual in His Family, An Adaptational Study*. Springfield, Ill.: Charles C. Thomas, Publisher, 1970.

33. Moore, Francis, *Metabolic Care of the Surgical Patient*. Philadelphia: W. B. Saunders Company, 1959.

34. Murphy, Juanita, ed., *Theoretical Issues in Professional Nursing*. New York: Appleton-Century-Crofts, 1971.

35. Murray, Ruth, and Judith Zentner, *Nursing Assessment and Health Promotion through the Life Span*. Englewood Cliffs, N.J.: Prentice-Hall, Inc., 1975.

36. National Institute of Mental Health, *Biological Rhythms in Psychiatry and Medicine*. Washington, D. C.: United States Department of Health, Education, and Welfare, 1970.

37. Parsons, T., *Structure and Process in Modern Societies*. Glencoe, Ill.: The Free Press, 1960.

38. Rahe, Richard H., Joseph D. McKean, Jr., and Ransom J. Arthur, "A Longitudinal Study of Life-Change and Illness Patterns," *Journal of Psychosomatic Research*, 10 (1967), 355-66.

39. Richter, Curt, *Biological Clocks in Medicine and Psychiatry*. Springfield, Ill.: Charles C. Thomas, 1965.

40. Romano, John, ed., *Adaptation*. Bingingham, N.Y.: Vail-Ballow Press, Inc., 1949.

41. Roy, Sr. Callista, "Adaptation: A Conceptual Framework for Nursing," *Nursing Outlook*, 18: No. 3 (1970), 42-45.

42. Schwartz, S., *Principles of Surgery*. New York: McGraw-Hill Book Company, 1967.

43. Secor, Jane, *Patient Care in Respiratory Problems*. Philadelphia: W. B. Saunders Company, 1969.

44. Seyle, Hans, *The Stress of Life*. New York: McGraw-Hill Book Company, 1956.

45. ———, and Gunnar Heuser, eds., *Fifth Annual Report on Stress, 1955-1956*. New York: MD Publications, Inc., 1956.

46. Toffler, Alvin, *Future Shock*. New York: Random House, 1970.

47. Wolf, Stewart, and Helen Goodell, eds., *Stress and Disease*. Springfield, Ill.: Charles C Thomas, Publisher, 1968.

48. Yamamoto, William S., "Homeostasis, Continuity, and Feedback," in *Physiological Controls and Regulations*, eds. William S. Yamamoto and John R. Brobeck. Philadelphia: W. B. Saunders Company, 1965.

49. Yousef, Mohamed, S. Horvath, and R. Bullard, eds., *Physiological Adaptation*, New York: Academic Press, Inc., 1972.

Section I

RELATIONSHIP OF BIOLOGICAL RHYTHMS TO MAINTENANCE OF ADAPTATION

DEFINITIONS

Self-sustaining, repetive, rhythmic patterns found in plants, animals, and man are termed **biological rhythms.** Biological rhythms are found throughout man's external and internal environment and are basic to the person's adaptation and survival. Man's biological rhythms may be exogenous or endogenous.

Exogenous rhythms are dependent on the rhythm of external environmental events, such as seasonal variations, lunar revolution, or night-and-day cycle, which function as time givers to man. These help man to synchronize his internal rhythms with external environmental stimuli and establish an internal time pattern or biological clock.

Endogenous rhythms arise within the organism, such as sleep-wake and sleep-dream cycles. Endogenous and exogenous rhythms are usually synchronized. However, many internal rhythms do not readily alter their repetitive patterns, even when the external stimuli are removed. For instance, when a person shifts to sleeping by day and waking at night, as frequently happens with nurses, a transient or temporary desynchronization occurs. Body temperature and adrenal hormone levels are usually low during the sleep cycle. With the shift in sleep and waking, the person is awake and making demands on his body during his usual sleep period. Three weeks may be needed before internal rhythms adapt to the shift. A similar period of desynchronization occurs when a person makes a flight crossing time zones[16].

Within any 24-hour period, physiological and psychological functions of man reach maximum and minimum limits. When a physiological function approaches a high or low limit, the body's feedback mechanisms attempt to counterregulate the action. *This form of endogenous rhythm which reoccurs in a cyclic pattern within a 20- to 28-hour period is a **circadian rhythm**.* Body temperature, blood pressure, urine production, and hormone, blood sugar, hemoglobin, and amino acid levels demonstrate this rhythmic pattern. Similar variations or rhythms in the levels of alertness, fatigue, tenseness, and irritability can also be demonstrated.

CIRCADIAN RHYTHMS IN ILLNESS

Much data is available that confirms an interrelationship between circadian rhythm and mental or physical illness. Also, the pattern of living taught by the culture affects body rhythms. Epidemiological research continues to seek further correlations among these factors. A few examples of how circadian rhythms influence illness are presented below. [For a more extensive discussion, refer to references 4, 13, and 16, listed at the end of Section I.]

Diagnostic Cues

Observing the integration of the body's rhythms (or lack of such integration) can be used to determine the person's health status. Diagnosis and treatment of some illnesses can be determined from the study of circadian rhythms or biological time. In some instances, the illness alters the pattern of the circadian rhythm. Other illnesses show exaggerated or decreased symptoms at a particular biological time. Blood pressure and temperature values, laboratory findings, and biopsy specimens for cell study are different according to the biological time of day. For instance, growth hormone levels in the blood are highest during the night hours; therefore, routine blood values taken at 8 in the morning will not give a total picture. Ambiguous laboratory findings and the need for repeated medical tests can be avoided if the person's normal biological rhythms are considered first.

Rhythmic time cycles appear to influence many aspects of human life. Births and deaths occur more frequently at night and during the early morning; persons with ulcers and allergies suffer more in the spring; there are certain yearly peaks in the number of suicides and accidents. Eventually, knowledge about circadian rhythms and biological time may serve as a major tool in preventive health programs.

Depression

A definite relationship is seen between health and the rhythmicity of depressed people. Altered biochemical rhythms, diurnal (daytime) mood swings, and altered sleep cycles have been noted. Although the exact relationship between mental health and sleep cycles is not known, the arrhythmicity of sleep in these persons is béing studied. Depressed persons usually experience insomnia or periods of predawn wakefulness. Their sleep cycles are shortened and fragmented, and they are easily disturbed by environmental changes. Successful treatment frequently comes in the form of antidepressant drugs that lengthen the sleep cycle.

Cancer

Cancer cells do not reproduce at the same rate as normal cells; abnormal mitosis (cell-reproduction) rhythms and, in many instances, a complete lack of circadian rhythm have been reported. X-ray therapy diminishes the noncircadian mitosis of cancer cells.

Normal cells show intervals of accelerated reproductive activity. For example, in man, skin and liver cells are more active at night. Experiments with hamsters and mice show that environmental light and the animal's activity pattern influence the rhythmic reproduction of cells. Further investigation may show a similar relationship in man, with both normal and cancer cells[16].

Adrenal Hormone Production

In persons on schedules of diurnal activity and nocturnal sleep, the blood and urine concentrations of adrenocorticosteroid hormones drop at night and rise to highest levels in early morning. The course of the adrenal cycle may also be followed by measuring the eosinophil (white-blood-cell) level; eosinophils decrease as the blood level of adrenal hormones increases.

Light is probably the synchronizer of the adrenocorticosteroid rhythm. This has implications for people who are night workers or who have varying degrees of blindness. Since adrenal hormones control other circadian rhythms within the body, knowledge of their cycle is important in the study and treatment of numerous conditions.

Low blood levels of adrenal hormones affect the nervous system and cause a person to be more sensitive to sounds, tastes, and smell. Sensory acuity reaches its maximum at the time of lowest steroid levels. A sudden drop in acuity occurs in the early morning as steroid levels begin to rise. A person is therefore better able to detect taste, smell, or sound at the end of the day. Daily fatigue from lack of sleep and neurologically-related symptoms associated with adrenal insufficiency (Addison's disease) may be related to low levels of adrenal hormones.

Adrenal rhythm is also important in handling certain allergies. Sensitivity to histamine follows a circadian rhythm: it peaks about the time of evening or night when adrenocorticosteroids are reaching their lowest levels. Nasal congestion from hayfever, skin reactions from drug sensitivity, and breathing crises in asthma patients occur more frequently during the evening or night[16].

Rhythm Alteration by Drugs

Circadian rhythms can be altered by drugs. Actinomycin-D (an antibiotic) can alter the rhythms of synthesis within the cell's DNA (deoxyribonucleic acid) and RNA (ribonucleic acid) molecules. This shift in rhythm may in turn alter the circadian rhythm of some central nervous system functions. Barbiturates such as sodium pentobarbital and sodium thiomylal may also shift circadian rhythms. These drugs suppress the normal rhythm of adrenal hormones, which may account for some of the hangover effect, mental blunting, and confusion that frequently accompany use of these drugs[1, 2].

Some drugs may be given deliberately to produce altered circadian rhythms. Certain enzyme inhibitors are being used experimentally to shift the circadian activity-sleep cycle. Other drugs, tricyclic antidepressants, extend the period of the sleep cycle. Attempts are also being made to discover if certain adrenal hormones will lessen the period of transient desynchronization which occurs when a person enters a different time zone[16].

IMPLICATIONS FOR NURSING

Altered Rhythms Resulting from Hospital Environment

Since the person's cyclic functioning is synchronized with environmental stimuli, physiological disequilibrium or maladaption occurs whenever he is confronted with environmental or schedule changes. Transient desynchronization may occur whenever a person is exposed to the hospital or nursing home stimuli. New noise levels, lighting patterns, schedules for eating, sleeping, and personal hygiene, and unfamiliar persons intruding upon the person's privacy may all contribute to this desynchronization. Disturbed mental and physical well-being and increased subjective fatigue reflect the conflict between the internal time pattern and external events. Several days are usually required before the person adapts to his environment and thereby regains synchronization—normal biological rhythms.

You can control some external factors, make them more nearly similar to the patient's normal (outside) routine, and lessen the stress to which the patient is subjected. Gathering and using a nursing history is one method of lessening this stress.

A nursing history is directed at getting information about the patient's pre-illness or prehospitalization patterns for sleep, rest, food and fluid intake, elimination, and personal hygiene (see Figure 7-1). Once this information has been obtained, nursing actions can be initiated that support the patient's established daily patterns and possibly prevent total disruption of body rhythms during hospitalization.

Circadian Rhythm Log

In addition to the postadmission nursing history, a daily log of sleep and waking hours, meal times, hunger periods, voiding and defecation patterns, diurnal moods, and other circadian rhythms recorded for 28 days prior to hospitalization can help determine the person's cyclic patterns. Diagnostic tests and certain forms of medical and nursing therapy can then be appropriately prescribed, using the person's own base line rhythm measurements. Determination of each patient's rhythms before, during, and after hospitalization or illness will eventually be possible when more simplified, economical, and accurate measurement devices are available.

Drug Response and Administration

People respond differently to drugs. Recent research indicates that the effectiveness of some drugs, such as penicillin, antihistamine, and aspirin, is influenced by the individual's biological clock. A specific drug dosage may be more or less effective, depending on whether the dose is administered when the person's physiological functions are at minimal or maximal levels. For example, the dosage of analgesics needed to relieve pain during the evening or dark hours is more than that needed during the activity period[12, 16].

Circadian rhythms are also important factors in determining drug toxicity. A distinct 24-hour rhythm of vulnerability or resistance to drugs has been identified. Part of the toxicity rhythm is due to the rhythm of the liver enzymes, which are responsible for most drug detoxification. Before setting a drug's toxic level, both the person's biological clock and the drug dosage must be considered [16].

Without the aid of suitable measurement devices, it is impossible to determine a person's biological clock. Drug administration is therefore usually based on other factors. Most medications are given before or after meals, at bedtime, or at the convenience of nursing personnel and patients. In the future, as knowledge of the internal clock increases, you, the nurse, will find yourself altering drug administration times to suit the person's biological time. Perhaps you will be in charge of a master computer that, after analyzing information about each person's biological clock, will send the appropriate medication dose at the appropriate time.

FIGURE 7-1
History of Pre-Illness Patterns

Patient's Name: Sociocultural data:

Diagnosis:

Admitting Date _____   Date of History_____

History obtained by _____

Habits of Daily Living:

1. Food habits: Diet:
   A. Meal patterns: Time   Usual Foods
      Breakfast

      Lunch

      Dinner

      Snacks
   B. Food dislikes:
   C. Food allergies:
   D. Foods which disagree or cause discomfort:

2. Fluid habits:
   A. Fluid preferences:
   B. Fluid dislikes:
   C. Usual amount of fluid intake prior to illness:

3. Sleep habits:
   A. Usual bedtime?
   B. Usual number of hours of sleep?
   C. Get up during the night?
   D. Nap habits:
   E. Number of pillows desired?
   F. Number of blankets desired?
   G. If unable to sleep at home, what things do you do that help you fall asleep?

4. General hygiene
   A. Bathing preference: Usual time
      Tub _____   _____
      Shower_____   _____
   B. Care of teeth: Usual time of cleaning
      Natural _____   _____
      Dentures_____   _____

190

FIGURE 7-1 (cont.)

---

5. Elimination
   A. Usual bowel habits:
      Frequency _____ Time _____
   B. Bowel irregularities
      Constipation? _____ Diarrhea? _____
      What usually helps regularity?
   C. Urinary habits:
      Frequency of voiding:
      Bladder irregularities:

Any questions from the patient:

Observations made during history-taking:

Temperature Routine

A person's internal and skin temperatures both show a systematic rise and fall over a 24-hour period, a cycle difficult to alter in normal adults. Body temperature usually peaks between 4 and 6 in the afternoon and reaches it lowest point around 4 in the morning in people who are active by day and sleep at night. When the internal temperature is normally peaking, other body functions such as pulse rate, blood pressure, and cardiac output (volume of blood pumped by the heart) are also changing. Pulse rate is high when the temperature is highest and drops during the night. Blood pressure shows a marked fall during the first hour of sleep, followed by a gradual rise during the remaining time. Cardiac output reaches minimum levels between 2 and 4 in the morning, the period of lowest temperature findings [4, 16].

The existence of a normal rhythmic temperature pattern has been known for almost 200 years. Yet this knowledge has not been applied by hospital personnel when establishing time schedules for routine measurements of body temperature. In most hospitals the schedule is based on considerations of tradition or convenience, such as the time of shift change. Since the primary reason for checking body temperature is to detect the presence of an elevation, the procedure should be done at the time when maximum temperature occurs [5]. The implications of this for nursing practice include the importance of establishing routines for temperature measurements with circadian rhythms in mind, considering the time of day when evaluating temperature measurements, and considering the person's preadmission rest and activity routine.

Work Schedule

Nurses as well as many industrial and law-enforcement personnel are frequently required to change shifts every week or month. Shift workers who rotate reportedly are more subject to anorexia, digestive disturbances, restless sleep patterns, and lowered work quality. Rotating shift assignments are thus relevant to these workers' health and quality of work performance[8]. Altering the sleep-wake sequence requires time for the person to make adjustments and regain synchrony.

If shift rotation cannot be eliminated, then nurses should be required to rotate not more frequently than once a month. Consistently working at night allows a person to acquire a new sleep-wake rhythm. Therefore, night work should be made more attractive to persons who can adapt to the shift and are willing to remain on it permanently. Those who cannot adapt should be exempt from rotation.

Health teaching of any rotating-shift worker concerning the possible consequences of such a routine should not be overlooked.

REFERENCES

1. Bolund, L., "Actinomycin-D Binding to Isolated Deoxyribonucleoprotein and Intact Cells," *Experimental Cell Research*, 63 (November 1970), 171-88.

2. Bunning, Erwin, *The Physiological Clock* (2nd ed.). New York: Springer-Verlag New York, Inc., 1967.

3. Colquhoun, W. P., ed., *Biological Rhythms and Human Performance*. New York: Academic Press, Inc., 1971.

4. Conroy, R. T. W. L., and J. N. Mills, *Human Circadian Rhythms*. London: J. & A. Churchill, 1970.

5. DeRisi, Lucy, "Body Temperature Measurements in Relation to Circadian Rhythmicity in Hospitalized Male Patients," *American Nurses' Association Clinical Sessions*. New York: Appleton-Century-Crofts, 1968, pp. 251-58.

6. Edelstein, Ruth, "The Time Factor in Relation to Illness as a Fertile Nursing Research Area: Review of the Literature," *Nursing Research*, 21: No. 1 (1972), 72-75.

7. Farrell, Barbara, and Margaret Allen, "Physiologic/Psychologic Changes Reported by USAF Female Flight Nurses During Flying Duties," *Nursing Research*, 22: No. 1 (1973), 31-36.

8. Felton, Geraldine, and Mary Patterson, "Shift Rotation Is Against Nature," *American Journal of Nursing*, 71: No. 4 (1971), 760-63.

9. Ferguson, Eugene, "The Measurement of the 'Man-Day,' " *Scientific American*, 225: No. 4 (1971), 96-103.

10. Halberg, Franz, E. Johnson, W. Nelson, W. Runge, and R. Sothern, "Auto-rhythmometry: Procedures for Physiologic Self-Measurements and Their Analysis," *The Physiology Teacher*, 1: No. 4 (1972), 1-11.

11. Harker, Janet, *The Physiology of Diurnal Rhythms*. Cambridge, England: The Cambridge University Press, 1964.

12. Murphy, Juanita, ed., *Theoretical Issues in Professional Nursing*. New York: Appleton-Century-Crofts, 1971.

13. Richter, Curt Paul, *Biological Clocks in Medicine and Psychiatry*. Springfield, Ill.: Charles C Thomas, Publisher, 1965.

14. Sollberger, A., *Biological Rhythm Research*. New York: American Elsevier Publishing Company, Inc., 1965.

15. Sutherland, V. C., *A Synopsis of Pharmacology* (2nd ed.). Philadelphia: W. B. Saunders Company, 1970.

16. United States Department of Health, Education, and Welfare, Public Health Service, *Biological Rhythms in Psychiatry and Medicine*. Chevy Chase, Md.: National Institute of Mental Health, 1970.

17. Yamamoto, W., and J. Brobeck, *Physiological Controls and Regulations*. Philadelphia: W. B. Saunders Company, 1965.

Section II

RELATIONSHIP OF MOBILITY AND BODY MECHANICS TO MAINTENANCE OF ADAPTATION

In the living organism, motion is the perpetual force of adaptation and is therefore synonymous with life. A person's degree of mobility determines his adaptive capacity at the cellular, systemic, and structural levels, as well as the degree to which he can make psychosocial adjustments.

DIMENSIONS OF IMMOBILITY

Immobility, *prescribed or unavoidable restriction of movement in any sphere of a person's life*, must be viewed in a broad context. Even normal physiological or psychosocial experiences have their dimensions of immobility. For example, a new student adjusting to college life feels a certain restriction of free movement as compared to the ease with which he could function in his former school environment. Likewise, pregnancy imposes varying degrees of physical, psychological, and social adaptation restrictive of free movement.

The dimensions of immobility can be identified as area, cause, extent, direction, duration, sequelae, and volition[4]. Nursing care based on these dimensions will provide support and promote adaptive responses when health is threatened.

Area. A person may be immobilized in any one or in several areas or facets of his life: physical, social, intellectual, or psychological. Physical immobility is not confined to loss of musculoskeletal function, the application of casts, or the use of traction. It may be restriction of movement for an elderly person who cannot go out to shop because there are too many stairs to climb, a lack of transportation, or no one to help carry a heavy load. Social immobility can occur in a number of ways. The widow may find that her ability to lead the life to which she has been accustomed is restricted because as a single woman alone she no longer fits into her group of friends. The person who migrates from one country or region to another may have difficulty establishing friendships. Intellectual immobility exists for those limited by a lack of mental development. Psychological restrictions can arise from maladaptation to stress. Physiological processes may be slowed or made nonfunctional by disease or injury.

Cause. Factors within the person or in his environment may cause limited mobility. Disease states are most usually considered as causes of immobility, but the therapy used in the treatment of the disease, such as traction or a cast, could be more immobilizing than the illness itself.

Extent. For a given person, immobility will vary in intensity at different times. Also, two people may have basically the same injury and treatment plan but will recover at different rates; this difference often reflects how each perceives his disability. Therefore, the extent of the immobility is relative.

Direction. Only in death is there no potential for change. In the living organism, immobility undergoes directional shifts as adaptation occurs. The interplay of organ systems, cell metabolism and body defenses, and the influence of psychosocial factors, mediate the direction of change toward improvement or regression.

Duration. The length of time during which degrees of immobility will occur under certain describable circumstances is to some extent predictable: The physician is able to predict the number of days that must elapse before sutures may be safely removed. The nurse plans for the possible duration of the patient's immobility in many ways: How frequently and for how long will it be necessary to check the obstetrical patient's fundus? When will the postoperative patient be able to help with his bath? What plans should be made for teaching the new diabetic or the new colostomy patient the ways in which each can take care of himself at home?

Sequelae. Maladaptive responses stemming from a primary disease process or disability may extend the duration of immobility or change its direction. Effective preventive measures designed to avoid harmful side effects must be part of every nursing care plan. You will need to predict the probable hazards associated with the particular area and degree of immobility with which you are dealing in order to avoid or minimize unfavorable effects.

Volition (Use of Will). The patient with a fractured bone, an abdominal incision, or arthritic joints may need help in accepting nursing care that provides necessary mobility within prescribed limits, especially when movement or a change in position causes pain. On the other hand, when a disability occurs that is not accompanied by sufficient discomfort to limit the patient's mobility, he may not easily accept prescriptions for needed rest and restricted activity. In either case, patient teaching should help shorten, or at least not prolong, the person's period of forced immobility.

EFFECTS OF IMMOBILITY ON FUNCTIONAL AREAS

Cardiovascular Function

Adequate exchange of respiratory gases and metabolic substances depends on the efficiency of the cardiovascular system, including the heart, arteries, venous channels, and lymph vessels. Physical immobility produces three critical changes in the adaptive ability of this system to carry blood to and from capillaries: in (1) vasomotor control, (2) blood return to the heart, and (3) venous stasis [2, 6].

Orthostatic hypotension is the inability of the autonomic nervous system to adapt readily to a sudden change from a recumbent to an upright position. Equalization of the blood supply throughout the body is affected adversely during prolonged bedrest. The valves within the veins require muscle action to assist them in opening to permit venous return of blood to the heart. Without adequate muscle contraction, tone is lost, muscles lose strength, and venous blood tends to pool in the lower extremities. The decrease in neurovascular reflex control of blood vessels during bedrest may be caused by the lower pressure, higher flow, and increased diameter of vessels in the supine position[2].

Though rest is considered an essential factor in the treatment of disease, a second major change in cardiovascular performance resulting from immobility has been identified: The heart suffers an increased work load in the resting supine position resulting from the altered distribution of blood throughout the body. Gravity provides downward pressure in the erect position, and when this is relieved by lying down, the circulating blood volume is increased, placing an additional load on the right side of the heart as more blood returns from the periphery to the heart[2].

Periodically, the patient on bedrest is required to exert strain on his heart in what is known as the *Valsalva maneuver*. This is the act of fixing the thorax, holding one's breath, and thereby forcing pressure against the closed glottis—the action one takes when straining to defecate. Intrathoracic pressure is increased and prevents venous blood from entering the large vessels. When the breath is expired, a sudden drop in the intrathoracic pressure occurs, resulting in a rush of blood to the heart. This maneuver may be used by a bedfast patient as often as 20 to 30 times per hour as he uses his arms and the muscles of the upper trunk to change his position in bed[6].

Thrombus formation is the third hazard associated with cardiovascular functions during immobility. Venous stasis occurs, leading to hypercoagulability of the blood. External pressure is exerted by the patient's position, the bedding, or both. Bed patients are often dehydrated, which contributes to an increased viscosity of the bood and may in turn lead to clotting. Also, the blood level of calcium is increased during rest. The calcium may combine with material from platelets to form thrombin (a precursor for the conversion of fibrinogen to fibrin), producing hypercoagulability[6].

The intima of blood vessels may be easily damaged by maintaining one position for a prolonged time, especially if one extremity rests on the other. Platelets will then form a matrix over the damaged area and may form a clot.

Range-of-motion exercises to assist in venous flow and the restoration or maintenance of muscle tone will be important to your care of any patient on bedrest. Consult a nursing fundamentals text for specific information on doing range-of-motion exercises. Self-care should be encouraged as much as possible within the limits set by the medical regimen. Frequent changes in position should be required, especially for providing a change from horizontal to vertical whenever possible. Patient teaching should help the patient learn how to move in bed with a minimum of effort; an overbed trapeze can be provided for this purpose.

One of the best examples of nursing support for adaptation is that of preventing constipation. Positioning the patient in a well-supported position on the bedpan or commode helps to relieve the strain that might otherwise put too much work load on the heart.

Respiratory Function

Certain adaptive responses are compensatory during immobility: basal metabolism decreases, cells require less oxygen for synthesis of proteins, and less carbon dioxide is produced as a by-product of cell metabolism. In addition, the rate of respiration decreases, there is less movement of secretions, and oxygen-carbon dioxide balance is altered[6].

Added to the compensatory decrease in respirations during periods of bedrest are a number of factors that are significant for nursing care. Chest expansion may be adversely affected. The bed may splint the chest by its pressure, especially if the patient maintains one position too long. Some postures may compress the thorax. Abdominal distention or a tight binder or dressing may prevent the normal descent of the diaphragm during inspiration. Drugs that depress the central nervous system will affect the respiratory center in the medulla, motor areas of the cerebral cortex, and the cells of the spinal cord.

Pooling of secretions follows respiratory embarrassment. Inflammation of the trachea and the bronchial tree leads to a further decrease in the ability to use normal cleansing mechanisms, such as coughing and deep breathing. Stagnant secretions provide a receptive medium for the growth of microorganisms, thereby increasing the chances of threatening sequelae.

Lack of respiratory movement and the pooling of secretions result in oxygen-carbon dioxide imbalance. The first adaptational response resulting from increased accumulation of carbon dioxide in the blood is temporary stimulation of the respiratory centers. Continuous stimulation causes the aortic and carotid bodies to react against the stimulus, and overadaptation to excessive stimulation causes the respiratory centers to become depressed. Respiratory acidosis follows and may lead to cardiac failure unless reversed.

Nursing measures for prevention of functional respiratory disabilities are those that preserve the patient's ability to breathe. This begins with astute observation of his respirations—their rate, depth, and quality. The way in which he uses his muscles to breathe is important. He may be using neck muscles to supply force. His position may give a clue to difficulty in breathing; or he may speak in partial, clipped sentences, indicating his inability to inspire sufficient air. Listening to his breathing and then using a stethoscope to auscultate breath sounds will provide a basis for accurate reporting of signs and symptoms.

Turning, coughing, and deep breathing are among the simplest and yet most effective methods for preserving the immobilized patient's respiratory function. Teaching the patient how to do this regularly and encouraging him toward as much self-care as his disability permits will provide support for cardiopulmonary function, which in turn promotes healthy adaptive responses in other systems.

Nutrition and Elimination

Because immobility reduces the energy requirements of cells and slows metabolic processes, gastrointestinal function is impaired, affecting both the ingestion of food and the elimination of wastes[2, 6].

At prolonged rest, nitrogen balance in the human is reversed to a negative state. Anabolic and catabolic activities are not equal—the balance is upset: catabolism is increased, and protein loss is accompanied by mechanical and psychological disturbances in gastrointestinal function as the desire for food diminishes.

Anorexia results in a loss of nutrients and is apt to prolong whatever disease process or dysfunction caused the immobilization in the first place. Though loss of appetite is an adaptive mechanism in response to decreased metabolic requirements, sufficient nutrients for basal metabolism and for compensation of catabolic losses must be maintained if healing is to take place.

Adequate amounts of the Basic 4 food groups served in small, frequent feedings may help encourage the patient to eat. Personal preferences and cultural variations in food habits may need to be considered, and food should be appetizing and served appropriately hot or cold. Food becomes for the immobilized person a source of comfort, a symbol of the caring of others for him, a welcome break in the day's routine.

Elimination is the other significant gastrointestinal function affected by prolonged rest. The combination of smooth and skeletal muscle activity with complex reflex action provides for successful defecation. Loss may occur in any of these mechanisms. Lack of muscle tone occurring during immobility is reflected in a weakening of the abdominal muscles needed for the expulsion of stool. Dehydration may cause fecal material to be dry and hard. Suppression of the urge to defecate often occurs. The patient is in an unfamiliar environment; privacy is minimal; his usual pattern of living has been disrupted. Often he must assume an unnatural position to defecate. If the gastrocolic reflex that moves the fecal contents from the sigmoid into the rectum is ignored repeatedly, it will become less strong until it possibly disappears altogether and chronic constipation develops.

Fecal impaction can and does frequently occur in immobilized persons, regardless of age, unless nursing intervention has been preventive rather than curative. Increased fluid intake, a daily serving of prune juice in anticipation of prolonged bedrest, and preservation of muscle tone are measures that will prevent constipation and mechanical intervention. The elderly patient with a stroke or fractured hip, the patient in casts or traction regardless of age, or anyone confined to bed for an extended period for any reason are all persons for whom an early assessment of bowel habits and a preventive plan of care are essential.

Patient teaching is important since many persons do not understand what constitutes a normal bowel pattern. Misconceptions regarding the frequency, amount, and characteristics of a normal stool must be clarified. What is normal for one person will not be for another. The idea that a daily bowel movement is necessary for all people may need to be explored with the patient, since cultural groups vary in their emphasis upon this and other body functions. It is not how often defecation occurs, but what its characteristics are, that determines healthy gastrointestinal function. If the stool is soft, formed, and easily expelled, the frequency is not significant. Evacuation twice a week in sufficient amounts and of soft consistency is considered to indicate normal bowel function in the immobilized patient[6].

Many pharmaceutical stool softeners are available for patients who may need help in getting a bowel pattern established, but the use of laxatives and enemas should be discouraged. In any bowel-training program, the patient's habits prior to his immobility should be investigated and incorporated into the plan. Peristalsis sufficient to move bowel contents into the rectum usually occurs most strongly after breakfast. Therefore, following that meal the patient should be encouraged to use the bedpan, commode, or lavatory, allowing about 15 minutes for the process. Sometimes digital stimulation of the anal sphincter or the use of a suppository may be helpful in establishing this pattern.

If an acceptable pattern for defecation has not been established and a fecal impaction occurs, the cardinal symptom will be the frequent passing of liquid fecal material from around the impacted stool. When this is suspected, a rectal examination should be done; and if there is an impaction, it must be dislodged and removed by gentle digital manipulation. Often this will be followed by an oil retention enema before cleansing enemas are used.

Locomotion

Maintenance of structural stability is essential for man's adaptation to his environment. Integrity of osseous (bony) structures, efficiency of muscle action, and an intact integument (skin) are the first lines of defense against physical trauma. Muscles, bones, and skin are coordinated with the nervous system to produce the complex process of locomotion. The element of stress is important to motor function. Without the normal stresses and strains of daily activity, strength is depleted as bones lose their solidity and muscles become too atonic to support the weight of the body and move its parts with ease. Cell nutrition suffers as the muscle pump activity cannot be maintained for adequate circulation of blood.

Immobility contributes to three major complications of musculoskeletal deterioration, and these are manifested in tissue changes and dysfunction of bones, muscles, and skin. Each complication contributes to the others[6].

Osteoporosis is one of the deteriorative processes resulting from immobility. Adaptive mechanisms and a balance of energy exchange are continually striving to maintain optimum strength in osseous tissue. A bone is a living structure. Its growth and development are built upon a vital matrix that carries the calcium necessary to give it strength and solidarity. Counterforces are constantly breaking down and replacing this matrix and its calcium throughout the life of the bone[6].

Osteoblasts are cells that form the bony matrix. Their function depends on the stresses and strains of movement; without this stimulus they cease forming new bone. Meanwhile, the *osteoclasts, cells that have the opposing function of absorbing and removing osseous tissue from the bone*, continue their destructive process. Decalcification occurs; phosphorus and nitrogen are removed; and *as this demineralization progresses the bone becomes porous, producing a condition known as osteoporosis.*

Weight bearing, which is unnoticed by normal, active persons, becomes painful for the person with osteoporosis. Bones may compress and become deformed, and they are easily fractured. Demineralization of bone cannot be diagnosed by X-ray until approximately 50 percent of the calcium is lost. Patients with this condition in which there has been a gradual onset are usually those beyond middle age. They may have a great deal of generalized pain on bearing weight and become less mobile as the disease progresses. This leads to further complications, with muscles losing tone from disuse, and the skin becomes susceptible to pressure from prolonged rest in one position.

The significance of osteoporosis is that it can occur in a relatively short time in any person, regardless of age, during prolonged periods of immobility. Nursing measures for prevention or decrease of mineral loss must be those directed toward maintenance of weight bearing and muscle strengthening. Stress on bones can be provided through exercises and the use of weight-bearing equipment such as a tilt bed or oscillating bed. If walking is difficult or limited, having the patient use a walker or parallel bars at regular intervals may be prescribed. One of the best nursing interventions is to encourage the patient to participate in his own care, to stretch, to reach, to exercise against resistance to his maximum ability.

Contractures of the muscles is the second deteriorative process. Prolonged disuse of any muscle produces *atrophy, the wasting away of muscle tissue*: the size of the muscle decreases and its strength ebbs. If weakness prevents the full range of muscle contraction or if there is *imbalance between the strength of opposing muscles, contracture* can occur: the weak muscle cannot contract adequately and its antagonist exerts an opposing pull, thereby flexing part of an extremity in a fixed, sometimes irreversible, position.

Proper body alignment in an anatomically correct position is important during bedrest and is the first step toward increased mobility and preservation of function. A firm mattress and perhaps a bed board are necessary when there is to be a prolonged stay in bed. The use of a properly placed footboard will prevent footdrop by assisting the patient to use the muscles of the lower legs. The board must be placed in such a way as to rest firmly against the patient's feet and not require him to stretch to reach it.

Frequent and regularly scheduled changes of position combined with full-range-of-motion exercises for all unaffected joints are essential. Again, the patient and his family should be taught how to help in these exercises so that they may participate in his care.

Skin breakdown also occurs frequently with osteoporosis or contracture formation and is the third deteriorative process.

The Integument

The moving and turning just referred to are directly related to the maintenance of skin integrity. Ordinarily, as a person sleeps or rests in bed, he turns and moves, changing position and avoiding pressure on any one area for very long. This shifting about occurs frequently even during sleep. The movement preserves the integument from assault that might deprive skin areas of an adequate blood supply over a period of time and thus break down.

Persons who are aged, paralyzed, obese, or immobilized because of disability are all prone to skin breakdown. Either sensation is not keen enough to warn of pressure, or there is lack of ability to turn without aid because of weight, weakness, or the pressure of restrictive mechanical devices. If no assistance is given to provide mobility, the skin suffers in two ways: (1) muscle disuse decreases the circulatory exchange in the soft tissues, and (2) the constant pressure obstructs the flow of blood to the part. *Ischemia*, or *local anemia* of the area, develops, and this leads to necrosis and ulceration. This is the classic decubitus ulcer that is so insidious in its onset and so difficult to heal. In addition to the threat of skin breakdown due to immobility per se there is the danger of malnutrition in the bedfast patient because he is in negative nitrogen balance. Unless the skin receives adequate nourishment it cannot survive the effects of constant pressure and embarrassment of its blood supply, a fact that emphasizes the interrelationship of the body's functional areas[2, 6, 7].

Nursing intervention is the primary preventive therapy in this area. Skin breakdown can and must be prevented through nursing, not medical, care. The development of an open area caused by pressure is unnecessary today. The responsibility for initiating prophylactic measures rests with you. In addition to frequent position changes, gentle massage over bony prominences, range-of-motion exercises, and mechanical aids may be used. An alternating-pressure mattress, a flotation mattress with its gel foam pad that protects the sacral area, oscillating beds, tilt boards, or even a simple measure such as a sheepskin under the hips can be used to protect the skin.

Position change must be accompanied by close inspection and meticulous care of the skin. The patient's linen should be dry and wrinkle-free at all times. Keep the skin clean and use an emollient lotion to keep it pliant. Make sure the lotion you use is thoroughly absorbed, or the excess removed, to prevent maceration of skin by too much moisture.

In essence, prevention insures an intact musculoskeletal system in the immobile patient. Provide as much movement as possible. Use anatomical positioning that avoids pressure points for long periods. Encourage the patient to participate in his care. Use patient teaching for optimum nutrition. And base your intervention on careful assessments of skin and muscle tone so that the direction of adaptation will be toward full function.

Urinary Excretion

Figure 7-2 shows that free drainage of urine from the calyces of the kidney to the bladder for excretion through the urethra is designed, in the human, for the upright position. When a person is supine, urine must leave the kidney against an upward gradient. Hence mobility for the bedfast patient preserves urinary function. Any stasis of urine in the renal pelvis for even a few days may lead to infection or the formation of *renal calculi, urinary tract stones*[2].

Protein breakdown, bone demineralization, and loss of muscle tone during prolonged immobility contribute to marked changes in urinary excretion. The nephron continues to be selective of constituents in the blood, excreting those in excess and preserving those in deficit. Minerals and salts are in excess in blood plasma as a result of bedrest, and thus the nephron increases excretion of these. These particles become ideal nuclei for the formation of renal calculi. Their precipitation is favored by stasis, alkaline urine, decreased volume of urine, and bacterial invasion[2, 6].

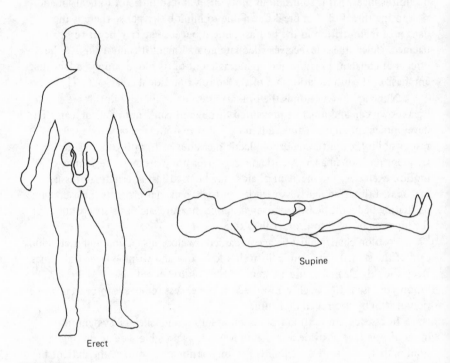

Supine

Erect

FIGURE 7-2
Urinary Drainage Related to Position

Nursing intervention can prevent urine stasis through frequently changing the patient's position and avoiding a supine position for too long a period of time. An alkaline urine occurs during bedrest because of a lack of muscular activity; acid end products decrease and the urine pH rises. Acid-ash between-meal snacks such as cranberry juice or cereals can help overcome this and should be a part of every immobilized patient's care plan.

Forcing fluids is perhaps the simplest and most effective means for preserving urinary function, yet it is often overlooked or given only lip service. Keeping a pitcher of water at the bedside and changing it faithfully is apt to be considered adequate provision of fluid intake, but unless you actually assist the patient in drinking the water, it will do no good. This assistance is different for every patient. It may mean keeping the water within easy reach or pouring it when strength is diminished. But two actions are essential: (1) *offer the water frequently* as you encourage its use, and (2) *carry out effective teaching* as to its importance for body fluids as well as for urinary excretion.

Prevention of urinary tract infection depends on nursing measures. Indwelling catheters should be used only when other measures to keep the patient dry and his bladder empty have failed. During their use, meticulous perineal care and cleansing of the catheter where it emerges from the meatus must be done at least once daily.

Metabolic Processes

The functional changes resulting from prolonged rest include the following: a decreased metabolic rate, tissue atrophy, protein catabolism, bone demineralization, altered exchange of nutrients and vital substances between the intracellular and extracellular compartments, fluid and electrolyte imbalance, and changes in gastrointestinal motility[6].

Some of the above changes resulting from immobility have been discussed: the decreased metabolic rate, protein breakdown, threat of renal calculi, decreased muscular use, and loss of stress to the skeletal system. Another important effect of bedrest is the loss of heat by conduction and radiation because of the pressure of the bed and its linens. Blood vessels are dilated in the supine position, and since much of the body's surface is covered with bedclothes, perspiration is increased, This adds to the fluid loss, and with perspiration the essential electrolytes, sodium, potassium, and chloride are lost.

Diurnal patterns are closely bound to metabolic response. Activity of body functions such as temperature, hormone secretion, and renal regulation is at its best during a person's waking hours; during sleep most body functions are reduced to a minimum. If a person is supine for long periods, whether asleep or awake, these physiological functions will decline to a minimal output.

Metabolic homeostasis is preserved through the nursing measures discussed in relation to all the functional body systems: around-the-clock exercise and movement, increased fluid intake, acid-ash foods, attention to nutritional and elimination needs, care and stimulation of the integument, and interventions that conserve heat loss and cardiac output.

Psychosocial Aspects

Ego identity is distorted by immobility. The integrated personality a person develops through socialization and the meanings he assigns to situations are threatened when he is confronted by restriction of free movement[6].

Learning and motivation are affected, and problem solving becomes less direct when a person is isolated or immobile. Drives, expectations, and emotional responses are altered: the first two are diminished, and the latter are expressed in behaviors not typical of the person's usual pattern. Withdrawal, apathy, aggressiveness, or regression may occur where no such behavior previously existed. Lack of self-determination in activities changes behavior.

The immobilized person views the environment, including people, from a different physical position; the feedback upon which he relies to tell him who and what he is may seem unfamiliar. He may incorporate the apparatus of hospitalization into his body image. Thus traction equipment, casts, intravenous or any other tubing attached to or inserted within him may alter his perception of self.

Changes in the way sensory stimuli are perceived occur because the sensory processes are slowed during prolonged bedrest or isolation. Form and substance, weight, pressure, and temperature may be perceived differently. Time is now ordered by others' activities. Direction often means one place—where he is. There is no east, west, north, or south.

The social institutions of the family, education, religion, work, and recreation ordinarily define a person's roles. During immobility, roles are reversed, changed, or eliminated according to the restrictions imposed. In American culture, youth, vigor, upward mobility, and energy expenditure are stressed as desirable attributes. During prolonged disability, the loss of or diminished capacity for these highly valued goals is interpreted by the patient, and sometimes by those with whom he associates, as a loss of personal worth. It is no wonder that under such circumstances a person develops behavior patterns misunderstood by and unacceptable to others.

Nursing intervention for psychosocial adaptation should concentrate on helping the patient move from dependency to independence, providing him with sensory stimuli, helping him adjust to a temporary or permanent body-image threat, orienting him to time and place, and supporting him during necessary role change.

Through your astute assessment, you can make a systematic and complete care plan that can be used by the entire staff. A clock and a calendar are necessary to a patient's orientation to reality, as even the short-term patient often misjudges the passage of time. Describing the location of his room in relation to the points of the compass and in relation to other parts of the unit can be extremely helpful. You might move the patient's bed to a courtyard or lounge when long-term disability precludes his being moved on a cart or using a wheelchair. In this way, the patient's environment is extended for him, and he experiences increased sensory input.

Patient teaching is essential for psychosocial as well as physical adaptation to immobility. Explain procedures and equipment to the patient and teach him ways of participating in his care and of making use of increased leisure time.

Work with the family or friends to help stabilize the patient's societal roles. Encourage those he loves and relies on to treat him with the same respect as in the past. As soon as possible he should be allowed to participate in the same decisions and role expectations that his family assigned to him before his illness.

Immobilization disability is one of today's major health hazards. Mobility supports autoregulatory processes. Through patient teaching and intervention based on scientific rationale, you can help each patient and family experiencing some immobility to adapt as fully as possible.

REFERENCES

1. Beeson, Paul B., and Walsh McDermott, eds., *Cecil-Loeb Textbook of Medicine*. Philadelphia: W. B. Saunders Company, 1971.

2. Browse, N. L., *Physiology and Pathology of Bedrest*. Springfield, Ill.: Charles C. Thomas, Publisher, 1965.

3. Brunner, Lillian Sholtis, et al., *Medical-Surgical Nursing* (2nd ed.). Philadelphia: J. B. Lippincott Company, 1970.

4. Carnevali, Doris and Susan Brueckner, "Immobilization: Reassessment of a Concept," *American Journal of Nursing*, 70: No. 7 (1970), 1502-7.

5. Metz, Edith A., "Development of a Standardized Test of Cognitive Aspects of Efficient Body Movement for Technical and Professional Nursing Students," *Nursing Research Conference*, 5 (1969), 196-207.

6. Olson, Edith V., "The Hazards of Immobility," *American Journal of Nursing*, 67: No. 4 (1967), 779-97.

7. Wessels, Norman K., "How Living Cells Change Shape," *Scientific American*, 225: No. 4 (1971), 77-82.

8. Winters, Margaret Campbell, *Protective Body Mechanics in Daily Life and in Nursing*. Philadelphia: W. B. Saunders Company, 1955.

9. Works, Roberta F., "Hints on Lifting and Pulling," *American Journal of Nursing*, 72: No. 2 (1972), 260-61.

CHAPTER 8

Crisis Intervention:
A Therapy Technique

Study of this chapter will help you to:

1 Differentiate between crisis and stress.

2 Identify the types of crises and give examples of each.

3 Describe factors that influence coping with and the outcome of a crisis.

4 List the phases of crisis and discuss normal behavioral responses in each phase.

5 Discuss examples of behavior that indicate a crisis was not adequately resolved.

6 Discuss the necessity of integrating crisis theory into your philosophy of care.

7 Relate the steps of the nursing process to crisis therapy.

8 Define *loss, grief,* and *mourning* and discuss the crisis of separation and loss as a part of life.

9 Describe the sequence of reactions and behaviors typical of the grief syndrome and mourning process.

10 List factors influencing the mourning process.

11 Explore your role in helping the person who has experienced loss.

12 Discuss factors contributing to the person's definition of and susceptibility to illness.

13 Identify the sick role and behaviors typical of the sick role.

14 Compare the reactions of the person who is ill at home to those of someone hospitalized for illness.

15 List and discuss the stages of illness and tasks of convalescence.

16 Define and discuss the characteristics of impaired role behavior.

17 Explore how you can help a patient and family resolve the crisis of illness.

18 Assess and care for a patient and family in a crisis.

"I remember all the feelings in my first semester of college. I never thought I'd make it! I was mad at my teachers. Then I realized it wasn't my teachers. It was me! In retrospect, realizing that I was in a crisis helps me understand what I was living through."

Crisis theory provides nursing with a theoretical model of the processes of adaptation that follow certain kinds of stressful, disquieting, unmanageable events in the person's life. The usefulness of the theory lies in its systematic organization of events that appear haphazard and unpredictable and in its potential to guide your intervention when working with persons in crisis.

DEFINITIONS AND CHARACTERISTICS

Crisis is any transient situation that necessitates reorganization of one's psychological structure and behavior, that causes a sudden alteration in the person's expectation of himself, and that cannot be handled with the person's usual coping mechanisms [11, 18].

The person's ordinary behavior is no longer successful emotionally, intellectually, or physically. Old habits are disturbed, and the person feels motivated to try new responses in order to cope with the situation at hand. Although the person's behavior is inadequate or inappropriate to the present situation and may be different from normal, it should not be considered pathological. The crisis may also reactivate old unresolved crises or conflicts, which imposes an additional burden to be resolved at the present time. However, the crisis is a turning point, and, with its resultant mobilization of energy, operates as a second chance for correcting earlier maladaptations or faulty problem solving. The time of crisis serves as a catalyst or opportunity for growth emotionally. There is a realignment of behavior that, if all goes well, will lead to a state of equilibrium or behavior that is more mature than the previous status. On the other hand, because of the stress involved and the felt threat to equilibrium, the person is also more vulnerable to regression and mental or physical illness. The outcome—either increased maturity or illness—depends on how the person handles the situation and on the help others give. Encountering and resolving crisis is a normal process that each person faces many times during his life.

Stress, defined and discussed earlier, must be differentiated from *crisis*. *Stress is the everyday wear and tear on the body, the effects of the rate at which you live at any moment, positive and negative, physical, emotional, or mental*[51]. All living things are constantly under stress, and anything, pleasant or unpleasant, that speeds up the intensity of life causes a temporary increase in stress or in the wear and tear upon the body. For example, a painful blow or a passionate kiss can be equally stressful. Stress does not consist merely of damage, but also of the adaptation to damage, and can be positive and life-promoting. During a stressful period, the person can use his normal coping mechanisms. The temporary upsets in equilibrium are solved by previously learned coping techniques and various mechanisms of tension discharge, such as talking. Stress, however, has a great potential for reducing the person's level of mental health, whereas crisis has a great potential for raising the level of mental health. Yet both may have either a positive or negative outcome[47, 51].

Not all persons facing the same hazardous event will be in a state of crisis. But some events or situations are viewed as a crisis by all persons, in that some behavioral adjustment must be made by anyone facing that situation. Crises also vary in degree; a situation may be perceived as major, moderate, or minimal in the degree of discomfort caused and the amount of behavioral change demanded.

Crisis in the person's life can be considered from the standpoint of adaptation theory discussed in Chapter 7. The total person responds to crisis in ways that affect adaptation or higher levels of integration of total body function. His response to crisis is also a way of adapting. Crisis, and one's reacion to it, affects physiological, intellectual, emotional, social, and cultural aspects of the person's life as well as of the family unit.

TYPES OF CRISES

There are two types of crises: (1) developmental, maturational, or normative, and (2) situational or accidental[11].

Developmental Crisis

Developmental crises are transition points, the periods that every person experiences in the process of biopsychosocial growth and development and that are accompanied by changes in thoughts, feelings, and abilities. These are times in development when new relationships are formed and old relationships take on new aspects. Others have new expectations of the person, and certain emotional tasks must be accomplished so that he is better equipped to move on to the next phase of development. The onset of the developmental or maturational crises is gradual because it occurs as the person moves from one stage of growth and development to another.

Why does normal development leave the person vulnerable to crisis? Spiegel's description of role theory is helpful for understanding[52].

Role is a goal-directed pattern of behavior learned within one's cultural setting and carried out by the person in his social group or situation because both he and the group expect this behavior. No role exists in isolation, but is always patterned to dovetail with or complement the role of another. When one person changes his role, his role partners—other persons in that system—undergo reciprocal role or behavioral changes. The times of maturational or developmental crisis are mainly periods of many role changes, although they may be slow and gradual and vary from one culture or class to another. A maturational crisis occurs when the person is unable to make role changes appropriate to his new level of maturity. The stressful events are the social and biological pressures on the individual to see himself in a new and different role and act accordingly[52].

There are three main reasons why someone may be unable to make role changes necessary to prevent a maturational crisis:

1. The person's inability to picture himself in a new role. Roles are learned; adequate role models may not exist.
2. The person may be unable to make role changes because of a lack of intrapersonal resources—for example, inadequate communication skills, his realization that with life passing he will not be able to achieve certain goals, or inability to realize alternatives to his present life style.
3. Refusal by others in the social system to see the person in a different role. For example, when the adolescent tries to move from childhood to the adult role, the parent may persist in keeping him in the child role[52].

The main developmental crises are entry into school, puberty, leaving home, engagement, marriage, pregnancy, childbirth, middle age, menopause, retirement, and facing death of others and of the self.

Situational Crisis

*The **situational crisis** is an external event or situation, one not necessarily a part of normal living, often sudden, unexpected, and unfortunate, which looms larger than the person's immediate resources or ability to cope and which demands a change in behavior.* There is a threat or danger to life goals; tension and anxiety are evoked; unresolved problems and crises from the past are reawakened. The amount of time taken for healthy or unhealthy adaptation to occur is usually from one to six weeks, since this type of crisis does not continue indefinitely. A situational crisis may be occurring at the same time as a developmental crisis.

Situational crises include natural disasters, such as a hurricane, tornado, or flood; loss through separation, divorce from, or death of a loved one; losing one's job, money, or valued possessions; and a change in job. Illness or hospitalization, a power struggle on the job, a sudden change in role responsibilities, or a forced geographical relocation are other examples.

FACTORS INFLUENCING THE OUTCOME
OF CRISIS

A variety of factors influence how the person reacts to and copes with crises situations[1, 11, 18].

1. *The person's perception of the event*. If the event or the consequences of it conflict with his value system or wishes for the future, he is likely to define the situation as hazardous. The perception of the event is reality for the person, regardless of how others might define reality. The person's perception rather than the actual event determines his behavior. For example, two persons live through the disaster of a flood. One loses his house and all his possessions; the other loses his boat, but everything else is intact. The latter may react with greater shock, denial, anger, or depression than the person who loses his home and possessions because of their different perceptions—the meaning to each of his loss.
2. *The physical and emotional status* of the person, degree of health, amount of energy present, age, genetic endowment, and biological rhythms.
3. *The coping techniques or mechanisms and the level of personal maturity*. If adaptive capacities are already strained, or the stress is overwhelming, the person will cling to old habits and his behavior will very likely be inappropriate to the task at hand. The person who has met developmental tasks all along will adapt more easily in any crisis.
4. *Previous experiences with similar situations*. The past serves as a model for present action. If a person resolved past crises by distorting reality or withdrawing, when similar crises arise he must attempt to cope with a new situation while also burdened with prior failure. Crises of any kind are often cumulative in effect. The most recent crisis revives the denial, depression, anger, or maladaptation that was left unsettled or unresolved from past crises.
5. *The objectively realistic aspects of the situation*, such as personal or material losses.
6. *Cultural influences*. How the person is trained and socialized in the home

to solve problems and meet crisis situations, his expectations of how the social group will support him during crisis, and the method established by the social system to provide help influence present behavior.

7. *The availability and response of family and close friends or other helping resources,* including professional persons. The less readily available the person's environmental or emotional support systems are to decrease stress or buttress his coping response, the more hazardous he will define the event. The family system, by its influence on development of self-concept and maturity, can increase or decrease one's vulnerability to crisis. When the person's involvement with others is concentrated on only a few family members—as, for example, in the nuclear versus the extended family support system—vulnerability is increased. The reaction to crisis is increased in today's mobile, urbanized society because traditional support systems of long-term family and friends have been disrupted. Thus the professional person is more likely to be needed and sought. Even a small amount of influence exerted by a significant person can be enough to decide the outcome for mental health and against mental illness. However, sustained mental health is in large measure a result of a life history of successfully resolving crises.

PHASES OF CRISIS

All crises require a sudden restructuring of biopsychosocial integration. The phases involved are: shock, followed closely by general realization of the crisis; then defensive retreat; acknowledgement; and finally, adaptation or resolution[11, 18].

In the Initial, Impact, or Shock Phase, the person feels a high level of stress, helplessness, anxiety, chaos, and possibly panic. He feels overwhelmed and depersonalized. Self-esteem is threatened, and thinking and behavior are disorganized. He is unable to plan, to reason logically, or to understand the situation. Judgment is impaired. Habitual or automatic problem-solving behaviors are used without success, although the person cannot perceive his inadequacy. He may suffer physical illness or injury and either focus attention on these or completely ignore his physical status. Socially, he is unable to function appropriately, becoming withdrawn, docile, or perhaps hyperactive and chaotic. The person is unable to meet basic needs without help.

The shock phase usually lasts a short time, perhaps a few hours or one or two days. As the person either perceives for himself or is told what has happened, he copes with the realization of the sudden discontinuity in his life through the second phase, defensive retreat.

In Defensive Retreat, the person tries previously used successful ways of solving problems and adjusting, but tension and discomfort are not reduced nor is the situation alleviated. He feels increasingly upset and ineffective. He will at first try to approach the problem directly, but his behavior does not work. Then he may try to redefine the problem (usually unrealistically), avoid the problem, or seek the support of others. Usually the person retreats into himself, avoiding reality, denying, fantasizing about what could be done or how well he used to handle problems. He may become disoriented, indifferent, apathetic, or euphoric. Usually because of repression, he will state that he feels all right; he does not perceive his anxiety. He is resistant to change suggested by others, maintaining a rigid manner of thinking and expressing the same ideas over and over. His behavior is ineffective and disorganized; he is unable to carry on daily activities. He cannot devise alternate courses of action nor predict accurately the effects of his behavior. Physical symptoms are usually minimal, and he may actually feel better than usual. Socially, he may be withdrawn or superficial and hyperactive, but unable to adequately maintain his social roles. The phase of defensive retreat may last for a brief or prolonged period of time, depending on circumstances.

Denial is a mechanism used in defensive retreat and involves use of three other mental mechanisms: (1) rationalization about discomfort or symptoms and the cause of the situation (for example, the person with chest pain says he has indigestion); (2) displacement of dangerous, disquieting, uncomfortable information onto the health team or family, often in the form of demands or complaints; and (3) projection of his own feelings of inadequacy onto others, saying how inept or neglectful others are. The purposes of these mechanisms are to protect the self from painful information.

The Third Phase, Recoil or Acknowledgement, begins when the facts impose themselves. The person realizes the objective reality of the situation and slowly begins to redefine it, attempting to do problem solving. Tension and anxiety again rise. Reality may seem harsh; and depression, agitation, apathy, self-hate, low self-esteem, and the process of mourning occur. His coping abilities and self-concept may disintegrate before he is able to direct energy toward coping. Thinking may at first be disorganized, but gradually the person can make appropriate plans and by trial and error find solutions for the situation. Physically, he may feel well, or tension may be somaticized. The person will give up certain goals as unattainable. He will recognize that he has been a social burden and make plans to resume his former roles to the degree possible.

The Fourth Phase, Resolution or Adaptation and Change, occurs when the person perceives the crisis situation in a positive way and integrates the painful event into his new self. He can do successful problem solving and express feelings about the event. He feels a new sense of worth, a firm identity, a gradual increase in satisfaction as he masters the situation, and a gradual lowering of anxiety. He is organized in thinking and planning, using appropriate resources and abilities. Physically, he is functioning at the optimum level. Socially, he resumes his status and roles and repatterns his behavior to cope and thus avoid future similar crises. In order to integrate the crisis into his personality, the person must have developed a different concept of himself and his life style. He does not feel bitter about the event encountered or changes made.

At this point, the person should be at a higher level of maturity and adaptation than earlier; he has acquired new coping mechanisms.

Difficulty in achieving resolution is compounded by the negative influences discussed earlier and by additional hardships or complications caused by the crisis itself. Ineffective mastery or problem solving or lack of expression of feelings associated with the crisis may cause a restricted level of functioning in one or all spheres of the personality. The problem may be repressed and permanently denied and unresolved, or major disorganization such as neurosis, psychosis, socially maladjusted behavior, or chronic physical disability may occur.

These are the predictable phases of crisis; however, each stage is not sharply demarcated. One stage may merge into another, particularly in developmental crisis, where the person's functioning may be appropriate in one sphere but less so in another aspect of his personality. In addition, the person may be at the beginning of one phase and then return to the previous phase behaviorally. Thus the person may demonstrate some behaviors indicative of one phase—such as defensive retreat—and simultaneously demonstrate a few behaviors of shock or of acknowledgement.

The family undergoes the same phases of crisis as the designated patient, although the intensity and timing may be different. Thus they will need the same nursing approach as the patient to help them work through these phases.

INEFFECTIVE RESOLUTION OF CRISIS

If there is no adaptive resolution or change in behavior to cope with the crisis, maladaptive or ineffective reactions occur as an attempt at resolution. There may be a delayed reaction in that the crisis event and its consequences are presently denied and repressed. A reaction will eventually be precipitated when a future crisis occurs that recalls the buried feelings and that then renders the person ineffective in functioning. Various other reactions of distorted or inappropriate behavior may occur, although neurosis, psychosis, or socially ineffective behavior occur only in a small percentage of people. The person may be euphoric if denial is prolonged. In the crisis of death of a loved one, the person may prolong identification with the deceased by developing symptoms like those in the last illness of the deceased. And eventually the organic pathological changes specific for the disease may occur[14, 21, 46]. Sometimes such illness occurs on the anniversary of the loss. Or the aggrieved person may develop a different disease, caused by the *mind-body relationship—in which physiological changes occur because of the effects of emotional states upon body parts and which eventually cause organ damage*[21]. *(Illness resulting from the effects of the emotional state is also called **psychosomatic illness**.)*

A study by Rees and Lutkins shows a relationship between loss and developing psychosomatic symptoms. Bereaved relatives were found to have a higher mortality rate during the first year of mourning, a rate that was even increased further for widowed persons. The risk of the close relative dying from the effects of anxiety, hostility, and guilt during that first year was significantly increased when the loved one had died at some place other than home[46].

A study by Parkes shows that medical office consultations for psychiatric symptoms and chronic somatic conditions, such as arthritis—increased by 63 percent the first six months after loss of a husband. Thereafter, the rate of consultation decreased, but still remained higher than the premourning period. The aged particularly express grief reactions through somatic symptoms: persons over 64 years had even higher rates of doctors' office visits. The psychic state may contribute to a number of disease processes through increasing biological vulnerability[46].

Sudden death has occurred in persons who feel depressed and acutely anxious or angry following a crisis situation, apparently from disequilibrium in the hormonal and autonomic nervous systems[24]. The phenomenon needs further study.

Maladaptation may include expressing hostility for an excessively prolonged time against authority figures—doctors, nurses, policemen, parents, or teachers. Prolonged sadness, apathy, lack of initiative, irritability, suspicion, and withdrawing from others because of internalized anger or shock can be equally detrimental to relationships with others and overall conduct. Feelings of isolation, worthlessness, hopelessness, and guilt may become magnified to the point of inducing suicide attempts. Then again, the person may suppress his own personality, taking on traits of the lost person.

The person who stays compulsively busy or is ritualistic may become ineffective in attempts to cope. Alcohol, drugs, or excessive eating may become a crutch or escape when activity no longer provides adequate tension release.

The person may engage in action detrimental to the self economically or socially through excessive generosity or foolish financial dealings (which represent self-punishment) or through delinquency. The latter invites apprehension, punishment, and, at times, someone else making decisions for him.

After loss of a loved one, the person through extreme denial may continue to act as though the lost person is still alive and present. For example, the survivor may continue to set a place at the table for the deceased or keep all the possessions of the lost one. Or the person may acknowledge the death but deny the significance of the loss emotionally or intellectually. He may not take care of business matters because the deceased person was the person who previously did this.

You have an opportunity to help prevent maladaptive resolution through appropriate crisis intervention. When assessing the patient in any illness situation, determine if his problems and needs could be the result of an earlier crisis now causing symptoms or inappropriate behavior.

Working with a person who has maladaptive behavior can be a slow process. You should not expect too much of yourself or of the person, for in your disappointment and frustration you may withdraw from him, thus preventing crisis resolution. Recognize your strengths and limitations and decide whether the patient can use help beyond what you can offer. Accept the fact that because this person is unique, available knowledge and techniques may not be sufficient to help him. On the other hand, knowing that there is a possibility of failure should not preclude trying to help.

Provide an environment in which the person can experience the phases of recovery from his maladaptive behavior or illness. Help him in reminiscing about what he used to do, expressing fear, looking forward optimistically but realistically to the future, and using appropriate rehabilitative measures.

THE NURSING PROCESS
AND CRISIS INTERVENTION

You will encounter crises in a variety of settings: in the emergency room, recovery room, coronary-care unit, surgical intensive-care unit, industrial or school dispensary, and in the obstetrical, pediatric, and psychiatric units. In most of these settings, you will collaborate with the physician and other health team members while doing crisis intervention. In the mental health clinic or neighborhood health center, you may function as primary therapist within the guidelines set down by the agency or with other health team members.

Your philosophy of care must include the concept of crisis. The person in crisis is at a turning point. He is ready for great changes in a relatively short period of time because of the felt tension, pain, and disequilibrium associated with crisis. These feelings motivate him to try to alter his situation. His distress creates an openness to assistance and change. He expects expert help and perceives the nurse as an expert. A minimal amount of support and help can influence the outcome of a crisis to a significant degree.

Crisis therapy is based on the theory that aid during crisis will help the person to adapt in a healthy manner. The minimal goal of therapy is psychological resolution of the immediate crisis and the restoration of coping mechanisms to at least the level of functioning that existed before the crisis event. The maximal goal is to bring about a change in behavior that is more mature than that of the precrisis level. Crisis work involves reinstating earlier stress-reducing behavior or developing new adaptive techniques. Underlying these goals is the assumption that the person seeking help has unused resources that, with minimum assistance, can be called upon to function effectively in everyday living.

Factors influencing the course of crisis therapy include the following: :

1. Attitude of the therapist and the value he places on crisis work.
2. Use of time, in that assessment is done as quickly as possible to ac-

curately define the nature of the crisis, identify the person's response to the event, and devise a course of action for resolving the crisis.

3. Use of nontraditional treatment practices, since appointment time and place are determined by the degree of stress and impaired functioning that the person is experiencing, the skill of the therapist, and the number and kind of resources in the community to assist the person.

4. Differences between the value systems of the therapist and the person. The therapist must be open to what constitutes a problem for another. The life style and values of the person may be foreign to or in conflict with those of the therapist, but the person needs acceptance in order to maintain his basic life style and value system.

Assessment

Collecting information must be systematic yet flexible, rapid enough to interrupt the crisis, but thorough enough to define the problem and identify and achieve the desired outcomes.

The following should be assessed: the anxiety level and feelings of the person; his ego functioning (perception, judgment, memory, problem solving); presence of symptoms; whether the person is suicidal or homicidal; and his usual living patterns, work arrangements, and interpersonal and social situation. Nonverbal behavior and the consistency between verbal and nonverbal behavior must be noted. The person does not always mean what he says, nor will he always act in a way that directly expresses his true feelings. If the person cannot identify the problem because of disorganized thinking, focus his attention on what was occurring just prior to the situation and onset of symptoms. Constructing a sequence of events helps him become reoriented.

After determining the extent of the problem, focus the person's perception on the event—for example, the illness or loss. What does this situation mean to him? How does he see its effect on his future? Does he see the event realistically? What hardships have been created by the crisis—for example, job loss due to depression or mental illness, which in turn causes financial and family problems and loss of self-esteem?

Ascertain if the person plans to kill himself or another person. If so, try to learn how and when. If the intention is carefully planned and details are specific, hospitalization and psychiatric evaluation must be arranged to protect himself and others.

Your next questions should be directed to the availability of help and supportive others or the extent of isolation from significant relationships. What is the person's relationship with supportive others? Crisis intervention is sharply limited in time. The more persons who are helping him the better. Then, too, when crisis therapy is terminated, if helpful others are involved, they can continue to give support to the person. Assess the adaptive capacities of the others involved in the situation who have not sought help but who might also be experiencing crises. If no helpful resources are available, you become a temporary support system while helping the person to establish a relationship with a person or group in the community or work setting.

Ascertain what the person usually does when he has an unsolvable problem. What are his coping skills? Has anything like this happened before? What did he do to decrease tension? If he is trying the same method now and it is not working, what does the person think *would* decrease stress symptoms? Activity that has been done in the far past to cope successfully could be tried again. Determine his strengths and not just his problems and limitations.

Through assessment, you can determine why this situation is a crisis to this person, why he is unable to alter his life style to cope with the situation, and what in his life style can be altered so the crisis can be resolved.

Planning Intervention

As you study the data collected in the preceding manner, the person should also be actively involved in seeking a potential solution. You cannot solve the problem for the person; you can only help him to help himself.

The problem should be clarified and the immediate situation put in focus. The plan for intervention is determined by assessing the nature of the crisis (whether it is acute or chronically recurring), the reactions of others significant to the person, and the strengths and resources of all persons involved. The plan for intervention must extend beyond the person to others involved less directly in the crisis. To understand the person's adaptive capacity in comparison to pre-crisis adaptation, some attention must be paid both to past experience and current personal and environmental resources.

Several alternate solutions should be explored. Positive guidelines for action should be given to the person when he leaves each session, including the first one, so that alternate solutions can be tested. This permits evaluation of coping behavior at each successive session so that additional solutions can be sought if necessary.

Intervention

Some help can be provided during the first interview by clarifying the problem with the person and encouraging his verbalization of feelings. Getting a hold on a problem by talking it through is the first step in problem solving. The person can begin to recognize what this situation means to him, his capacity to cope with it, and what or who can help him. The resultant increase in self-confidence motivates further coping behavior.

Employ primary, secondary, or tertiary preventive intervention, depending upon the person and the crisis.

Primary prevention, or preventing a crisis, can be achieved by helping the person work through developmental periods or anticipated situations.

The anticipation of life crises is an important concept in health promotion and therefore has broad implications in nursing. If the person can prepare for what is potentially in store for him, he will be less vulnerable to physical or mental illness, as shown in studies by Janis on the "work of worrying" or anticipatory grieving. The more thorough the thinking, planning, or "work of worry" before a crisis, the more adequate the subsequent adjustment and the less severe the impact felt. Persons with either excessively high or excessively low levels of fear or worry, however, are ineffective in preparing for crisis. The high-level worrier feels so much fear that something bad will happen that he cannot effectively plan ahead. The low-level worrier does not adequately contemplate impending stress and feels anger and resentment when it comes. The moderately worrisome person can express tension physically, emotionally, and verbally, but maintains self-control and thus can rationally plan and adjust his behavior to the situation[25].

You can help the person do the "work of worry" or anticipatory grieving in the following ways: through premarital counseling to increase the chance of healthy resolution of stressful marital events and the achievement of appropriate developmental tasks; teaching and counseling in prenatal classes to prepare for childbirth and child care; talking with a mother whose child will soon enter school or be married; preretirement counseling to help the person plan ahead to meet the problems and developmental tasks associated with retirement; counseling the family of a terminally ill patient; and talking preoperatively with the person who is undergoing major surgery and body-image changes. Can you think of other situations in which primary prevention can promote health?

Preventive intervention is not designed to bring about major changes in the maturity or personality structure of the person, but rather to maintain his usual level of functioning or equilibrium. The intervention for health promotion described by Murray and Zentner[40] is thus most apt to work with well persons.

Secondary prevention involves early identification of the crisis so the person can avoid maladaptive behavior. The person is helped to adapt to the crisis, thereby reducing the intensity and duration of reaction to it. He is quickly given support, encouraged to use his energies and available resources constructively, and helped to understand that his feelings and behavior are a normal response to the situation.

Examples of secondary prevention in crisis therapy are working with women who have not resolved the crisis of motherhood and extending help to the person who is mourning the loss of a significant person, object, or role.

Tertiary prevention is aimed at preventing further decompensation or impairment, after the person has partially resolved a crisis, so that he can continue to live a useful role in the community. The person's behavior may initially interfere with rehabilitation. When he can resolve the meaning or implications of the crisis and his feelings about it, he will be able to become involved in rehabilitation. His progress depends strongly upon the counseling role of the nurse and upon continuity in the nurse-patient relationship. Through this kind of intervention the person may eventually rework the crisis and become behaviorally more effective. Examples of tertiary prevention are group therapy with chronically ill or disabled persons to help them cope with their health problems, counseling to help a person work through delayed mourning, and remotivation techniques to prevent further disengagement in the aged (outlined by Murray and Zentner [40]).

Crisis therapy is basically brief and specific to the present situation and involves placing attainable goals directly before the person. Thus the principles of crisis intervention are relevant to all persons, including people who are concerned primarily with the here-and-now, who prefer brief, concrete intervention, and who seek assistance for specific problems.

The person or family in crisis becomes more susceptible to the influence of significant others. A little help directed purposefully and with the right timing is more effective than more help given at a period of less emotional accessibility. View yourself as intervening in a social system, into a network of relationships, and not as a single resource to the person. Use the skills of other health team members—the doctor, social worker, chaplain, psychologist, and occupational therapist—either directly or for consultation.

Principles of Intervention, stated below, can be accomplished by using your knowledge of crisis theory, therapeutic communication (discussed in Chapter 3), and establishment of a nurse-patient relationship (discussed in Chapter 4).

Show acceptance of the person and establish a positive, concerned relationship so that he feels a sense of hope, self-worth, and lessened anxiety.

Often during crisis you are confronted by an angry, bitter, or accusatory person or family who berate you, other health team members, or the agency for negligence. Keep two things in mind: their statements may be accurate and justified, or they may serve as the only way they can cope with their own aggression, helplessness, or guilt at the time. Provide the best care possible, show genuine concern, and do not become verbally involved in the dispute. Do not take the behavior personally if it does not apply to you.

Help the person confront the crisis by talking about his present feelings of denial, anger, guilt, or grief. Catharsis lowers tension, clarifies the problem, promotes comprehension of the reality and of the consequences of the situation, and mobilizes energy for constructive action.

Help the person confront the crisis in amounts or "doses" he can manage, being cautious not to overly soften the impact of the event. The reality of the situation must be kept in the foreground, although periods of relief from facing the whole situation are needed. Help him first gain an intellectual understanding of the crisis; then encourage an emotional understanding and adjustment. In this way, he can more objectively handle the real situation.

Recognize denial as a normal reaction. Cope with personal feelings about his behavior and situation; observe his behavior objectively; avoid reinforcing denial; and gently represent reality to him. Work with other resource persons for information, collaboration, maintenance of support, and representation of reality.

Explain to the person the relationship between the crisis situation and his present behavior and feelings. The person feels less overwhelmed and better able to manage when he understands that his emotions are normal in the context of crisis.

Help him find facts, since facts are less awesome than speculations or fantasies about the situation or the unknown.

Explore past life occurrences only in relation to the existing crisis, particularly if feelings aroused in past crises have been unresolved and are influencing the present behavior. The present experience can bring forth defensive behaviors used in the past that are no longer useful.

Avoid giving false reassurance. Acknowledge the validity of fears and other feelings. Show faith in the person's ability to manage, but do not reduce his motivation to cope and adapt by saying that everything will be fine.

Do not encourage the person to blame others for the crisis event, since this process avoids the truth, reduces his motivation to take responsibility for his behavior, and discourages adaptation. Listen initially to his rationalizations; then raise doubt about such statements through questioning.

Anticipate that people facing loss may behave in a grossly maladaptive way and need to be treated with tact, patience, warmth, and empathy, as well as encouraged to express feelings without feeling guilty about doing so. Set limits on behavior that would be destructive to the person or to others.

Explore coping mechanisms to assist the person in examining alternate ways of coping and in seeking and using new behaviors or alternate ways of satisfying needs. Help him to learn or relearn basic social skills as necessary and to fit his personality to the demands presented by the crisis.

Strengthen or reinforce previously learned behavior patterns that can be effective but are not presently being used.

Clarify and reemphasize the person's responsibility for his own behavior, decisions, and way of life. For example, the person in crisis from illness and hospitalization should be assisted in learning the patient role. Then he can replace his uncertainty about expectations for self and others with the feeling that he is a participating member of the treatment team. Therefore, he needs orientation to the hospital division's policies and routines, his room (and roommate, if any), personnel, diagnostic procedures, and preoperative and postoperative care. When the patient is conversant about the possible outcomes of his illness, he can make decisions about his present care goals and future health needs. When he knows what to expect from the health team members, his behavior can be adaptive. He can use the health care workers as resources to improve his health status.

Help the person establish necessary social relationships and change his personal behavior accordingly. If he has lost or is otherwise removed from all significant persons, as might be true for the elderly or new immigrants, introduce him to new people to help fill the void and to obtain support and gratification.

Assist the person in seeking and accepting help. By acknowledging that trouble exists, he is more likely to use his own resources and the help offered by others. If necessary, encourage him to accept help with the everyday tasks of living and to mobilize inner strengths as well as concerned others in his environment.

Although you work with a person or family in crisis therapy, some crises may upset an entire community, such as natural disasters. Use of support systems and role redistribution is then more complex.

Crisis Resolution and Anticipatory Planning terminate crisis intervention. Crisis work is then reviewed, and the accomplishments of the person in working through his predicament should be emphasized. Adaptive coping mechanisms and appropriate behavior that he has successfully used should be reinforced. Positive changes in behavior should be summarized to allow reexperiencing and reconfirming the progress made. Give assistance as needed in making realistic plans for the future, and discuss with the person ways in which the present experience may help him cope with future crises. The person should leave with self-confidence in managing his life and with the awareness that assistance will be available in the future if necessary.

Evaluation. In order to continue to do effective crisis intervention, the step of evaluation in the nursing process must be carried out as discussed in Chapter 4.

A Case Study

Consider the following case. Some of the details are omitted, but the significance of crisis intervention is obvious.

The police in a Midwestern city of 60,000 picked up a 15-year-old boy for burglary. The Juvenile Department learned this was the boy's first offense and wanted to help avoid a future offense. A juvenile officer contacted the boy's school about his attendance and general conduct; both were reported to be within normal limits. The juvenile officer then asked the school principal to send the boy to the school counselor for psychological testing.

The principal first asked the school nurse to make a home visit. He asked her to gather as much information as possible about the boy's emotional health and background. Then proper referral would be made for psychological testing.

The school nurse found the mother and the rest of the family in an acute situational crisis. The husband had recently left his wife and four children. There was no hope of reconciliation. There was little food and almost no money. Additionally, each child was in developmental crisis. The oldest, the boy who had burglarized, was expected to take over the father's role. He was having a struggle just being an adolescent. But he had stolen to get money for the family. The next oldest child, a 12-year-old girl just entering puberty, was having personal problems at school. She had been especially close to her father and now cried much of the time about his departure. The 5-year-old child was having difficulty adjusting to kindergarten. The 1-year-old baby had just learned to walk and was unusually active and demanding, possibly because of the emotional state in the home.

The nurse acted rapidly. She saw the opportunity for intervention at the secondary prevention level. The mother was somewhat apathetic and appeared to be in the defensive-retreat phase of crisis. But she soon responded to the concern and warmth of the nurse, who listened attentively to the story.

The nurse decided that their need for food and money was primary. She transported the mother first to the Emergency City Aid Department, which provided temporary supplies and cash, and then to the Welfare Department to arrange for more permanent aid. The next day she contacted the Big Sister program at a local college to secure a "big sister" for the 12-year-old girl. The college student was majoring in counseling, so with an understanding of the situation she was able to give immediate companionship and support. The nurse notified the kindergarten teacher of the 5-year-old's family situation.

After the results were received from the recommended psychological testing, the nurse sent the 15-year-old boy to Project Alter, an organization with staff specially trained to help alter lawbreaking tendencies in adolescents. The organization worked with other community agencies to set up a network of supportive help for the boy.

Because of this immediate help, the mother was able to move quickly to the third stage of crisis acknowledgement. She could now begin crisis resolution and anticipatory planning while giving more attention to the 1-year-old child.

The key figure in this case is the *nurse* who made a quick and valid assessment. She intervened effectively because she understood crisis therapy and because she knew her community's resources. She would evaluate her crisis intervention after resolution of the crisis.

THE CRISIS OF SEPARATION AND LOSS

The crisis of separation and loss can be either developmental or situational in origin, and both kinds of losses may occur simultaneously.

Life—A Series of Losses

Loss and the universal reaction to loss, grief and mourning, are experienced by everyone at some time in their lives, and you are frequently the one most involved with and available to the person who is experiencing loss.

As one's interdependence with others grows, the likelihood increases that separation, loss of something valuable, or death of a loved one will induce a crisis. The capacity to have warm and loving relationships also leaves one vulnerable to sadness, despair, and grief. The more one has emotionally invested in that which is lost, the greater the threat felt to the self.

Every person is also subjected to separations or losses that are subtle and may not be recognized. Any crisis, developmental or situational, involves some degree of loss. If nothing else, there is a loss through change in old behavior patterns and the addition of different coping mechanisms. The process of achieving independence in psychosocial development in the course of normal upbringing involves a whole series of separations. The way these early separations are dealt with affects how later separations and loss, including death, will be resolved. Examples of loss situations, either partial or total, temporary or permanent, throughout the life span include the following:

1. Period of weaning in infancy; learning to wait.
2. First haircut, even when it involves pride and anticipation.
3. Period of increasing locomotion, exploration, and bowel and bladder control and resultant loss of dependency.
4. Loss of baby teeth, baby possessions, toys, clothes or pets during development.
5. Change in the body, body image, and self-attitude with on-going growth and development.
6. Change in body size and shape and in feelings accompanying pregnancy and childbirth; loss of body part or function, external or internal, through accident, illness, or aging.
7. Departure of children from the home when they go to school or marry.
8. Menopause and loss of childbearing functions.
9. Loss of hearing, vision, memory, strength, and other changes and losses associated with old age.
10. Changes and losses in relationships with others as the person moves from childhood to adulthood—loss of friends and lovers; separation from or death of family members; changes in residence, occupation, or place of business; promotions and graduations.
11. Losses that have symbolic meanings, such as the loss of a symptom that attracted others' attention, a loss or change that necessitates a change in body image, or "loss of face," honor, or prestige.
12. Loss of home due to natural disaster or relocation projects; loss of possessions or money.
13. Loss experienced with divorce or incapacitation of a loved one.

Thus the person brings to any major crisis a backlog of experience that predisposes him either to successfully integrate a personal tragedy or to fail to absorb into himself another loss or change. The significance of the present reaction may become clear only when you understand his earlier separations and losses.

Definitions

Loss can be defined as *giving up external or internal supports required by the person to satisfy basic needs.* In regard to loss, the term *object may mean a person, thing, relationship, or situation.*

Grief is a sequence of subjective states, a special intense form of sorrow and depression caused by loss, either through separation or death of a loved person or loss of an object that is felt to be a part of the self or that provides psychological gratification. Grief is the emotion involved in the work of mourning. Absence of that which is lost is felt as a gap in one's sense of continuity and self-concept.

Grief reaction differs from depression in that cognitive disorders, such as gross distortion of events, are not normally present in grief; also, the reaction is more directly proportional to the amount of loss. In depression, the feeling of sadness and self-depreciation affects the person physically, intellectually, cognitively, emotionally, socially, and spiritually; it is out of proportion to the apparent situation, and is more greatly influenced by developmental and symbolic changes[5].

Mourning is a broad range of reactions, a psychological process that follows either loss of a significant or valued object or person or realization that such a loss could occur. It is the process whereby the person seeks to disengage himself from an emotionally demanding relationship and reinvest emotionally in a new and productive relationship.

Grief and the Mourning Process

A review of the grief syndrome described by Lindemann and the stages of grief and mourning described by Engel provide an understanding of the dynamics involved when any crisis results in a grief and mourning reaction[36, 16].

Upon becoming aware of the loss, the person is likely to feel somatic distress and an altered sensorium. The somatic symptoms last from 20 minutes to a few days, and may include shortness of breath, choking, sighing, hyperventilation, chills, tremors, fatigue, anorexia, tightness in the throat, emptiness in the abdomen, and loss of strength. The altered sensorium exists during the stages of shock and disbelief or defensive retreat. Included may be feelings of unreality, emotional distance from people, intense preoccupation with the image or occasional hallucination of the lost object or person, helplessness, loneliness, and disorganization. In spite of apparent intellectual and verbalized acceptance of the loss, the implications of the loss are not comprehended. The person may overtly behave as if nothing happened or may be unable to carry out ordinary activities of living, lacking energy, organization, and initiative in doing daily tasks. The person may at times seem out of contact with reality and express feelings of despair and anguish as the reality of loss penetrates awareness.

Increased preoccupation with the lost object, a heightened desire to talk about the loss, a search for evidence of failure "to do right," verbal self-accusation, and ambivalence toward the lost object become manifested with increasing awareness of loss.

The greater the ambivalence felt toward the lost object or person, the greater the feelings of guilt and shame. With any love relationship, the person will also at times feel anger or dislike toward, or desire to be rid of, the person, along with love feelings toward him. In addition, the grieving person may feel angry at the lost (deceased, divorced, or separated) person for having left him. Guilt and anger feelings, a normal part of grieving, are frequently displaced onto others: the doctor, nurse, employer, family member, or God. If guilt is not resolved, self-blame for the loss and preoccupation with it, with future losses, or with his own death will occur. Unsuccessful attempts at expiating guilt and anger may be made by blindly identifying with the lost object, by quickly seeking a substitute relationship or object, by absorbing oneself in work, by overindulging in alcohol or drugs, or by literally fleeing from the situation. The person may fear he is going crazy because of felt despair, helplessness, hopelessness, and guilt. (Early crisis therapy can reduce the intensity of some of these reactions.)

Crying (the intensity of which depends on the culture) helps to express some of the anguish and is a form of communication that engenders support from others. In America, loss through death is one situation in which adult tears, even in the male, are acceptable and cause no loss of respect.

The Importance of Ceremonies. Restitution for or adaptation to the loss, the actual work of mourning, is assisted by religious, cultural, or legal ceremonies.

For example, the funeral ceremony, with the gathering of people who share the loss of the dead person and who either need or can give support to the grieving survivors, serves several purposes. It helps to emphasize the reality of the death, to minimize the expression of anger, and to expiate guilt. In addition, support is sought from a more powerful figure (God, Allah). Emphasis is placed on the possibility of life and reunion after death in some religions, and the process of identification with the deceased is initiated. Through the ceremony the person symbolically expresses triumph over death and denies fear of death. The shared fellowship of a meal before or after the funeral, common in some subcultures, symbolically expresses return to life through the oral incorporation of eating and talking. The ceremony is the public way of adapting to the loss. But the persons closest to the deceased will continue to suffer for some time after the ceremony.

Other ceremonies dealing with separation or loss and involving the work of mourning may not be as extensive, obvious, or sad as a funeral. However, each culture provides ways to help the person acknowledge separation or loss. In fact, some of these ceremonies are joyous occasions, for the loss or separation means leaving behind old ways and behavior and being promoted or progressing to a new stage of life or adopting new behavior. For example, consider the baptism or circumcision; the birthday or graduation party; the first communion, confirmation, or Bar Mitzvah; the engagement or baby shower; and the retirement party. Although these ceremonies vary in degree of overt expression and intensity of feeling, they each represent essentially what the funeral represents after the death of a loved one.

Stages in the Mourning Process. Resolving loss, whether the death of a loved one or the loss of a significant object, status, or job, involves a number of steps.

The loss is first felt as a defect in the psychic self as the mourner becomes aware of innumerable ways in which he was dependent upon the lost object as a source of gratification, for a feeling of well-being, for effective functioning, and for his sense of self. He is not ready to accept a new object in place of the old one, although passively and transiently he may accept a more dependent relationship with remaining objects, roles, or persons.

The mourner becomes increasingly aware of his own body. In addition to developing symptoms that are a normal part of grieving, he may develop symptoms similar to those suffered by a deceased loved person. This identification process maintains a tie with the deceased loved one and appeases some of the guilt felt for harboring earlier aggressive or angry feelings toward the dead person. How such symptoms are expressed depends on the person's constitutional factors as well as on past learning about which symptoms are most likely to get attention or to be defined as illness by the self and others.

The person is preoccupied with the lost object; there is a strong wish to have a continuing experience with the lost object. The mourner frequently talks about that which is lost, the pleasant memories and events associated with it. Constantly talking about the loss and its meaning is one way of reinforcing reality as well as of expiating guilt through repeated self-assurance that all possible action was taken to prevent the loss. This repetitious talking continues until the person forms an image in his mind almost completely devoid of negative characteristics of the lost object to replace that which no longer exists in the real world. This process of idealization follows the difficult and painful experience of alternating guilt, remorse, fear, and regret for real or fantasied past acts of hostility, neglect, and lack of appreciation, or even for personal responsibility for the loss or death.

Through identification following idealization, the mourner consciously or unconsciously adopts some of the behavior and admired qualities of the dead person. He changes his interests in the direction of activities formerly enjoyed by the lost loved one, adopts that person's goals and ideals, or even takes on certain mannerisms of the deceased. As this final identification is accomplished, preoccupation with the deceased, ambivalence, guilt, and sadness decrease and thoughts return to life. If strong guilt is present, the person is more likely to take on undesirable characteristics, including the last disease symptoms, of the deceased. This negative identity may lead later to psychopathology.

Feelings are gradually withdrawn from the lost object. A yearning to be with the lost person is replaced by a wish to renew life. The person gradually un-learns old ways of living and learns new life patterns. The lost object becomes detached from the person and is enshrined in the form of a memory, memorial, or monument. At first, the person's renewed concern for others may be directed toward other mourners or other persons in crisis. It is easier to feel closeness with someone who has experienced a similar loss.

Finally, the person becomes interested in new objects and relationships, and he allows himself new pleasures and enjoyments. At first the replacements must be very much like the former object, but eventually new relationships are formed and objects acquired that are equally or even more satisfying.

Acceptance—the Successful Work of Mourning—may take 6 to 12 months. Complete resolution of or adaptation to the crisis of loss is indicated by the ability to remember comfortably and realistically both the pleasures and disappointments of the lost relationship. When the mourning process is adaptive or successful, the person is capable of carrying on his life with new relationships without mental or physical illness.

This syndrome of feelings, thoughts, and behavior, although varying somewhat in sequence or intensity from person to person, is characteristic of grief and mourning.

Factors Influencing the Outcome of Mourning

In addition to the factors mentioned earlier that affect the resolution of any crisis, the duration of reaction and manner in which the person adjusts to the changed social environment after loss also depend on the following factors:

1. Degree of dependency for support from the lost object. The greater the dependency, the more difficult is emancipation from the lost object and resolution of loss.
2. Degree of ambivalence toward the lost object. Since ambivalence in a relationship determines the amount of felt guilt, this emotion slows the processes of idealization, identification, and reinvestment of emotional energy in new objects.
3. Preparation for loss ("anticipatory grieving"), whether the loss was expected or had only been briefly thought of some time in the past.
4. Number and nature of other relationships. If prior to his loss the person derived satisfaction from a variety of other objects, persons, or roles, he now has more bases of support and can more readily form new relationships.
5. Age of the mourner or of the deceased person. The death of a young person generally has a more profound effect on mourners than the death of an aged person in American culture. There is the feeling of great social loss for the young person who has had inadequate time to fulfill himself. Among mourners, children generally have less capacity for resolving loss

than adults because of their relative inexperience with crisis and abstract thinking.

6. Changes in the pattern of living necessitated by loss of a person, money, job, pet, valuable possessions, role, or status.
7. Social and cultural roles of the mourner as defined by society. In American culture, mourning dress, fasting, and sacrifice are indefinitely prescribed. The role of mourner may also conflict with other roles—for example, with masculine or wage-earner role. Society makes little provision for replacement of the loss or for discharge of hostility and guilt created by loss.

In general, obstacles to the normal progression of grieving arise when the person tries to avoid the intense distress connected with the grief experience and the expression of related emotions.

Nursing Process for the Person Experiencing Loss

The nurse's role with the person experiencing any kind of significant loss is essentially the same as with the person and family experiencing the greatest loss, death. For a thorough account of these nursing measures, see Murray and Zentner's chapter on death as the last developmental stage[40].

Reactions to loss are not always obvious. In assessing the patient who is admitted for a medical or surgical illness following a serious loss, direct your assessment and intervention to the mourning process as well as to the illness. Recognize the necessity of grief work for this patient if he is to achieve his optimum level of wellness.

The principles of crisis intervention described earlier and the concepts of primary, secondary, and tertiary prevention are applicable to the person experiencing loss.

You can help the person finish the mourning process by supporting him as he disengages himself from the significant object and seeks new and rewarding relationships and patterns of living. The person cannot be hurried through mourning to resolution of the crisis. He will need encouragement as well as a time and place to talk, weep, and resolve grief. He will need help in developing his philosophy about life to the point where he can again tolerate stress, changing his behavior to meet the situation rather than using behavioral mechanisms excessively to protect himself from reality. Encourage the person to do what he can for himself. Help him experiment with new modes of living and behaving and with new relationships. At times you may be a source of anxiety to this person as you attempt to encourage change and growth, but your simultaneous support will aid his resolution.

The person who has been in mourning for some time may exhibit inappropriate behavior. Denial, feelings of emptiness, self-depreciation, anger at self and others, self-pity, somatic complaints, hopelessness, and helplessness may be expressed. Although such behavior may be disturbing, this person needs respect and acceptance from you and others before he can again respect himself and accept his life situation.

ILLNESS: A SITUATIONAL CRISIS

In order to further relate crisis theory to nursing practice, the most common type of family crisis, illness, will be discussed. Chapter 1 furnishes a basis for the discussion in this section.

Illness may be defined as *an experience, manifesting itself through observable or felt changes in the body, that interferes with the person's capacity to carry out minimum functions appropriate to his customary status* [64].

The sensory quality of the illness experience is the result of nerve receptors. Exteroceptors include the organs of reception for visual, gustatory, olfactory, and auditory sensations. Interoceptors include organs of reception for sensations of pain, touch, pressure, warmth, and cold. Proprioceptors transmit impulses for tension, position, and movement. Illness can be experienced as a change in the intensity, extension, preciseness, or duration of sensation from any of these receptors, accompanying various pathological states [64].

Influences on Illness Susceptibility

In addition to the influences on health and illness discussed in Chapter 1, the difference in illness susceptibility from person to person may arise from differences in perception and evaluation of the environment, or from innate constitutional differences, or both. There is usually a relationship between the frequency of a person's illness episodes and the manner in which he perceives life situations. Those who perceive their life experiences as challenging, demanding, and conflict-laden suffer more disturbances of bodily processes, mood, thought, and behavior. Susceptibility to illness may also be influenced by actions taken to avoid illness and by age, since adaptive defenses are not well developed in the very young and are less effective in the very old. Developmental level also influences perception and response to environmental demands [21].

Every person is active in a number of social roles that place various demands upon him and call for shifts and flexibility in attitude and behavior. However, at times the kinds and nature of the roles in which the person is involved are demanding or stressful to the point of contributing to illness. For example, the occupational role is important. Whether the person is a farmer, nurse, steel-mill worker, or an office clerk predisposes him to different kinds of illness.

The family contributes not only to genetic predisposition but also to the actual etiology of specific diseases through the transmission of social values, the socialization process of the child, and the family pattern of daily living and behavior.

Since health is a multidimensional concept involving varying degrees of feelings, performance, and symptoms, the family places a certain value on health as well as a definition, often unspoken, of what they consider to be illness. For the person from a low socioeconomic background, symptoms are important only if they interfere with his everyday functions and work. Therefore he goes to the doctor only when he is severely ill. Perhaps only after the symptoms are corrected does he admit how ill he was, since previously the pressure to earn a living wage kept him going. For some people, health is so highly valued that they are acutely aware of many body sensations, and any unusual ones are considered symptoms of illness and reported promptly to the doctor. While the latter value system can signal hypochondria, it is also the system that permits early diagnosis and a greater degree of health promotion. The family attitude toward money and spending indirectly affects their value on health. For some, the new car or television set is more important than the elective surgery or treatment that can be postponed.

The definition of illness is learned by the child through family values. For example, if the father is a construction worker who uses his back muscles considerably on the job, he and his wife are likely to express concern verbally and nonverbally when he suffers backache. His back represents a job, status, money, and masculinity to him. The child perceives the situation; later, if he feels uncomfortable, he may also complain of backache. He soon learns he will get his parents' attention because of their value on this part of the anatomy. Backache is defined as illness in this family, while other symptoms or signs of equal or greater intensity or potential severity may go unattended. The child is likely to keep this orientation into adulthood. Likewise the pianist, minister, and editor will emphasize their hands, voice, and eyes, respectively. Such attitudes have to be recognized and worked with in health teaching and care. Just telling the person which symptoms are regarded as a threat to health is useless. The person's behavior depends upon his own definition of illness.

The family pattern of living and the socialization of family members are influential in contributing to and defining illness—for example, through eating and rest habits, housing and sanitation standards, leisure-time pursuits and hobbies. The family that places a high value on food or has learned to use food for tension release is more likely to contain obese members who develop illnesses related to obesity. The athletic family is more likely to suffer sprains, bruises, and fractures. A tension-filled family life may contribute to mental illness, and indirectly to physical illness or socially maladjusted behavior.

Factors Determining the Definition of Illness

People in American society perceive illness as an obstacle to goal achievement, an interruption in the rhythm of life, a personal crisis, a frustration of normal life patterns and enjoyments, a disruption in social relations, or a punishment for misdeeds[64]. Thus illness is considered a deviant role because the culture enforces an unusually high level of activity, independence, and responsibility on the person. Illness is closely related in people's minds to the role of childhood dependency. Moreover, resorting too frequently to illness as an escape poses a threat to the stability of social systems. Thus the institutionalized role of illness involves important mechanisms of social control: during illness certain behaviors are expected of the sick person and his caretakers.

Being ill involves more than being admitted to a health center or visiting the doctor. When you first see the patient during the diagnostic process, the disease may be at midpoint. The diagnosis or definition of illness does not usually occur until after the symptoms are felt and described by the person to someone, usually in his family; both the person and family agree that he is ill; and a course of action is planned.

The person recognizes himself as ill from the cues given by the illness, such as his own uncomfortable sensations, or the statements, facial expressions, or actions of others. Recognition of illness is usually made when present cues are seen to agree with past experience. In the absence of familiar cues, the person may fail to recognize his illness or become so apprehensive that he denies it. Even familiar cues may cause sufficient anxiety so that the person denies them and his illness experience[64].

Whether or not the family or others validate the person's definition of his illness depends on their pattern of interaction with him, their expectations of him, and their past experience with his being ill. Does he "cry wolf" too often? Does he malinger? Is he acting "like a baby" now? Such interpretations are likely to cause the family to prod the person to persevere in his independent, healthy role. The person's role within the family is also crucial. The breadwinner of the family may feel that he cannot afford to recognize illness unless it is severe enough to interfere with his ability to work.

Hence the family can either accept or reject the person as ill. In turn, the person will accept or reject the family definition of the situation, depending upon how he feels. If he continues to define himself as ill, he will seek help. When he declares himself to be ill, he enters the sick role.

The person's course of action is dependent upon previous illness and health care experience, the kinds of help traditionally sought by his family, his knowledgeability about illness and the health care system, his value system, his religion, and a variety of other factors. Such factors include the nature, visibility, seriousness, and intensity of the illness; the body part involved; the extent to which symptoms interfere with daily patterns of living; the anticipated consequences of the illness; the person's tolerance for abnormality; his tendency to be concerned about self; and the availability, cost, and convenience of treatment facilities. Social class, culture, age, sex, and occupational status are additional determinants of this behavior[64].

The person may seek help for his illness from any one of a number of resources: a family member, neighbor, local pharmacist, chiropractor, osteopath, a medical "quack," soothsayer, religious advisor, herbalist, midwife, nurse, or medical doctor.

Perhaps the best way to insure that a patient will seek a qualified health care worker in any *future* crisis of illness is to treat and care for him in a way that he perceives as helpful in his *present* one.

The Sick Role

Illness forces the person to assume a social posture to which he is unaccustomed, called the *sick role* by Parsons and Lederer[44, 33]. In the sick role, he comes into contact with the caretakers—doctors, nurses, or other health workers—whose jobs are defined by society. In addition, society defines who is sick and who is well. What is considered illness in one culture is not so considered in another.

In the sick role, the person has declared himself to be in a position where he must be taken care of. Society and the health care system reinforce that he is not competent to care for himself. He cannot do—nor supposedly, does he know— what needs to be done. Thus he must follow the orders of others and let others make decisions for and about him. The sick role frees the person from responsibility for his illness, but it carries the obligation to cooperate with caretakers and to get well. Medical workers get frustrated, angry, or judgmental when it appears that the person will not or cannot get well. While the person is "working" to return to an independent, healthy status, society frees him from his ordinary duties, obligations, and responsibilities. Thus the sick person's two rights are: (1) exemption from usual responsibilities, and (2) absolution of blame for illness. His three obligations are to: (1) view his illness as undesirable, (2) want to get well, and (3) seek competent help from and cooperate with his caretakers.

Certain Adaptive Behaviors normally unacceptable to society are common during illness and are considered helpful in promoting rest and recovery. By accepting illness, the structure of the person's world becomes simpler and more constricted. He becomes somewhat dependent and regressed, either because of the unpleasant sensations, physical weakness, and helplessness caused by the illness; because of society's expectations; or from egocentricity, feelings of helplessness, and concerns about his body functions and routines administered for his welfare. Withdrawal into self rather than interest in others, a focus on the present rather than on the past or the future, and a reduced ability to concentrate and to think abstractly are all typical behaviors of the sick person. Routines may seem too burdensome, so that daily activities such as taking a bath and personal grooming may be avoided, if possible, by the sick person. Through social, emotional, and physical regression and in compliance with the medical plan, the sick person redistributes his energies to encourage the healing process.

The patient is simultaneously in a position of great power and of extreme weakness. This combination of domination and dependence provokes a difficult inner conflict, a certain ambivalence similar to what young children feel at times. The patient in essence loves the authority figure (the nurse or doctor) for taking care of him, while simultaneously feeling angry toward him or her for being powerful while he is essentially helpless.

Certain Deviant or Maladaptive Behaviors in the sick role may occur and be so labeled by the medical team because the behaviors do not assist the person in getting physically well or regaining independence. When the person uses illness for secondary gain, attention, escape from responsibility, control, or manipulation of others in his environment, he does not move through the sick role to return to health at the expected pace or in the expected way.

The health team also considers the patient deviant if he is unable to accept the dependent sick role. Often this pattern occurs when the person has unresolved dependency-independency conflicts. The patient may fear becoming dependent, or he may actually long to be dependent and feel guilty about this urge. Strongly independent behavior such as protracted denial of illness, unwarranted physical activity, or refusal to cooperate with health care workers may be a signal of such inner conflicts. Recognize, however, that in some cultures the ill person may refuse a dependent role because of expectations of himself and others[60]. On the other hand, excessive dependency, using illness as a refuge, and refusing to engage in self-care activities within one's strength limitations are as detrimental to getting well as is excessively independent behavior.

The patient may hinder his progress by becoming apathetic or uninterested in his recovery. Overly compliant, submissive, docile behavior should not be mistaken for cooperation with the treatment plan. Rather, the person's feelings of powerlessness and hopelessness, the lack of initiative and enthusiasm, signs of physical and emotional depression, or an apparent retreat as if waiting for death appear to diminish natural body responses for recovery[64].

In addition, any maladaptive response noted in this chapter's discussion of crisis may occur and can hinder progress to recovery, at least from the viewpoint of the medical team.

The Culture of Illness

Although the prescribed medical care may be identical, a person acts and is treated differently if he is sick at home or sick in the hospital. In his home, the person is in a familiar environment; he can retain his sense of dignity, rights, and privileges and can insist on being treated on his own terms. He is reinforced by family and friends, who accord him special concessions. These prerogatives are generally disregarded when the sick person enters a hospital in the American health care system.

Hospitalization may be defined as *confinement of a person to an institution, away from his family, for a varying amount of time. Its purposes may be diagnosis; care or treatment that is palliative, rehabilitative, or curative in nature; or restoration of the person to a previous state, such as return to a non-pregnant state after delivery.*

Upon hospitalization, personal possessions are stripped from the person. Gone are familiar surroundings that afford a sense of security. Instead there are various strange, disquieting, and bothersome odors, noises, and sights. At home the health care worker rings the bell and waits for the door to open. In the hospital the patient rings the bell and waits for a nurse to come. At home the doctor is on call, the nurse is a visitor, and the relatives belong. In the hospital the patient is admitted and discharged, the health care workers perform their duties, and relatives are the visitors. At home everyone present acknowledges the patient's every whim. In the hospital all health care workers are in a distinct position to grant or withhold small and very precious favors from him, often depending on their personal judgment of him and his behavior[9].

Reactions to Hospitalization

In the best of settings, the patient is overwhelmed with many strange, foreboding, conflicting, or frightening feelings. In spite of the many people around, he feels isolated and lonely. In fact, lack of privacy, with the intrusion of these many workers into his room, often unannounced, is a frequent complaint. Compartmentalization of care, bureaucracy, and other characteristics of the hospital within the health care system discussed in Chapter 2 combine to strip the patient of his individuality and identity. He is robbed unnecessarily of decision-making power and any sense of responsibility by a rigid schedule and ritualistic routines. Moreover, his body rhythms are disrupted.

The hospital often means separation from valued persons, objects, and activities. It may seem to be a place where one is sent in retaliation for inappropriate behavior or at least a place that inflicts undesirable controls and forced conformity. There is endless waiting and the feeling of boredom, aimlessness, and sameness every day. On the other hand, some patients may consider the hospital more as a source of relief. It may seem a secure place, with its emergency equipment and trained concerned personnel, where basic needs can be met without effort of the self. For still others, the hospital is a place to go to die[64].

Health team members should consider some of the possible undesirable side effects of hospitalization on the patient:

1. Enforced dependency on strange authority figures.
2. Dramatic changes in the physical environment.
3. Disruption of daily routines and preferences.
4. Separation from family.
5. Different behavioral expectations imposed by the sick role.
6. Forced adjustment to and interaction with a variety of strangers at a highly vulnerable time.
7. Depersonalization, loss of privacy and freedom, and fostered regression.

8. Increased anxiety from all of these effects, which may cause further physical and mental changes and further impede progression toward wellness.

Thus illness, especially if it necessitates hospitalization, is a crisis. The person is moving from familiar into strange territory, and his usual patterns of behavior are not adequate to cope in the strange situation. The crisis becomes greater in its impact when, as a result of the illness, the person must thereafter live with a chronic debilitating or disabling condition or when a structure or function of the body has been altered.

Stages of Illness

The crisis of illness does not occur as an isolated event in the life of the person. The psychological states that occur during illness do not represent a change or difference in the person so much as temporary adaptive behaviors that maintain or promote restoring the presickness self. The reactions to illness must be understood in terms of the person's prior personality organization. Thus adopting the sick role and going through the phases of crisis during the stages of illness are maladaptive only when the person is *not* sick by commonly accepted standards.

The stages of illness described by Janis, and listed next, fit into the phases of crisis described earlier[25].

Transition from Health to Illness, the First Stage, lasts from the time the person first considers that he might be ill until he and others around him acknowledge that he is. During this period he may show signs of emotional shock if the illness is acute or severe and the disruption to normal life is considerable. Then denial is used, at least briefly, to minimize or ignore the symptoms. If denial is strong, the person has a feeling that nothing can happen to him, that he never felt better, and he may engage in more than the usual amount of activity. Denial is usually impossible to maintain for a prolonged time because of pressure from others, feelings of extreme discomfort, or manifestation of more symptoms when the person tries to maintain normal behavior.

Acceptance of Illness, the Second Stage, occurs when the person feels the reality and impact of his illness, acknowledges the illness, seeks validation from significant others, seeks help from a caretaker, and enters into the sick role with all the related behaviors previously described. During illness the patient may go through a mourning process for loss of body function or structure, even if such loss is temporary. During this time the patient has many worries—job, finances, ability of the family to manage without him (or her), fidelity of the spouse, child care, and loss of status. He may become aggressive or haughty, displacing anger on others, even though he feels weak or inadequate. Or he may be passive in order to control his fears and anger.

The stigma, embarrassment, or shame felt because of illness begins to be worked through along with the emasculating or defeminizing effects felt as part of the illness. Feelings of rejection, of being abandoned, and self-pity gradually diminish.

Different body parts and certain body functions may have great significance to the patient. If these have been altered by illness or the treatment plan, the distortion in body image that occurs must be resolved before the patient can enter the last stage of illness, convalescence. Gradually the coping mechanisms are reorganized and perception becomes more realistic.

Convalescence, the Last Stage, is analogous to the adaptation or resolution phase of crisis. Now the patient returns to health. Or, in the case where there is a permanent disability and no further physical improvement is possible, convalescence marks a gradual increase in satisfying experiences. The patient's new sense of worth and reduced anxiety enable him again to utilize those abilities typical of health. This period is like moving from adolescence to adulthood. The person is reassessing the meaning of his life and is becoming increasingly independent, stable, outward-looking, and involved in decision making[41].

There are many variations in convalescence. Physical convalescence frequently occurs before emotional convalescence or resolution of the illness. The person's level of maturity, the kind of crisis intervention given, and the environment in which the person must function combine to determine progress. Whether others encourage constructive activity or passive, less adaptative behavior influences how thoroughly the person will resolve his feelings about having been ill. Then again, health may represent more of a threat than illness due to the pressures of life. If illness justifies irresponsible behavior, provides an escape from obligations, or satisfies emotional or financial needs, then the person may actively (although perhaps unconsciously) resist convalescence.

Tasks of Convalescence

Certain tasks must be accomplished, in addition to solving the practical problems of returning home from the hospital, in order to go from illness to full emotional and physical health. The minor adaptations in the physical environment of the home and in the daily routine can usually be easily made. Then the family and friends expect the newly discharged patient to be grateful for recovery and for what they have done for him, to be cheerful about rejoining his loved ones, and to be eager to return to his usual way of life. However, they may soon find he is unable to live up to these expectations.

Before the patient can resume his usual activities and make the transition back to health, he must first accomplish the three tasks of convalescence described by Norris[41]. Only then will he have resolved his crisis.

Reassessment of Life's Meaning is one of the primary tasks for the convalescing patient. He thinks about his goals and purposes and perhaps even the meaning of death, and redirects his energies toward development of his full potential for living.

Reintegration of Body Image becomes a second major task after the acute phase of illness, when the patient is less concerned about any threat to his life. Scarring, deformity, impaired functioning, or removal of valued organs must be dealt with and integrated into himself. The person must work through feeling dependent, "dirty," repulsive, unattractive, or possibly totally unacceptable to certain others. Moreover, he may not feel the same even if there has been no actual change in his body structure or function.

Moving from the dependent patient role to independent adult status takes time and help. The person must feel self-interest, assertiveness, and persistence. Independence cannot be demanded from the patient; it is the result of work, usually nurse-patient work.

Resolution of Role Changes or Reversals that have occurred during the illness is a third major task and must be worked out within the patient and in relation to family members. After illness, there are no prescribed behaviors for convalescence, but the person usually does not fully assume his normal responsibilities for some time. Seeing the family members carry out some of his responsibilities may be difficult for him, and family members themselves usually look forward to a return to the normal pattern of living with less burden.

Added to the problem of continued role changes are the mood swings and other unpredictable responses of the convalescing patient—behavior that may be quite unlike his pre-illness personality. Some distance still exists between the convalescing person and the rest of the activities going on around him.

Today, the sick person often returns early to his home for convalescence or rehabilitation. Before the patient's discharge, you must learn if he has a family to care for him or at least a place to go, whether he has transportation to get home, and how he will manage within specific limits, such as restrictions on mobility or diet. Every patient comes from a culture and a community and returns to the same. Do not make assumptions; rather, ask the patient what his situation is so that realistic plans can be made. If you listen and use nondirective interviewing techniques, you can help the patient and family reexamine their lives, marshal their strengths, and focus their energies on convalescence.

The person who has a fatal illness will not truly convalesce, yet he may enjoy periods of essentially good physical health. The reaction of the person who is terminally ill must be understood in terms of numerous and sometimes conflicting factors, taking into account previous relationships and previous experiences with crisis, particularly illness and loss. There must be an understanding of the significance of family, social group, occupation, and religion as well as of the external sources of love, comfort, and support. The person's self-concept and body image, his ability to recognize and cope with reality, and his responses to dependency, pain, and uncertainty will influence his overall reaction. Other crucial factors are the nature of the specific illness; the organ or body system affected, along with its symbolic as well as real significance to the person; the type of treatment required; and the degree of functional loss and disfigurement.

Impaired Role Behavior Related to Illness

Following illness or surgery, the person may not regain complete health; he may remain chronically ill. He then reaches a state where he gets neither better nor worse, but is no longer viewed by himself or by society as being ill. He may even be disabled by a condition that imposes a restriction on activity and provokes social prejudice and stigma[63]. Examples of such conditions include blindness, deafness, and cases where some body part or function is congenitally or surgically absent or malfunctioning. The disability may or may not be obvious, but the person considers himself well most of the time. He has emotionally resolved the crisis that surrounded his disability, but he has limited ability to carry on usual roles and responsibilities. For the disabled person who is not experiencing illness, social pressures serve to aid him in maintaining normal behavior within the limits of his potential. This situation is called impaired role behavior[20].

The behavior of the person depends on his perception of his disability as well as on the perceptions of others around him. Some persons who are chronically ill or congenitally or surgically disabled will remain in the sick role indefinitely. Such persons have not resolved the crisis of illness; the person with impaired role behavior has.

Characteristics of Impaired Role Behavior differ from those of the sick role. Thomas suggests that **impaired role behavior** *is an extension of the sick role. The disabled person, however, is not considered by society to be exempt from normal behavior or responsibilities within the limits of his conditon.* He is expected, as far as possible, to improve or modify his life situation in the light of his disability, to make the most of his remaining capabilities to overcome the disability, and to accept his limits realistically. He is then considered rehabilitated and no longer in the sick role[56].

The behavioral responses of the disabled person also depend on his feelings of being accepted or rejected. Schutz describes the basic human need to be included rather than excluded from others, to feel lovable, worthwhile, significant, competent, and responsible. The disabled person desires and needs to have some close relationships with nondisabled persons and needs to be accepted by others for what he is, in spite of his disability[50].

Disability often forces the person to modify his self-concept and self-image. New and different body sensations, changed appearance or body functions, and changed or reduced abilities challenge the person's self-confidence. He may feel shame, worthlessness, and inferiority, often to a degree not justified by the condition. Negative responses from others then intensify low self-esteem, and a negative self-image results, for everyone learns to incorporate the image that others have of him into his self-concept.

The disabled person is expected to learn to adjust and respond to being dependent on the aid of others to complete tasks or meet his needs, in spite of the American cultural emphasis on self-reliance and independence. He is expected to share in the management of his medical condition and be involved in decisions regarding his treatment and care. He will be asked to explain his disability to others, often revealing considerable personal information, and accept that he is an object of curiosity medically and socially. He recognizes that by means of these explanations, he is helping to reduce social stigma, pity, and prejudice, and this will eventually permit him greater opportunities to realize his potentialities.

The primary reason for considering impaired role behavior is that some people are neither ill—and therefore governed by sick-role norms—nor healthy in the usual sense. The well-adjusted disabled person views himself as physically or psychosocially restricted rather than ill.

In contrast, not accepting one's disability and its attendant limitations results in behavior that interferes with maintenance of health, prevention of further illness, and performance of social roles. Such a person is considered deviant in his behavior in that he remains in the sick role.

Nursing Responsibility

The Nursing Process and Principles Described Earlier in this chapter and in Chapter 4 are applicable to the care of the sick person and his family. The principles of crisis intervention combined with the necessary physical care will help the person reach his maximum potential.

The Meaning of the Illness and Related Care Determine Behavior. Diagnostic and treatment activities that the ill person encounters can be classified into four categories, according to the amount of threat perceived in each activity. Since these activities carry certain meanings, you can predict with some degree of certainty the person's behavior. Diagnostic, treatment, or care activities may involve the following feelings[63]:

1. Intrusion or forceful entry into a body orifice, such as in an enema, catheterization, irrigation, gastric intubation, or injection.
2. Invasion of privacy, as in a probing interview, a vaginal or rectal examination, or undue exposure of the body during care.
3. Threat of pain, suffering, or annihilation, such as presented by surgery or any other care procedure that threatens to distort, alter, or destroy the person's body image.
4. Little or no threat, as in taking routine vital signs or bedmaking.

Surgery may have any or all of the following meanings to a patient: pain; the unknown; fear of not being told the truth; mutilation and changes in the body image caused by incisions and removals; fear of death; disruption of life plans, including occupational and recreational; and fear of loss of control under anesthesia[13].

Establishing a Frame of Reference is helpful in preparing the patient for diagnostic, treatment, or care measures. If he can compare a familiar event or sensation to the event he is about to experience, the event will seem less strange to him. He will feel less threatened and more in control of the situation, and illness can be better tolerated and perceived more realistically. Of course, the frame of reference must have meaning for the patient. For example, a breast biopsy could be compared to the removal of a mole. If a procedure is going to hurt, the sensation should be described to the patient—for example, as feeling like the pain of a burn from a hot stove, a needle prick, a toothache, or abdominal pressure from having overeaten. A patient usually will not engage in a comparison of the sensation or experience of illness without prompting; his main concern is to get relief from it.

If the person has been prepared intellectually to expect certain consequences, such as the possible outcome of a diagnostic procedure or the complexity of a tentative treatment plan, his emotional reaction will be less disorganized when he learns that the possibilities have become reality. He needs help in thinking about the possibilities of what might happen so that he can utilize certain behavioral mechanisms that help him cope with potential and actual danger. His behavior will become more cooperative with the health care team, whereas when the person's perception of the diagnostic or treatment plan is anxiety-laden and negative, his behavior is likely to be negative and uncooperative[25, 27]. You will be the health team member best qualified to do this preparation.

Consider the Less Obvious but Equally Important Needs of Patients, such as esthetic needs. Eliminate or at least control unpleasant sights, sounds, and odors whenever possible. Consider the likes and dislikes of the patient and his family. Let the family or patient make decisions about "the little things that count" as long as they do not interfere with the treatment plan. Help the person maintain his identity by addressing him by his proper title and name. Encourage bringing some personal possessions from home, and instruct patient and family about hospital routines and policies in order to reduce feelings of strangeness, isolation, and powerlessness. Flexible visiting hours can reduce loneliness and anxiety related to separation from loved ones.

As a nurse, you will coordinate various activities of other health care workers as well as perform the unique functions of care called *nursing*. Many times you are the only care giver prepared to understand the total person and his many unique needs while engaging in a therapeutic process with the patient.

The Tasks of Convalescence can best be accomplished when patient, family, and nurse collaborate, with the patient doing most of the work. Promote realistic adaptation by explaining to the patient and family the meaning of the crisis of illness and the tasks of convalescence. With shorter hospitalization the rule today, some resolution of feelings traditionally accomplished in the hospital must now be done at home. Be supportive and accepting, and help family and patient prepare for the tasks of convalescence to be managed at home after discharge. This preparation is as important as the discharge planning that helps the patient make necessary physical adaptations or learn self-care. The person may never be able to do the latter satisfactorily if he is given no help with the former.

Therapeutic communication is essential in helping the person resolve convalescence. Pick up his verbal cues. Reflect back pertinent statements. Do not feel you must give answers. Encourage him to talk about his thoughts and feelings so that he will arrive at his own answers.

Much of the physical care given in the hospital, such as bathing, changing dressing, guiding range-of-motion exercises, and positioning, could be done with greater thought directed toward helping the person acquaint himself with and accept his changed body. Preserve and emphasize his strengths, but do not ignore or minimize his problems. Realistic, pertinent teaching is essential for the patient to adapt to a changed body. Further information on assessment of and intervention for an adult with a changed body image is discussed by Murray and Zentner[40]. Recognize the signs of independence and promote it—without forcing the patient to be independent before he is ready.

Final discharge planning and preparing for termination of the nurse-patient relationship should be started long before the day of discharge. When you and the patient jointly work through feelings about termination, both of you feel less cheated or rejected when he leaves the hospital.

You can evaluate the effectiveness of care and preparation for convalescence best through follow-up home visits or interviews with patient and family upon their return to the clinic or doctor's office. Convalescence and the crisis of illness have been resolved when the person can talk about his illness or surgery with equanimity and acceptance. Convalescence is not resolved when the person needs to talk continuously about his illness experience or states that he "never did get over it!" You can help to prevent or minimize such responses.

By intervening as a crisis therapist, you are involved in promoting the health of the person and family in the present situation as well as in future crises. In turn, the health and functioning of the community is indirectly enhanced.

REFERENCES

1. Aguilera, D., J. Messick, and M. Farrell, *Crisis Intervention: Theory and Methodology*. St. Louis: The C. V. Mosby Company, 1970.

2. Baumann, Barbara, "Diversities in Conception of Health and Physical Fitness," *Journal of Health and Human Behavior*, 2 (1961), 39-46.

3. _____, and G. Kassenbaum, "Dimensions of the Sick Role in Chronic Illness," *Journal of Health and Human Behavior*, 6: No. 1 (1965), 16-27.

4.   Baziak, Anna, and Robert Dentan, "The Language of the Hospital and Its Effect on the Patient," in *Social Interaction and Patient Care*, eds. J. Skipper and R. Leonard. Philadelphia: J. B. Lippincott Company, 1965, pp. 272-77.

5.   Beck, Aaron, "Etiologies of Depression," in *The Medical Management of Depression*, eds. Denis Hill and Leo Hollister. New York: Lakeside Laboratories, 1970, pp. 17-20.

6.   Berliner, Beverly, "Nursing a Patient in Crisis," *American Journal of Nursing*, 70: No. 10 (1970), 2154-57.

7.   Blackwell, B., "Stigma," in *Behavioral Concepts and Nursing Intervention*, coord. C. Carlson. Philadelphia: J. B. Lippincott Company, 1970, pp. 317-30.

8.   Broden, Alexander, "Reaction to Loss in the Aged," in *Loss and Grief: Psychological Management in Medical Practice*, eds. B. Schoenberg, A. Carr, D. Peretz, and A. Kutscher. New York: Columbia University Press, 1970, pp. 199-217.

9.   Brown, Esther Lucille, *Newer Dimensions of Patient Care*. New York: Russell Sage Foundation, 1965.

10. Brown, H. F., V. Burdett, and C. Liddell, "The Crisis of Relocation," in *Crisis Intervention: Selected Readings*, ed. H. Parad. New York: Family Service Association of America, 1965, pp. 248-60.

11. Caplan, Gerald, *Principles of Preventive Psychiatry*. New York: Basic Books, Inc., 1964.

12. Carlson, C., "Grief and Mourning," in *Behavioral Concepts and Nursing Intervention:* coord. C. Carlson. Philadelphia: J. B. Lippincott Company, 1970, pp. 95-116.

13. Carnevali, Doris, "Preoperative Anxiety," *American Journal of Nursing*, 66: No. 7 (1966), 1536-38.

14. Carr, A., and B. Schoenberg, "Object Loss and Somatic Symptom Formation," in *Loss and Grief: Psychological Management in Medical Practice*, eds. B. Schoenberg, A. Carr, D. Peretz, and A. Kutscher. New York: Columbia University Press, 1970, pp. 36-48.

15. Christman, Luther, "Assisting the Patient to Learn the Patient Role," *Journal of Nursing Education*, 6: No. 2 (1967), 17-21.

16. Engel, George, *Psychological Development in Health and Disease*. Philadelphia: W. B. Saunders Company, 1962.

17. Evans, Frances Monet Carter, *Psychosocial Nursing*. New York: The Macmillan Company, 1971, chapter 2.

18. Fink, Stephen, "Crisis and Motivation: A Theoretical Model," *Archives of Physical Medicine and Rehabilitation*, 48: No. 11 (1967), 592-97.

19. Gebbie, K., "Treatment Drop Outs and the Role of the Crisis Therapist," *Journal of Psychiatric Nursing and Mental Health Services*, 6: No. 6 (1968), 328-33.

20. Gordon, Gerald, *Role Theory and Illness*. New Haven: College and University Press, 1966.

21. Hinkle, Lawrence, W. N. Christenson, F. D. Kane, A. Ostfeld, W. N. Thetford, and H. W. Wolff, "An Investigation of the Relation between Life Experience, Personality Characteristics, and General Susceptibility to Illness," *Psychosomatic Medicine*, 20: No. 4 (1958), 278-95.

22. Hollingshead, August, and Frederick Redlich, *Social Class and Mental Illness*. New York: John Wiley & Sons, Inc., 1958.

23. Jackson, Edgar, *Understanding Grief*. New York: Abington Press, 1967.

24. Jaco, E. Gartly, ed., *Patients, Physicians, and Illness* (2nd ed.). New York: The Free Press, 1972.

25. Janis, Irving, *Psychological Stress*. New York: John Wiley & Sons, Inc., 1958.

26. Johnson, Dorothy, "Powerlessness: A Significant Determinant in Patient Behavior," *Journal of Nursing Education*, 6: No. 2 (1967), 39-44.

27. Johnson, Jean, "Effects of Restructuring Patients' Expectations on Their Reactions to Threatening Events," *Nursing Research*, 21: No. 6 (1972), 499-504.

28. Joselson, Maurice, and Ruth Joselson, "Do Perceptual Changes Occur in Crisis? A Case Study," *Journal of Psychiatric Nursing and Mental Health Services*, 10: No. 5 (1972), 6-10.

29. Kasl, Stanislav, and Sidney Cobb, "Health Behavior, Illness Behavior, and Sick Role Behavior," *Archives of Environmental Health*, 12 (1966), 531-41.

30. Keining, Sr. Mary Martha, "Denial of Illness," in *Behavioral Concepts and Nursing Intervention*, coord. C. Carlson. Philadelphia: J. B. Lippincott Company, 1970, 9-28.

31. King, Joan "The Initial Interview: Basis for Assessment in Crisis Intervention," *Perspectives in Psychiatric Care*, 9: No. 6 (1971), 247-56.

32. Larson, Virginia, "What Hospitalization Means to Patients," *American Journal of Nursing*, 61: No. 5 (1961), 44.

33. Lederer, Henry, "How the Sick View Their World," *Journal of Social Issues*, 8 (1952), 4-15.

34. Lee, J., "Emotional Reactions to Trauma," *Nursing Clinics of North America*, 5: No. 4 (1970), 577-87.

35. Lewis, Garland, "Communications: A Factor in Meeting Emotional Crisis," *Nursing Outlook*, 13: No. 3 (1965), 36-39.

36. Lindemann, Eric, "Symptomology and Management of Acute Grief," *American Journal of Psychiatry*, 101 (1944), 141-48.

37. Maloney, Elizabeth, "The Subjective and Objective Definition of Crisis," *Perspectives in Psychiatric Care*, 9: No. 6 (1971), 257-68.

38. Messick, Janice, "Crisis Intervention Concepts: Implications for Nursing Practices," *Journal of Psychiatric Nursing and Mental Health Services*, 10: No. 5 (1972), 3-5.

39. Morley, W., "Crisis: Paradigm of Intervention," *Journal of Psychiatric Nursing*, 5: No. 6 (1967), 531-44.

40. Murray, Ruth, and Judith Zentner, *Nursing Assessment and Health Promotion through the Life Span*. Englewood Cliffs, N.J.: Prentice-Hall, Inc. 1975.

41. Norris, Catherine, "The Work of Getting Well," *American Journal of Nursing*, 69: No. 10 (1969), 2118-21.

42. Ossenberg, Richard, "The Experience of Deviance in the Patient Role: A Study of Class Differences," *Journal of Health and Human Behavior*, 3 (1962), 277-82.

43. Parad, H., ed., *Crisis Intervention: Selected Readings*. New York: Family Service Association of America, 1965.

44. Parsons, Talcott, *The Social System*. New York: The Free Press, 1951.

45. Peretz, David, "Development, Object-Relationships, and Loss," in *Loss and Grief: Psychological Management in Medical Practice*, eds. B. Schoenberg, A. Carr, D. Peretz, and A. Kutscher. New York: Columbia University Press, 1970, pp. 3-19.

46. _____, "Reaction to Loss," in *Loss and Grief: Psychological Management in Medical Practice*, eds. B. Schoenberg, A. Carr, D. Peretz, and A. Kutscher. New York: Columbia University Press, 1970, pp. 20-35.

47. Rapaport, Lydia, "The State of Crisis: Some Theoretical Considerations," in *Crisis Intervention: Selected Readings*, ed. Howard Parad. New York: Family Service Association of America, 1965.

48. Reeves, Robert, "The Hospital Chaplain Looks at Grief," in *Loss and Grief: Psychological Management in Medical Practice*, eds. B. Schoenberg, A. Carr, D. Peretz, and A. Kutscher. New York: Columbia University Press, 1970, pp. 362-72.

49. Robischon, Paulette, "The Challenge of Crisis Theory for Nursing," *Nursing Outlook*, 15: No. 7 (1967), 28-32.

50. Schutz, William, *FIRO: A Three Dimensional Theory of Interpersonal Behavior*. New York: Holt, Rinehart & Winston, Inc., 1960.

51. Selye, Hans, "The Stress Syndrome," *American Journal of Nursing*, 65: No. 3 (1965), 97-99.

52. Spiegel, John, "The Resolution of Role Conflict Within the Family," in *A Modern Introduction to the Family*, eds. Norman Bell and Ezra Vogel. Glencoe, Ill.: The Free Press of Glencoe, 1963.

53. Tarnower, William, "Psychological Needs of the Hospitalized Patient," *Nursing Outlook*, 13: No. 7 (1965), 28-30.

54. "The Sick Poor," *American Journal of Nursing*, 69: No. 11 (1969), 2424-54.

55. Thomas, Betty, "Clues to Patient Behavior," *American Journal of Nursing*, 63: No. 7 (1963), 100-102.

56. Thomas, Edwin, "Problems of Disability from the Perspective of Role Theory," *Journal of Health and Human Behavior*, 7: No. 1 (1966), 2-14.

57. Turner, Ralph, "Role Taking: Process Versus Conformity," in *Human Behavior and Social Process*, ed. Arnold Rose. Boston: Houghton Mifflin Company, 1962, pp. 20-38.

58. Ujhely, Gertrude, "What is Realistic Emotional Support?" *American Journal of Nursing*, 63: No. 7 (1963), 758-62.

59. ____, "Grief and Depression: Implications for Preventive and Therapeutic Care," *Nursing Forum*, 5: No. 2 (1966), 23-25.

60. Vincent, R., "Factors Influencing Patient Non-Compliance: A Theoretical Approach," *Nursing Research*, 20: No. 6 (1971), 509-16.

61. White, R., "The Scientific Limitation of Brain Death," *Hospital Progress*, 53: No. 3 (1972), 48-51.

62. Williams, Florence, "Intervention in Maturational Crisis," *Perspectives in Psychiatric Care*, 9: No. 6 (1971), 240-46.

63. Wright, Beatrice, *Physical Disability: A Psychological Approach*. New York: Harper & Row, Publishers, 1960.

64. Wu, Ruth, *Behavior and Illness*. Englewood Cliffs, N.J.: Prentice-Hall, Inc., 1973.

FACTORS INFLUENCING HEALTH IN A PLURALISTIC SOCIETY

CHAPTER 9

Man's Relationship
to His Environment

Study of this chapter will help you to:

1 Explore the scope of environmental pollution and the interrelationship of the different kinds of pollution with one another and with man.

2 Observe sources of air pollution in your community and identify resulting hazards to human health.

3 List types of water pollution and describe resultant health problems.

4 Describe substances that cause soil pollution and the effect of these substances upon the food chain as well as upon other facets of health.

5 Discuss the types of food pollution and ways to prevent food contamination.

6 Listen to sound pollution in various settings and discuss its long-term effects upon health.

7 Contrast the different types of surface pollution and resultant health problems.

8   Discuss and practice ways that, as a citizen, you can reduce environmental pollution.

9   Discuss your professional responsibility in assessing for illness caused by environmental pollutants and in taking general intervention measures.

10 Demonstrate an ability to help establish a therapeutic milieu for a patient.

Often the physical environment in which we live is taken for granted, overlooked as a direct influence on the person and his health, although ecology is a well-publicized subject. You may wonder why a unit discussing major influences on the developing person and his health begins with a chapter about man and his environment. Yet where we live and the condition of that area—its air, water, and soil—determine to a great extent how we live, what we eat, the agents of disease to which we are exposed, our state of health, and our ability to adapt.

Some environmental factors external to and inside of the person that affect health status are discussed in Chapter 1. This chapter focuses primarily on noxious agents in the external environment to which many people in the United States are exposed and that are detrimental to health. Because of the interdependence of people, only those living in isolated rural areas escape the unpleasant effects of our urban, technologically advanced society. Yet even the isolated few may encounter some kind of environmental pollution, whether it be through groundwater contaminated from afar, food shipped into the area, or smog blown from a nearby city.

In the past, nursing was concerned primarily with the patient's immediate environment in the hospital or home. Increasingly, you will extend the nursing process to include assessment of and intervention measures directed toward promoting a healthy environment for the person and his family, well or ill. Understanding some specific environmental health problems, their sources and effects, will enable you to work both as a citizen and professional nurse to help prevent or correct those problems.

HISTORICAL PERSPECTIVE

The natural components of the environment were once considered dangerous. In most instances, man dealt successfully with the environmental problems that he encountered. In his quest to conquer nature, early man discovered fire and the wheel. Fire was essential to survival; but with its advent, natural or man-made, sparks and pollutants were sent into the atmosphere, the beginning of environmental pollution.

The fire and the wheel played major roles in the early civilization and industrialization of the world. With the Industrial Revolution came many technological advances that gave man increased power and comforts. These advances also introduced artificial, chemical, and physical hazards into the environment.

Soon after the start of the Industrial Revolution, the population of cities grew; disease spread with the crowding of people, and food distribution became more complex. It became apparent that the natural components of the environment were not as dangerous as the man-made components.

Antipollution legislation in the United States can be traced back to the early 1900s. In 1906 the first federal Food and Drug Act was passed, and in 1914 drinking water standards were enacted to serve as guides for water supplied on interstate carriers. In 1948 Congress passed the federal Water Pollution Control Act. However, most of these legislative moves were poorly funded and supported and therefore had little effect on growing pollution problems. Finally in the early 1960s Congress began taking a firm and leading role in combatting environmental pollution. The Clean Air and Solid Waste Disposal Act of 1965 and the Clean Water Restoration Act of 1966 are examples of this new attempt to fight pollution[33].

All of the environment has been and is a vital part of man's existence. Man's skill in manipulating the environment has produced tremendous benefits; but none of these has been without a price, the high price of pollution. Pollution of our environment is not only a health threat but may also offend esthetic, spiritual, social, and philosophic values. Epidemiological studies have identified environmental pollution as a complex, significant problem requiring multiple solutions (See Figure 9-1.)

The following discussion is divided into categories of air, water, soil, food, noise, and surface pollution. Keep in mind, however, that these categories overlap. For example, when man inhales harmful particles from the soil that have become airborne, soil pollution becomes air pollution. And soil or surface pollution becomes water or food pollution if these harmful particles are swept into the water, consumed first by fish and then by man.

AIR POLLUTION

...This most excellent canopy, the air, look you, this brave o'erhanging firmament, this majestical roof fretted with golden fire—why, it appears no other thing to me than a foul and pestilent congregation of vapors.

Hamlet (II, ii, 311-315)

Problems of Air Pollution

Air pollution, "aerial garbage," is not a new problem. Natural processes such as forest fires and volcanic eruptions, or burning cities set afire during war, have long contaminated the air. Smog and the by-products of coal burning have long been recognized as irritating disturbances plaguing many areas and clouding the skies. As long ago as 1272, King Edward I of England proclaimed an edict forbidding the use of a certain coal that was making London's air smoky and sooty.

Air and water pollution act interchangeably; together they present a world

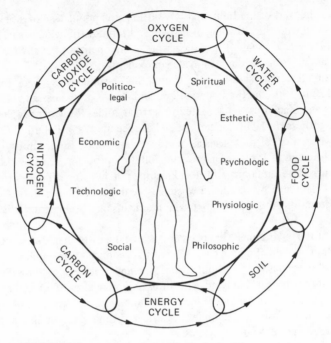

FIGURE 9-1
Man's Interrelationship with His Environment

problem. All people on the earth share the oceans and the air. Significant local pollution of either can greatly affect distant areas, especially if the oceans cannot by the processes of precipitation, oxidation, and absorption cleanse the atmosphere before harmful effects occur. Given enough time the ocean can cleanse the atmosphere. But if the amount of pollution exceeds the ocean's capacity to neutralize the waste, then the harmful effects are dispersed into the atmosphere and we realize the effects by breathing contaminated air[4].

Sources of Air Pollution

The sources of air pollution vary. The National Air Pollution Control Administration gives the following percentages[31]:

Transportation (cars and buses)	42.3%
Fuel Combustion	21.3
Industrial Processes	13.7
Solid-Waste Disposal	5.2
Miscellaneous (agriculture, forest fires)	17.5

Many of these sources involve imperfect combustion, a major cause of air contamination. *Perfect combustion* exists only in the chemistry books and is *the result of hydrogen and carbon uniting completely with oxygen, thereby relinquishing heat, water vapor, light, and carbon dioxide to the air. Imperfect combustion refers to the additional liberation of carbon monoxide, sulfur oxides, and nitrogen oxides into the air.* Car exhausts in heavy traffic produce a significant amount of *carbon monoxide, a colorless and odorless poisonous gas produced during the incomplete combustion of carbon.* This gas combines with the hemoglobin of red blood cells in place of oxygen, and can produce a *hypoxic state, a decreased amount of oxygen* in the body. The severity of this state depends on the ratio of carbon monoxide to oxygen in the air inhaled. Guyton states that an alveolar concentration of carbon monoxide of 0.1 percent is lethal. In smaller amounts, it can cause dizziness, headache, and fatigue. Carbon monoxide pollution can be especially dangerous for persons who suffer from heart disease, respiratory disease, or anemia, for they already have a physiologically impaired oxygen-carrying capacity [20].

Sulfur oxides are poisonous gases that come from factories and power plants that burn coal or oil-containing sulfur, eventually producing dangerous sulfur dioxide. *Sulfur dioxide combines with water to form sulfuric acid H_2SO_4, a heavy, corrosive, oily colorless liquid* that irritates the sensitive mucous membranes of the eyes, nose, and throat and injures the mucous membrane that lines the lung and the delicate structures accessory to the lung tissue. Besides directly affecting the health of man, sulfur dioxide and its by-product, sulfuric acid, indirectly jeopardize health by damaging plant life and by contributing to rust on metals. In the process of trying to control these harmful effects through technological means, man has sometimes created new industrial pollution. For example, rust-proof cans may contain some elements that contaminate the environment, and they add to waste-disposal problems too.

Other gaseous end products from burning fuels are the nitrogen oxides, especially nitrogen dioxide. While this gas hovers in the air, producing an unpleasant, characteristic odor, it causes irritation to the mucous membranes and creates a haze that destroys the view and blocks out necessary and helpful rays from the sun.

A second type of air contaminant is *smog, a noxious mixture of fog and smoke* [19]. Smog can be produced when sulfur compounds in smoke react with atmospheric moisture, relinquishing sulfuric acid. Smog can also be produced by *hydrocarbons and nitrogen compounds uniting through energy from the sun, forming a type of photochemical smog.* Smog often produces a more intense irritation to the mucous membranes than does nitrogen dioxide.

A third type of air contaminant is *particulate matter, minute particles such as dust, dirt, smoke, and fly ash.* Particulate matter, suspended in vapors and fumes, may stay hovering for annoying and dangerous periods of time, depending on atmospheric conditions. These pollutants may soil surfaces, scatter or distribute light rays unevenly, and, most dangerously, enter the lungs of people breathing the air. The severity of the lungs' response depends on the percentage of particulate matter or fumes and vapors in the air mixture and on preexisting lung disease. Sufficient exposure to any type of air pollution may lead to pulmonary emphysema (a condition in which the alveoli of the lungs become distended or ruptured). However, cigarette smoking is still the main factor contributing to this serious debilitating condition, according to the U.S. Environmental Protection Agency[51].

Radioactive substances are produced by mining and processing radioactive ore and by nuclear-fission and radiation procedures employed in industry, medicine, and research. Pollution from radioactive materials poses a serious threat to man's ability to reproduce and to his gene structure. It is also related to an increase in leukemia, as demonstrated in persons working with radioactive materials over long periods without adequate safeguards and in survivors of Hiroshima and Nagasaki. Overexposure to a radioactive substance requires intensive care—for a person, group, or entire community.

Breathing in asbestos particles released into the atmosphere from certain construction industries and from the wearing of brake linings and clutch facings in cars can cause cancer. Inhaled beryllium, used in making metal alloys, also is known to cause a debilitating form of lung infection[46].

With all these components circulating in the atmosphere, with harmful radioactive and disease-producing effects from our technology, and with waste in rivers and streams at levels that cannot be detoxified, air pollution exists. All forms of air pollution are physically irritating and present a potential hazard to our long-range health either by direct harm to the mucous membranes of the respiratory tract or by the indirect effects of continuously breathing contaminated air. Only as we become aware of these specifics as a *personal health threat* will we seriously consider alternatives to using two or three cars, seek to know the serious hazards in our jobs, and become concerned about our house downwind from an industrial site. Then we will work for clean-air-protection bills.

WATER POLLUTION

Pollution of the water from the natural processes of aquatic animal and plant life combined with man-made waste constitutes another hazard to the delicate state of man's health. The water-pollutant list is long: phosphates in laundry detergents; acid contamination from mine drainage; and industrial effluent of toxins, acids, radioactive substances, and mineral particles such as mercury. Less obvious causes are salinization of water from evaporation in the arid West, land erosion, heat from industrial processes, and oil spills[46].

Types of Water Pollution

Water pollutants causing much of the problem can be categorized as either common sewage, infection-causing organisms, nutrients, synthetic chemicals, inorganic chemicals, sediment, or heat.

Common Sewage, traditional waste from domestic and industrial sources, is a significant problem because oxygen is required to render this waste harmless. This waste thus uses up oxygen needed by aquatic plant and animal life. With increasing amounts of sewage, the problem is becoming ever more serious because of the inability of the water to deal successfully with the waste. When bacteria in the water can no longer decompose the waste, widespread aquatic death results. Waste will then accumulate, and the water becomes useless as a personal or industrial resource.

Infection-Causing Organisms pollute water when sewage carrying these bacteria enter a river or stream. A man or animal drinking this water can become ill. Microbiology and pharmacology have done a great deal in helping prevent and treat such diseases by identifying the responsible microorganisms and developing appropriate vaccines and antibiotics. However, occasionally a whole community or area may be negatively affected because of a gross error that contaminates a large body of water with diseased microbes. These microbes may spread infectious hepatitis or typhoid fever, especially in rural and urban fringe areas where population density is high and public utilities limited.

Nutrients that nourish plant life, particularly phosphates and nitrates, are produced by sewage, industrial wastes, and soil erosion. These nutrients are not easily removed by treatment centers because they do not respond to the usual biological processes. Moreover, treatment centers may inadvertently change these substances into a more usable mineral form that stimulates excessive plant growth. This growth in turn becomes a problem by interfering with treatment processes, marring the landscape, producing an unpleasant odor and taste in the water, and disturbing the normal food chain in a body of water. Because man depends on many lower forms of life for food, this process could eventually affect man's well-being if it occurred on a large scale. (See Figure 9-2.)

Synthetic Chemicals that are used in everyday household chores, especially chemicals found in detergents, pesticides, and other cleaning agents, affect the water. Even in small proportions they may be poisonous to aquatic life. Where they are resistant to local treatment measures, they can produce an unpleasant taste and odor in the water. The extent of the long-term problem is not known, but there might be a possibility of human poisoning over a long period by the consumption of small doses of these chemicals taken in drinking water. Further discussion of this problem follows later in the chapter.

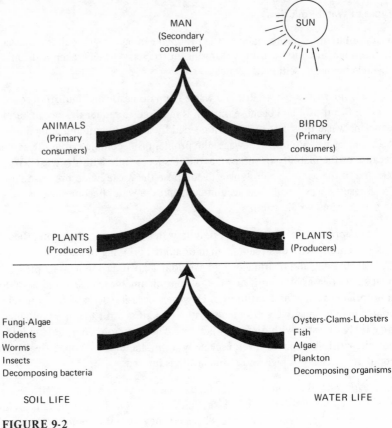

FIGURE 9-2
Food Chain

Inorganic Chemicals or mineral substances from mining or manufacturing processes can destroy land animals, (including people) and aquatic life when they are ingested. Industries sometimes improperly and illegally empty large quantities of toxic materials into sources of local water supply. This group of pollutants corrodes water-treatment equipment and makes waste treatment an even more expensive problem.

Sediment, particles of earth such as dirt and sand, composes a group of pollutants that is becoming a problem because of the magnitude of its debris. Sediment causes a nuisance and a hazard by covering food sources for aquatic life (and thereby eventually reducing sources for other life), by filling streams, and by preventing natural reservoirs from filling during rainy seasons. Resultant floods destroy animal and plant life and property, and can cause epidemics of such water-borne diseases as typhoid and salmonellosis. Sediment also increases the cost of water treatment because of its sheer volume.

Heat becomes a problem because it reduces the ability of the water to absorb oxygen. If significant amounts of water are heated through industrial use, the water becomes less efficient in providing oxygen for aquatic life and in assimilating waste. Even more dangerous, the ecological balance of lakes and rivers can be permanently upset through prolonged alteration of water temperature. The food man eats either comes directly from water or has fed upon aquatic life somewhere in the food chain. Faced with an expanding world population, we must increasingly be aware of the significance of every organism in the food chain (Figure 9-2) and its relationship to us.

Containing such a variety of pollutants in ever-increasing amounts, water, an essential to life, becomes a threat to the integrity of man's health. It poses a threat first, because of its increasing unavailability for consumption, and second, because of the harmful proportion of dangerous pollutants contained in what does remain.

We can become diseased from drinking the contaminated water; we can no longer enjoy polluted water for recreational purposes. The odor of decay and the unsightliness of polluted water most certainly destroy the beauty of any natural setting. This problem does not have an easy answer. But if the abuse of water resources exceeds purification, we will need more water than will be available. Our existence will then be threatened by one of the essential components of life.

Problems in Water Purification

The natural water-purification process involves the action of bacteria using oxygen to decompose organic matter. If too much waste is dumped into a given body of water, this natural cleansing process cannot take place, or at least does not take place fast enough.

The ultimate problem of water pollution stems from our using natural resources in greater and greater amounts because of additional industrialization, population growth, a greater dependence on appliances, and from a subsequent increase in the need for sewage disposal. The problem of dissolving waste has put a real strain on waste-disposal systems. Even excessive amounts of treated waste now obstruct the waterways. Current engineering research is attempting to solve some of the problems of water pollution by developing different types of waste-disposal systems.

Misuse of our water has far-reaching consequences, threatening man all over the world from every age group and culture. Therefore, we must take definite personal responsibility for stopping needless pollution of the water by exercising careful personal use of agents that can ultimately destroy it and by utilizing legal procedures to prevent undue dumping of wastes into streams. Some of the health problems associated with contaminated water would be eliminated with proper legislation, and needless sickness and death could be avoided. More importantly, the health of future generations and their chance to enjoy the beauty, taste, and power of the water depend on us who are so carelessly polluting it.

SOIL POLLUTION

As early as 1950, the federal Food and Drug Administration announced that the potential health hazards of compounds containing chlorinated hydrocarbons such as dichloro-diphenyl-trichloroethane (DDT) had been underestimated[13]. However, it was not until the late 1960s that the general public became really aware of and alarmed by the hazards of these and other soil pollutants.

Substances used to kill weeds, rats, mice, worms, fungi, and insects are called pesticides. Soil pollution can occur as a result of excessive or improper use of pesticides (insecticides, herbicides, fungicides) or crop fertilizers. Many of the chemicals used in these preparations are highly toxic and can remain in the soil for long periods of time without being degraded, thus setting the stage for pollution of food, water, and ultimately man himself.

Although farmers are the largest users of pesticides, they are also used by industry, by federal, state, and local governmental agencies, and by individual people in their homes and gardens. Actual toxic effects of the different compounds vary, and some of the effects occur before the chemicals reach the soil. Vertebrates will not usually suffer acute poisoning from these substances except through accidental ingestion, direct skin contact, or inhalation of the dust or spray of the more toxic pesticides. Workers in pesticide manufacturing plants, agricultural workers, and commercial pest-control operators applying the chemicals to crops or soil can all inhale pesticide dust or spray. At times, inhalation exposure can occur in a subtle manner—for example, by inhaling the dust from storage bags during the filling and emptying process or from cultivated soil previously treated with pesticides. Symptoms occurring as a result of such exposure may not be attributed to the pesticides. Therefore, many episodes of acute poisoning go undiagnosed. Direct skin contact can occur when solutions are spilled accidentally or when the moist spray touches exposed skin[4, 35]. An occupational history aids early diagnosis of such problems.

Effects of Soil Pollution

Recent reports from epidemiological studies being conducted in Iowa and California indicate that a variety of acute illnesses and physiological changes have been observed in farmers after handling agricultural chemicals. Such effects on the central nervous system as forgetfulness, decreased attention and interest span, hyperirritability, anxiety, depression, nervousness, and insomnia have been reported. Skin diseases, eye and respiratory conditions, and digestive disorders have also been identified. In some instances, these problems occurred after a single exposure to a toxic chemical[35].

Pesticides have an immediate toxic effect on birds, bees, and rodents, thus curtailing the necessary natural agents of cross-pollination and insect destruction, which in turn can affect food supply. Surface water may be contaminated during spraying or dusting; or rain may wash pesticides or fertilizers into streams and lakes, again affecting food supply.

Edwards shows that earthworms are capable of concentrating toxic chemicals from the soil and storing these chemicals in their fatty tissues. Since earthworms provide food for other animals that are also capable of concentrating these chemicals, they may prove to be an important source of undesirable chemical residues in higher animals and man[16].

The effects on man of long-term exposure to pesticides by inhalation or by ingestion of food and water containing residual chemicals are unknown. However, lower activity values of serum lactic dehydrogenase (an enzyme present in large amounts in liver tissue), inhibited cholinesterase activity, and altered hemoglobin, hematocrit, and amino acid levels have been shown to exist in people occupationally exposed to pesticides[35]. Experimentally, small doses of pesticides have caused such metabolic changes as lowered estrogen levels, altered glucose metabolism, and inhibition of adenosine triphosphatase (ATP) in a wide variety of vertebrates, including man[43]. In addition, potent *herbicides, substances used to kill weeds or plants,* such as 2,4,5-T, have produced birth defects in animals and humans[46].

Much of the present pesticide problem is directly related to misuse. The Environmental Protection Agency has set limits on the amount of allowable pesticide residue in food crops. It has canceled the production of certain products and has set up studies to determine if there is a buildup of pesticide residues in human body tissue after prolonged exposure[14].

FOOD POLLUTION

Some of the same chemicals used in pesticide preparation are used as *food additives*. These purposely used additives are not designed to be toxic, but rather *to preserve, to improve, and to protect nutritional value.* The average person in the United States consumes approximately three pounds of these additives every year. Determining their potential health hazard over a life span is difficult[30].

Some food additives, however, have resulted in unexpected side effects due to antibiotic residues from drugs given to animals for growth promotion and disease prevention. In people these residues have resulted in (1) allergy and increased drug toxicity or resistance to pathogens when the *same* family of antibiotics is later administered therapeutically; and (2) change of normal bacterial flora in a body area so that invasion by pathogens is more likely, causing infection or disease[3]. In the future, diseases from food additives may assume as much significance in man as do the *zoonoses, diseases transmitted between ani-*

mals and man, such as trichinosis, brucellosis, tuberculosis, psittacosis, and salmonellosis.

Other food-pollution hazards are radioactive materials such as strontium-90, which has been traced in milk; mercury found in swordfish; worms; and mold, which may be present without noticeable change in the food's appearance, taste, or smell. Food handlers may introduce their infectious diseases into food by touching it or the equipment with soiled hands or by coughing onto it.

Because of the endless contamination possibilities from bacteria, toxins, viruses, parasites, and protozoa, the Food and Drug Administration and the Department of Agriculture enforce laws passed by Congress, impose various regulations of their own, and in general monitor the food industry nationwide. Various state and local authorities also attempt to regulate standards within their respective jurisdictions[4]. Yet these agencies cannot possibly determine every breach of regulation. Astute observations must be made about standards in the food store. Demanding to know the growing, cleansing, processing, and handling procedures is not out of line. Reporting suspected breaches is your responsibility for health.

NOISE POLLUTION

Sensory stimulation plays a major role in psychological and physiological development and is therefore directly related to physical and mental health. Sound is but one form of sensory stimulation. *Sound overload, unwanted sound that produces unwanted effects,* as well as sound deprivation, can be hazards to health [17, 27, 46].

Sound overload can produce temporary or permanent hearing loss by affecting the tympanic membrane and by slowly deteriorating the microscopic cells that send sound waves from the ear to the brain. The effects produced on each person's hearing vary, depending on the sound intensity and pitch, the location of the source in relation to the person, the length of exposure, and the person's age and history of previous ear problems. Surveys have shown that at least 20 million Americans have measurable hearing deficits and still another 16 million are exposed to occupational noise levels capable of producing permanent hearing loss[45, 60].

One means of determining the potential hazard of any sound is to measure its loudness. *The measurement of sound loudness is stated in decibels.* The faintest audible sound is designated 1 decibel; ordinary conversation, measured at 60 decibels, is considered adequately quiet. Studies have shown that moderately loud sounds of 80 decibels, such as those produced by a clothes washer, tabulating machine, or home garbage-disposal unit, can be discomforting to human ears and can produce temporary or permanent hearing loss. The following are examples of common sound pollutants and their decibel readings:

Heavy city traffic	90-95 decibels
Food blender in home	93
Pneumatic hammer	95
Air compressor	95
Power lawnmower	95
Farm tractor	98
Outboard motor	102
Jet flying over at 1,000 feet	103
Riveting gun	110
Motorcycle	115
Live rock music	120
Jet plane at takeoff	150
Rocket engine	180

Sound louder than 140 decibels, such as that produced by a nearby jet plane, gunshot blast, or a rocket at the launching pad, may cause actual pain [17, 45, 46, 60]. Persons who work regularly with any of the machines listed should realize the potential long-range effects of such noise levels.

Effects of Noise Pollution

Sound overload affects nearly everyone at some time by intruding on privacy and shattering serenity. It can produce impaired communication and social relationships, irritability, depression, fatigue, and tension, in addition to hearing loss. Recent research reports indicate that less obvious physiological changes can also occur. These changes include involuntary responses in the digestive, vascular, and nervous systems. They can produce blood vessel constriction, pallor, dilated pupils and visual disturbance, increased and irregular heart rate, hypertension, headache, gastrointestinal spasm with nausea and diarrhea and eventual peptic ulcer, hyperactive reflexes, and muscle tenseness. These responses do not subside immediately but continue up to five times longer than the actual noise. Noise has also been associated with elevated blood cholesterol levels, atherosclerosis, and accident proneness [17, 46, 60].

We do not adapt to excessive sound, as was once thought; rather, we learn to tolerate it. Even when a person is asleep, noise cannot be shut out completely. We are exhausted by our efforts to remain asleep in the midst of this external stimuli. Perhaps being aware of these environmental stress factors can aid in reducing or coping with them [17, 46, 60].

Although not every harmful form of sound can be avoided, measures such as wearing protective ear coverings, shortening exposure time, having regular hearing examinations, and seeking immediate medical attention for any ear injury or infection will decrease the possibility of permanent damage or hearing loss. Noise can be brought under control without excessive cost. You can educate the public about the hazards of excess noise.

SURFACE POLLUTION

Until recent years, Americans were not concerned with problems of waste disposal or recycling. Raw materials were plentiful, and the open-dump method of disposal was convenient and economical. Now, however, people are becoming more concerned about the decreasing supply of natural resources and the health problems being created by open dumps.

Over 4 billion tons of solid household, municipal, industrial, agricultural, and mineral wastes are produced yearly in the United States[57]. Most of the present disposal methods for this waste pollute either land, air, or water. We can see this pollution everywhere: in open air, foul-smelling dumps, smoking incineration centers, junkyards, and poorly covered landfills.

Solid-Waste-Disposal Methods

Solid waste is discarded in four basic ways: (1) open dumps, (2) sanitary landfills, (3) incineration, and (4) salvage. Of these methods, the *open dump* (now illegal in most states) is the oldest, most convenient, and most economical. However, this method creates many health problems and is esthetically undesirable. Dumps serve as breeding areas for rodents, flies, and other insects such as cockroaches; they also attract seagulls, notorious as thieves and litterers. Houseflies carry poliomyelitis, tuberculosis, diarrhea, dysentery, hepatitis, and cholera. Rats carry plague, tapeworm, Rocky Mountain spotted fever, and rat-bite fever. Water running off from these dumps pollutes local streams and lakes. Rain and surface water can seep through the wastes and pollute underground water. Any attempt to burn the surface waste in the dumps emits large quantities of foul-smelling fumes that increase air pollution and thus respiratory problems among local inhabitants. Dumps also invite accidents and fires as well as lower the value of surrounding property[33].

Landfills, when handled properly, can be economical, sanitary, and esthetically acceptable. These areas should be placed far from water sources. Even with this precaution, underground or surface water may become polluted. The waste should be quickly covered to avoid foul smells, spontaneous combustion, breeding of rats and flies, and scavenging by rodents[1, 39].

Approximately 80 percent of household solid wastes are combustible and therefore suitable for *incineration*. Decentralized incineration is usually poorly controlled and frequently produces gaseous emissions and particulates that pollute the air and damage man's health. Central incineration conducted by federal, state, or local governmental bodies is expensive, although necessary for large urban areas. The controlled-combustion process used in these centers prevents the emission of harmful gases and utilizes the by-product heat for an energy source. Through incineration, the volume of waste can be reduced to one-fifth of its original bulk. The remaining material can be removed to landfills or compressed for use in soil conditioners or construction material[4].

In the last ten years the composition of solid waste has changed, and now includes larger amounts of paper, plastics, aluminum cans, and other packaging and wrapping materials. Many of these materials will not decompose or rust; therefore, they present new problems in disposal. If these products are *salvaged*, they can be **recycled**, *treated by mechanical, thermal, or biological means so that they can be used again,* thus promoting resource recovery and reuse[6].

Hospital Waste

The amount of solid waste being produced by hospitals should be a primary concern to health workers. The average citizen accumulates and disposes of 5.5 pounds of solid waste daily, while the average hospital patient accumulates 24.16 pounds daily. This increase in hospital wastes can be attributed to the increase in disposable products: syringes, needles, surgical supplies, dishes and utensils, linens, uniforms, and medication containers. Many hospitals use disposable products because they consider them cheaper, easier to store, and less likely to produce cross-infection. However, hospitals often fail to consider the cost or inconvenience of transporting or discarding large quantities of these contaminated objects. Much of a hospital's solid waste, often contaminated by infectious organisms, is removed to open dumps or sanitary landfills without proper initial sterilization, thus spreading pathogens to land and water[34]. Most hospital workers don't consider the implications of casually using disposable items.

One study conducted in an urban area with 16 participating hospitals revealed that the nurse influences decisions regarding the purchase of patient care items more than does any other hospital worker. If these decisions are largely your responsibility, know how much trash your hospital creates, where the waste goes, the type of decontamination procedures used before disposal, the cost of disposal, why your agency uses disposable products, and how much your agency contributes to environmental pollution. Form an interdepartmental committee, perhaps of administrators, nurses, doctors, and patients. Report your findings to them, and together consider all the advantages and drawbacks of various products. Consider cost, convenience, infection control, and quality. Give each new product a careful clinical trial and adopt it for use only after careful consideration about contributions to patient care. Avoid using disposable items if nondisposables will do the job as well. Pass this information on to the patients and families. Encourage health workers in homes to demonstrate and teach proper disposal of such items as syringes and dressings. Work to reduce the huge volume of solid waste that is taking space and depleting natural resources[28]. And work for disposal of infectious wastes in nonair-polluting incinerators, which many cities and hospitals do not have.

Lead Poisoning

Lead is another surface pollutant. Man inhales lead as an air pollutant and ingests traces of lead daily through a normal diet. Because lead wastes have increased during the past century, particularly from industry and automobile use, exposure and intake into the body have increased. Consequently, the rate of absorption by soft tissue exceeds the rate of excretion or storage by bone[9]. An urgent problem is controlling the lead exposure that occurs from drinking or eating from improperly lead-glazed earthenware, using leaded gasoline, consuming lead-contaminated "moonshine," or working in industries where lead exposure is not controlled.

Another urgent problem arises when young children, mainly in urban slums, form the *habit of eating nonfood substances, including peeling paint, plaster, or putty containing lead. This behavior is called pica.* The precise cause of pica is not completely understood, but may be related to nutritional, cultural, and emotional factors. Acute or chronic lead poisoning, an insidious disease, results from this eating pattern and is a major source of brain damage, mental deficiency, and behavior problems. The pathological changes that occur affect the nervous, renal, and hematopoietic systems. Kidney damage is usually reversible, but chronic lead poisoning in childhood may lead to gout or kidney disease later in life. Damage to the hematopoietic system is evident by the reduction in the number and quality of red blood cells produced, thus leading to severe anemia. The most serious effects are on the nervous system. The mortality rate from lead encephalopathy (disease of the brain) is 5 percent. Of the children who survive acute lead poisoning, 40 percent have convulsive disorders and another 20 percent have significant neurological deficits[44].

NURSING RESPONSIBILITY

Personal Responsibility

Environmental problems are a concern to everyone and are of equal consequence to every part of the world. Each of us shares the earth, and thus we are all responsible for its well-being. Environmental pollution is our collective fault requiring our collective solutions.

Linton describes a fourfold environmental-protection system for continuously identifying, analyzing, and controlling environmental hazards:
(1) surveillance—maintaining an awareness of what man is doing to the air, water,

and land, and of the effect of these actions on his health; (2) development of criteria for the detection of pollution; (3) research; and (4) compliance—getting local government and industry to accept and implement new standards[33]. An informed public can help establish such a system, but the financial support and legislative and administrative guidance of federal, state, and local governments seem to be the most feasible solution. Chanlett, Rogers, and Hurst speak strongly of the need for environmental health planning on a widespread scale, involving the citizen and the government[8].

Personally, you should conserve natural resources to the best of your ability and learn about the environmental pollution in your own area. Avoid unnecessary use of water, electricity, and fuel; save cans and papers for recycling; avoid littering. Walk or bicycle instead of driving an automobile when feasible. Avoid cigarette smoking in closed, crowded areas. Avoid contact with pesticides by thoroughly scrubbing or peeling foodstuffs, and, if possible, maintain your own garden without use of pesticides. Quiet surroundings are a natural resource, too. Take it upon yourself to make yours quieter through personal habits. Help plan for local recreation sites that offer natural surroundings. Campaign for adequate acoustical standards in homes, apartments, hospitals, and industrial buildings, and for noiseless kitchen equipment. Participate in local governmental planning to decrease town and city noise in relation to transportation routes, zoning, and industrial sites. Develop a philosophy against the one-time-use concept and planned obsolescence. Buy beverages in returnable bottles when possible. Contribute to a natural resource, soil, by composting plants or organic content in garbage. Plant a rooftop or patio garden to contribute to the oxygen cycle. Join citizens' crusades for a clean environment or a conservation organization, and attend workshops given by the Cancer Society, Sierra Club, Conservation Foundation, and League of Women Voters to learn more about problems, preventive measures, and means of strengthening legislation. Support antipollution and noise-control laws. Be an involved citizen!

For more information on specific measures for wasting less and practicing ecologically sound living, see Saltonstall, *Your Environment and What You Can Do about It* [46]. Share the information with family and friends.

Professional Responsibility

Although nursing responsibilities have been interwoven throughout this chapter, consider that your primary responsibilities are thorough assessment, detection through epidemiological methods, suggestion, and health teaching. For example, you can play a significant role in the early detection of lead poisoning. Assessment of a child's health should include observation for physical signs such as tremors, abdominal discomfort, decreased appetite, and vomiting, as well as questions related to pica behavior. Ask the mother about her child's interest in play, ability to get along with playmates, coordination, and level of developmental skill attainment. Phrase your questions and comments carefully, in a nonjudgmental manner so the mother will not feel that her fitness as a parent is being judged. If the persons for whom you are caring live in unsatisfactory, low-income housing, work for improvement through local legislation. Emphasis must be placed on repair and deleading of dwelling places, not just on moving the present dweller to a new house or apartment. You can encourage the formation of screening and case-finding programs, already started in many cities, and you can assist with their activities.

Natural or man-made chemical pollution in soil, water, and food products can produce a variety of adverse effects in man, ranging from slight health impairments to death. For example, higher-than-normal concentrations of nitrates in water can cause acute methemoglobinemia (a type of anemia) in infants[13]. Although local public health officials are responsible for maintaining safe nitrate levels in the water supply, your responsibilities are to aid in the education of the public concerning the health hazards of such pollutants and to use the epidemiological method in your work. Be aware of such symptoms as fatigue, listlessness, and sleepiness that might indicate an untoward reaction to this particular form of pollution.

Another dangerous problem associated with chemical pollution is its possible carcinogenic effect. Incidence of specific forms of cancer can be higher or lower depending on exposure to particular compounds, a common example being the high incidence of lung cancer in the United States and England because of heavy tobacco use. Be aware and knowledgeable of the incidence of chemically produced cancer in your particular locale. Health teaching can then be directed at trying to eliminate or control the responsible carcinogenic chemical.

The biochemical response to chemical pollution or radiation can influence the cell in a variety of ways. *Teratogenic* (producing malformations) and *mutagenic* (producing hereditary changes) are two such changes in cells. Be aware of these possibilities and encourage prenatal care from the moment pregnancy is known. Genetic counseling might be indicated for particular couples. Citizens should know of the possibility for dealing effectively and therapeutically with biochemical changes, whether prenatally or in any stage of growth and development[21].

In the past 100 years, disease and death have been reduced because of preventive public health measures in the form of environmental control such as water and waste management, rodent and insect control, and development of housing codes. Now we are again faced with problems and diseases that have an environmental relationship. Prevention can begin with informed consumer groups who have educational and work projects as their goals. It can begin with your responsibility for the patient's environment.

The Patient's Immediate Environment

While you should feel responsible for the community and physical environment in which the patient lives, you also have a responsibility for his immediate environment while he is receiving health care. His *surroundings should constitute a* ***therapeutic milieu*** *free of hazards and conducive to his recovery, physically and emotionally.*

The patient's surroundings should be clean and adequately lighted, ventilated, and heated. Precautions should always be taken during care to prevent injury, such as burns from a hot-water bottle. Falls should be prevented by removing obstacles from walking areas and having the person wear well-fitted shoes and use adequate support while walking. Lock the bed or wheelchair while the patient is moving to and from them. Be sure that electrical cords and scatter rugs are not so placed that the patient could fall. Wipe up spilled liquids immediately. Use sterile technique and proper handwashing methods to insure that you bring no pathogenic organisms to the patient.

The esthetic environment is also important for rest. Arrange the articles on the person's bedside table in a pleasing manner if he is unable to do so himself. Keep unattractive equipment or supplies out of sight as much as possible. Minimize offensive odors and noise. Place the person's bed or chair by a window or door so that he can watch normal activity rather than be forced to stare at the ceiling and walls. As a nurse, involve yourself in making the entire ward as well as the patients' rooms look pleasing. Consider color combinations and the use of drapes, furniture, clocks, calendars, pictures, and various artifacts to create a more homelike atmosphere. The committee in charge of decorating and building should include at least one nurse. You may need to volunteer to assure that nursing and, indirectly, patients are represented in such programs.

The patient's surroundings should not only be safe and pretty. In addition, the emotional climate of the unit and entire institution affects patients and staff. The patient and family are quick to respond and react to the attitudes and manner of the staff caring for him. Questions you might ask yourself are: How do I treat delivery workers who bring gifts and flowers to patients? Do I participate in the joy such remembrances bring to the patient? Do I help arrange the flowers into a pleasant pattern, or just stick them quickly into whatever can be found? Do I treat visitors as welcome guests, or as foreign intruders? The emotional climate should radiate security and acceptance. A sense of warmth should prevail that promotes a feeling of trust, confidence, and motivation within the patient as he and the staff work together to cope with his problems. The emotional relationship between the patient and the health care staff should help the patient reach his goal of maximum health.

In a truly therapeutic milieu, the staff also feel a sense of harmony among themselves. There is mutual trust and acceptance between staff and supervisors, and supervisors recognize work well done by the staff. As a result, staff feel motivated to continue to learn and to improve the quality of patient care. Staff members are not likely to give individualized, comprehensive, compassionate care in an agency where they are not treated like individuals or where their basic needs are not met.

Specific ways of meeting the patient's environmental needs differ for various developmental stages. The components of a therapeutic milieu are different for the baby than for the middle-aged man. However, a safe, secure environment, physically and psychologically, must be present for both. Accurately determining the factors that compose the environment and making appropriate changes may be the first step in promoting health.

It is past time for all of us to ask ourselves some very basic questions: How much energy and natural resources do we need to sustain life, to maintain the high standard of living in the United States? How much are we willing to pay for benefits that will not poison us with side effects? How does population growth affect the use and abuse of natural resources? Will strictly controlled energy allocation be necessary because people refuse to abide by suggested limits? Must people continue to grow up with strontium-90 in their bones, DDT in their fat, and asbestos in their lungs? What more can each of us do personally and professionally to maintain a health-fostering environment?

REFERENCES

1. Anderson, Linnea, M. Dibble, H. Mitchell, and H. Rynbergen, *Nutrition in Nursing*. Philadelphia: J. B. Lippincott Co., 1972, pp. 108-16.

2. Beland, Irene, *Clinical Nursing: Pathophysiological and Psychosocial Approaches* (2nd ed.). New York: The Macmillan Company, 1970.

3. Brandley, C. A., and Charles Cornelius, eds., *Advances in Veterinary Science and Comparative Medicine*. New York: Academic Press, 1971, pp. 67-132.

4. Brubaker, Sterling, *To Live on Earth*. New York: New American Library, 1972.

5. Burnside, I., "Clocks and Calendars," *American Journal of Nursing*, 70: No. 1 (1970), 117-19.

6. Burton, Lloyd, and Hugh Smith, *Public Health and Community Medicine*. Baltimore: The Williams & Williams Company, 1970.

7. "Cancer and Ecology," *Newsweek*, July 10, 1972, p. 72.

8. Chanlett, Emil, D. Rogers, and G. Hurst, "The Necessity for Environmental Health Planning," *American Journal of Public Health*, 63: No. 4 (1973), 341-44.

9. Chisolm, Julian, "Lead Poisoning," *Scientific American*, 224: No. 2 (1971), 15-23.

10. Commoner, Barry, *Science and Survival*. New York: Viking Press, 1969.

11. ____, *The Closing Circle*. New York: Alfred A. Knopf, Inc. 1972.

12. Cooley, Richard, and Geoffrey Smith, eds., *Congress and the Environment*. Seattle: University of Washington Press, 1970.

13. De Bill, Garreti, ed., *The Environmental Handbook*. New York: Ballantine Books, Inc., 1970.

14. Division of Pesticide Community Studies, *Pesticides*. Chamblee, Ga.: Environmental Protection Agency, Pesticides Office, March 1971.
15. Drummond, David, and Eric Mood, "Actions of Residents in Response to Environmental Hazards in the Inner City," *American Journal of Public Health*, 63: No. 4 (1973), 335-40.
16. Edwards, Clive, "Soil Pollutants and Soil Animals," *Scientific American*, 220: No. 4 (1969), 88-99.
17. Goldsmith, John, and Erland Jonsson, "Health Effects of Community Noise," *American Journal of Public Health*, 63: No. 9 (1973), 782-93.
18. Goldwater, Leonard, "Mercury in the Environment," *Scientific American*, 224: No. 5 (1971), 15-21.
19. Guralnik, David, ed., *Webster's New World Dictionary of the American Language* (2nd college ed.). New York: The World Publishing Company, 1972.
20. Guyton, Arthur, *Textbook of Medical Physiology*. Philadelphia: W. B. Saunders Company, 1966.
21. Hamilton, Michael, ed., *The New Genetics and the Future of Man*. Grand Rapids, Mich.: William B. Eerdmans Publishing Company, 1972, pp. 179-228.
22. Haslam, P., "Noise in Hospitals: Its Effect on the Patient," *Nursing Clinics of North America*, 5: No. 4 (1970), 715-24.
23. Hawker, Lilian, and Alan Linton, eds., *Microorganisms: Function, Form, and Environment*. New York: American Elsevier Publishing Company, Inc., 1971.
24. Hitchcock, Stephen, and William Curtsinger, "Fragile Nurseries of the Sea: Can We Save Our Salt Marshes?" *National Geographic*, 141: No. 6 (1972), 729-65.
25. Hunter, John, "Shortcomings and Remedies for the Water Quality Improvement Programs of the United States: A Brief Summary," *American Journal of Public Health*, 63: No. 4 (1973), 345-51.
26. Izaak Walton League's Citizen Workshops for Clean Water for America, *Clean Water: It's Up to You*. New York, 1970.
27. Jamann, Joann, "Health Is a Function of Ecology," *American Journal of Nursing*, 71: No. 5 (1971), 970-73.
28. Jennings, Betty, and Susie Gudermuth, "Hospital Solid Waste: A Challenge for Nurses," *Missouri Nurse*, 47: No. 2 (1973), 5-7.
29. Jones, K., L. Shainberg, and C. Byer, *Dimensions: A Changing Concept of Health*. San Francisco: Canfield Press, 1972.
30. Kermode, G. O., "Food Additives," *Scientific American*, 226: No. 3 (1972), 15-21.
31. League of Women Voters of The United States, Fund Publication No. 393, *A Congregation of Vapors*. Washington, D.C., 1970.
32. _____, Who Pays for a Clean Stream? Washington, D.C., 1969.
33. Linton, Ron, *Terracide*. Boston: Little, Brown and Company, 1970.

34. Litsky, Warren, Joseph Martin, and Bertha Litsky, "Solid Waste: A Hospital Dilemma," *American Journal of Nursing*, 72: No. 10 (1972), 1841-47.

35. Long, Keith, "Pesticides: An Occupational Hazard on Farms," *American Journal of Nursing*, 71: No. 4 (1971), 740-43.

36. Medalia, Nahum Z., "Air Pollution as a Socio-Environmental Health Problem: A Survey Report," in *Patients, Physicians, and Illness* (2nd ed.), ed. E. Gartly Jaco. New York: The Free Press, 1972.

37. Minckley, Barbara, "Space and Place in Patient Care," *American Journal of Nursing*, 68: No. 3 (1968), 510-16.

38. National Commission on Community Health Service, *Changing Environmental Hazards: Challenges to Community Health, Report of the Task Force on Environmental Health*. Washington, D.C.: Public Affairs Press, 1967.

39. National Tuberculosis and Respiratory Disease Association, *Air Pollution Primer*. New York, 1969.

40. Neylan, Margaret, "The Nurse in a Healing Milieu," *American Journal of Nursing*, 61: No. 4 (1961), 72-74.

41. Oates, William, D. Snellings, and E. Wilson, "Microwave Oven Survey Results in Arkansas During 1970," *American Journal of Public Health*, 63: No. 3 (1973), 193-98.

42. Parrish, Henry, "Animal-Man Relationships in Today's Environment," *American Journal of Public Health*, 63: No. 3 (1973), 199-200.

43. Peakall, David, "Pesticides and the Reproduction of Birds," *Scientific American*, 222: No. 4 (1970), 72-78.

44. Reed, Jane, "Lead Poisoning: Silent Epidemic and Social Crime," *American Journal of Nursing*, 72: No. 12 (1972), 2181-84.

45. Rockefeller, Nelson, *Our Environment Can Be Saved*. Garden City, N.Y.: Doubleday & Company, Inc., 1970.

46. Saltonstall, Richard, *Your Environment and What You Can Do about It: A Citizens' Guide*. New York: Walker and Company, 1970.

47. Smith, Dorothy, "Patienthood and Its Threat to Privacy," *American Journal of Nursing*, 69: No. 3 (1969), 509-13.

48. Stephens, Gwen, "Clinical Research in Human Ecology," in *Current Concepts in Clinical Nursing*, eds. B. Bergersen, E. Anderson, M. Duffey, M. Lohr, and M. Rose. St. Louis: The C. V. Mosby Company, 1967, pp. 76-88.

49. Stevens, Leonard, "What Makes a Ward Climate Therapeutic?" *American Journal of Nursing*, 61: No. 3 (1961), 95-96.

50. Sutterly, Doris, and Gloria Donnelly, *Perspectives in Human Development*. Philadelphia: J. B. Lippincott Company, 1973, pp. 266-302.

51. The Conservation Foundation, "Your Right to Clean Air." Washington, D.C., 1970.

52. "The World and How We Abuse It," *National Geographic*, 138: No. 6 (1970), 782-83.

53. Trainer, Daniel, "Wildlife as Monitors of Disease," *American Journal of Public Health*, 63: No. 3 (1973), 201-3.

54. United States Environmental Pollution Panel, United States President's Science Advisory Committee, *Restoring the Quality of Our Environment*. Washington, D.C., 1965.

55. United States Environmental Protection Agency, *A Primer on Waste Water Treatment*. Washington, D.C.: U.S. Government Printing Office, 1971.

56. ———, *Environmental Protection, 1971*. Washington, D.C.: U.S. Government Printing Office, 1971.

57. ———, *Let's Dump the Dumps*. Greenfield, Mass.: Channing L. Bete Company, 1971.

58. ———, *Noise and You*. Greenfield, Mass.: Channing L. Bete Company, Inc., 1970.

59. ———, *Toward a New Environmental Ethic*. Washington, D.C.: U.S. Government Printing Office, 1971.

60. Van Sickle, Derek, *The Ecological Citizen*. New York: Harper & Row, Publishers, 1971.

61. Walker, Bailus, "Environmental Quality and the Local Health Agency: A Re-examination," *American Journal of Public Health*, 63: No. 4 (1973), 352-57.

62. Ward, Fred, "The Imperiled Everglades," *National Geographic*, 141: No. 1 (1972), 1-27.

63. Yen, Harry, "The Fragile Beauty All Around Us," *National Geographic*, 138: No. 6 (1970), 785-95.

64. Young, Gordon, "Pollution Threat to Man's Only Home," *National Geographic*, 138: No. 6 (1970), 738-81.

CHAPTER 10

Cultural Influences
on the Person

Study of this chapter will help you to:

1 Define *culture* and *subculture* and describe various types of subcultures.

2 Discuss the general characteristics of any culture and how these affect the persons you care for.

3 Identify the dominant cultural values in the United States and how they influence you as a health care worker as well as the patient and family.

4 Compare the cultural values of the traditional Greek, the Spanish American living in the southwestern United States, and the Japanese in relation to the family unit, male and female relationships, childrearing patterns, the group versus privacy, time orientation, work, and use of leisure, education, and change.

5 Contrast the attitudes toward health and illness of persons living in the main cultures of the United States, Greece, Spanish American neighborhoods in the southwestern United States, and Japan.

6 Interview a person from another culture and contrast his values to those described in this chapter.

7 Discuss influences of culture upon the health status of the person and group.

8 Describe how knowledge of cultural values and attitudes toward daily living practices, health, and illness can influence the effectiveness of your health care.

9 Discuss ways to meet the needs of another with cultural values different from your own.

10 Apply knowledge about the teaching-learning process to a health education program for a person or family from another culture.

11 Assess and care for a patient from another culture and identify your own ethnocentric tendencies.

When someone talks or acts differently from you, consider that to him you may also seem to talk or act differently. Many such differences are cultural and should be understood rather than laughed at.

The great divide between man and animals is culture. Culture includes using language, art forms, and games to communicate with others; cooperating in problem solving; deliberately training children; developing unique interpretations; forming organizations; and making, saving, using, and changing tools. Humans are heir to the accumulation of wisdom and folly of preceding generations and in turn they teach others their beliefs, feelings, and practices. The patient, his family, and you are deeply affected by the culture learned during the early years, often more so than by that learned later. An understanding of culture and its influence upon behavior is essential to understanding yourself and the person for whom you are caring.

DEFINITIONS

Culture is the sum total of the learned ways of doing, feeling, and thinking, past and present, of a social group within a given period of time. These ways are transmitted from one generation to the next or to immigrants who become members of the society. Culture is a group's design for living, a shared set of socially transmitted assumptions about the nature of the physical and social world, goals in life, attitudes, roles, and values. *Culture is a complex integrated system that includes knowledge, beliefs, skills, art, morals, law, customs, and any other acquired habits and capabilities of man. All provide a pattern for living together.*

A subculture is a group of persons, within a culture, of the same age, socioeconomic status, ethnic origin, education, or occupation, or with the same goals, who have an identity of their own but are related to the total culture in certain ways[24]. Spanish Americans, American Indians, and American blacks represent subcultures. Regional, social-class, religious, and family subcultures also exist. A description of each follows.

Regional culture refers to the local or regional manifestations of the larger culture. Thus the child learns the sectional variant of the national culture—for example, rural or urban, Yankee, Southerner, Midwesterner, or Westerner. Regional culture is influenced by geography, trade, and economics; variations may be shown in values, beliefs, housing, food, occupational skills, and language.

A social class also has its own culture. *A social class is a cultural grouping of persons who, through group consensus and similarity of occupation, wealth, and education, have come to have a similar status, life style, values, ideas, interests, feelings, attitudes, language usage, and overt forms of behavior.* The people belonging to this group meet each another on equal terms and have a consciousness of cohesion[24, 48]. Social class is not only economic in orgin, for other factors also contribute to superior status, such as age, sex, and personal endowment.

The more a class as a group becomes fixed, the more predictable is its patterns of attitudes and behavior. The child learns the patterns of his own class and his class attitude toward another class. These attitude patterns make up a culture's *value system, its conception of how people should behave in various situations as well as which goals they should pursue and how.* The value systems of the general culture and of the subculture or social class may at times conflict. Additional discussion about social classes can be found in Chapter 12.

Religious culture also influences the person, for a *religion constitutes a way of living and thinking and therefore is a kind of culture.* Religious influences on values, attitudes, and behavior are discussed in Chapter 11.

Family culture refers to the family life, which is part of the cultural system. The family is the medium through which the larger cultural heritage is transmitted to the child. *Family culture consists of ways of living and thinking that constitute the family and sexual aspects of group life.* These ways include courtship and marriage patterns, sexual mores, husband-wife relationships, status of men and women, parent-child relationships, childrearing, responsibilities to parents, and attitudes toward unmarried women, illegitimate children, and divorce[7].

The family gives the child status. The family name gives the child a social position as well as an identity, so the child is assigned the status of the family and the reputation that goes with it. Family status has a great deal to do with health and behavior throughout life because of its effect upon self-concept.

Family rituals are the collective way of working out household routines and using time within the family culture. *Ritual is a system of definitely prescribed behaviors and procedures, which provides exactness in daily tasks of living and has a sense of rightness about it.* The more often the behavior is repeated, the more it comes to be approved and therefore habitual. Thus rituals inevitably develop in family life due to the intimacy of relationships and the repetition and continuity of certain interactions. Rituals change from one life cycle to another—for example, at marriage, after childbirth, when children go to school, and when children leave home. Rituals are important in child development because: (1) They are group habits that communicate ways of doing things and attitudes related to events, including family etiquette, affectionate responses between family members, organization of leisure time, and education for group adjustment. (2) They promote family solidarity and continuity by promoting habitual behavior, unconsciously performed, which brings harmony to family life. Many rituals will continue to the next generation, increasing the person's sense of worth, security, and family continuity or identity. (3) They aid in maintaining self-control through disciplinary measures. (4) They promote feelings of euphoria, sentimentality, or well-being—for example, through holiday celebrations. They also dictate reactions to threat, such as at times of loss, illness, or death[7]. You must consider the person's standard rituals as you plan care. Family influences are dealt with more extensively in Chapter 13.

CHARACTERISTICS OF CULTURE

Culture as Learned

There are three basic characteristics of culture. First, *culture is learned*. People function physiologically in much the same way throughout the world, but their behavior is learned and therefore relatively diverse. Because of his culture, a child is ascribed or acquires a certain *status or position of prestige*. He also learns or assumes certain *roles, patterns of related behaviors expected of him by others, and later by himself, that define his behavior and adjustment to a given group.* His behavior, values, attitudes, and beliefs, learned within his culture, become a matter of tradition, even though the culture allows choices within limits and may even encourage certain kinds of deviancy. The way in which a person experiences his culture and society and what he learns as he grows are of great significance. Culture determines the kinds of experiences the person encounters and the extent to which his responses to life situations will be either unhealthy, maladaptive, and self-defeating, or healthy, adaptive, constructive, and creative[10, 45]. What the person has learned from his culture determines how and what you will be able to teach him, as well as your approach to him during care.

Culture as Stable But Changing

The second characteristic of culture is that *it is subject to and capable of change in order to remain viable and adaptive, although it is basically a stable entity.* The culture of a society, like a human body, is dynamic but maintained at a steady state by self-regulating devices. *Stabilizing features are traditions and the ready-made solutions to life's problems* that are provided for the group, enabling the person to anticipate the behavior of others, predict future events, and regulate his life within the culture. Behavior, carefully defined by the culture, is hard to change because of group pressure. Norms and customs that persist may have a negative influence on the group. Food taboos during pregnancy, a high-animal-fat diet, or crowding of people into a common dwelling that provides an apt incubator for spread of contagious disease are examples[40].

Another stabilizing, limiting aspect of culture is the use of language. Although language forms vary from culture to culture, the terms for *mother* and *father* sound very much alike across cultural lines, perhaps because certain vocalizations are easy for a child to articulate and learn.

Learning cultural and family language is primarily by ear and can affect the child who learns better by sight. In addition, use of language is determined considerably by age and sex—for example, baby talk, child talk, adult talk, girl talk, and boy talk. Subcultural groups, particularly the family, differ in conversational mores—that is, permitted topics of conversation; proper situations for discussing certain topics, such as during mealtime or before bedtime; level of vocabulary used; reaction to new words used; number of interruptions permitted; who can be interrupted; and who talks most[7].

The meeting ground between cultures is in language and *dialect, a variety of a language spoken by a distinct group of people in a definite place.* All immigrants to the United States brought their own ethnic and cultural heritage and language. No doubt all had problems being acculturated to mainstream America, but generally their different life styles and accents were considered interesting and eventually accepted. Until recently, the least accepted and understood group of "immigrants" have been the blacks, brought to America not by choice and separated from their culture and awareness of their past in Africa. They were expected to express their cultural and racial identity through the white man's culture and image of what it meant to be black. Thus English was superimposed on the many African languages that were forced together. An artificial subculture characterized by Aunt Jemima and Uncle Remus was created.

With the movement of the black American minority to express their identity, dialect, as well as other components of their subculture, has received attention[16, 17, 41, 65, 66]. Understanding of the black subculture and dialect can help you to talk with, understand, and care for the black person, just as understanding of subculture and dialect of any ethnic group enhances acceptance and care of that person. Nonblacks often do not understand black dialect. While it often coincides with "standard American English," it has its own grammatical rules (and errors), slang, cadence, and intonation. Black dialect will vary from region to region and with the age, sex, and economic status of the user. Some blacks avoid using black dialect, especially those more highly educated and in the higher social classes. And keep in mind that dialect usage changes, as all language usage changes, with time. A word that is first specific to a minority ethnic group can later be adopted by members of the mainstream culture.

Black dialect has words for which there are no analogies in "standard

American English," such as the *hawk*: a severe, bone-chilling wind (originally blowing off the Great Lakes). The verbs *am, is,* and *are* are often omitted in dialect, being unnecessary for a complete sentence. The verb form *be* can indicate extended or repeated action, and *been*, completed or past action: "He be hurtin' " means "He has been in pain for some time." "He been hurtin' " means "He was in pain." A sentence without an auxiliary verb indicates an activity going on now that does not usually occur—for example, "She workin'," or "She *be* workin' " indicates the person is doing the work she usually does. Possession can be expressed without the use of *'s*—for example, as in "my baby clothes," instead of "my baby's clothes." The letter *g* is commonly dropped as an end sound; two syllables may be shortened into one, and *th* pronounced like *v* or *d*. To avoid grammatical redundancy, the *s* is omitted in plural noun forms if some other word in the sentence indicates plural—for example, "She have three brother." *Man* may be used instead of the name of the person addressed or to convey emphasis. The word *ain't* can be used to negate verbs in the past tense: "Dey ain't like dat" can mean "They *didn't* like that" rather than "They *aren't* like that." An undifferentiated form of the possessive pronoun occurs—as in "He a nice girl."

You will find a variety of regional dialects in the United States—for example, "Brooklynese," southern mountain, Texas cotton country, Missouri Ozarkian, and Pennsylvania Dutch. Language differences may give a false impression about the intelligence of the person, since some people have difficulty switching from dialect to "standard American English." Listen carefully to the language spoken, be accepting of the dialect, and validate meanings of words when necessary.

Von Bertalanffy discusses how language emphasizes the values of a culture. For example, neither the language of the Nootka Indians on Vancouver Island nor that of the Hopi has a separate subject and predicate or parts of speech, as does English. These languages instead describe an event as a whole with a single term. He points out that Americans are complex, abstract, and fragmentary in their descriptions of the world around them. The Indo-European languages, of which English is one, emphasize time. Cultures using these languages keep records, use mathematics, do accounting, use clocks and calendars, and study archeology to learn of their historical past. In contrast, past, present, and future tense do not exist in the Hopi language; the validity of a statement is not based on time or history but on "fact," memory, expectations, or customs. The Navaho language also has little development of time and instead emphasizes type of activity, duration, or aspects of movement. Further, von Bertalanffy shows how Indo-European languages, like English, describe nonspatial relationships with spatial metaphors—for example, *long* and *short* for duration; *heavy* and *light* or *long* and *short* for intensity; *rise* and *fall* for tendency. In the Hopi language, psychological metaphors are used to name mental processes; for example, *heart* can be used for *think* or *remember*. Thus various cultures have different conceptualizations with which to perceive the same matter or reality.

The kinds of conceptualizations influence the values, behavior, stability, and progress of a culture[71].

Analyses of the habits and practices of various peoples show that traditional language and behavior patterns practiced between parent and child within a culture are related to the interactions within that culture between employer and employee, among peers, and between nurse and patient, making for predictability and stability. Stability of culture promotes adaptability and economy of energy[45].

Cultures also change, sometimes imperceptibly, so that norms, the usual rules for living, are modified to meet the group's needs as new life challenges arise. Cultures change primarily in response to technological innovation or by borrowing from another culture. For example, the harnessing of electrical power and the subsequent invention and use of electrical appliances and tools have changed the way of life in America: in work, recreation, food preservation, communication, education, vocabulary, women's roles, health care, and the entire value system.

Each culture is a whole, but not every culture is integrated in the same way to the same extent. Some cultures are so tightly integrated that any change threatens the whole. Other cultures are characterized by traditional patterns that are easy to manipulate and change.

When significant numbers of people begin to respond differently than usual to one or more facets of a culture, this may cause others in the society to realize that a particular custom or norm is no longer useful. Such customs might pertain to marriage, burial, childrearing, or moral codes. If a group of people (or isolated persons) can consistently adapt while at the same time following the norm imperfectly, they may establish a new norm, which may be gradually adopted by others until it becomes the generally established pattern. Thus the culture and the people in it can be changed, in spite of initial resistance. Such changes can have a positive or negative influence on health[45].

Cultural Components and Patterns

The third characteristic of culture is that *there are certain components or patterns present in every culture*, regardless of how "primitive" or "advanced" it may be[48, 75]. Understanding these can help you understand yourself, your patient, and the health care system in which you work.

A Communication System, which may include only the language itself or the complexities of mass media, computers, and satellites, is the basis for interaction and cohesion between persons and a vehicle for the transmission and preservation of culture[7]. In addition to vocabulary and word taboos, there are gestures, facial expressions, and voice qualities—intonation, rhythm, speed, pronunciation—that vary among families or groups within a culture and carry specific meanings. Since 100 million Americans nightly watch television, it has become the most powerful cultural communication force in the United States today. Television could be used more effectively for mass health teaching, just as it is used now for mass advertising[29].

Methods and Objects Are Used by a Culture to Provide for Man's Physical Welfare. Methods include getting food; establishing personal care habits; making, using, saving, and improving tools; and manufacturing. Objects include instruments and machines used to change land terrain for farming, home building, or industrialization, and equipment used to diagnose and test disease.

Means or Techniques of Travel and Transportation of Goods and Services are particularized to a culture. Whether these are walking, use of dog or horse, or a complex system of cars, trucks, railways, and airplaines, they will affect the person's ability to obtain health care, among other services and goods.

Exchange of Goods and Services may occur through barter, trade, commerce, involve occupational roles, and affect work and payment in a health care system.

Forms of Property, real estate and personal, are defined by the culture in terms of their necessity and worth. Respecting the person's property in the hospital or home shows that you respect him personally.

Sexual and Family Patterns, which may vary considerably from culture to culture, affect how you care for and teach the person. Such patterns include wedding ceremonies, divorce proceedings, forms of kinship relationships, guardianship roles, inheritance rights, the family's division of labor, and roles assigned men, women, and children.

Societal Controls and the Institution of Government include *mores, morally binding attitudes, and* **customs**, *long-established practices having the force of unwritten law.* Other controls include public or group opinion, laws, political offices and the organization of government, the regulation of time, and institutionalized forms of conflict within the society or between tribes, states, or nations, such as war. These factors all influence the health care system in which you work. Increasingly, the nurse must become familiar with the political system and skilled in using it for improving health care.

Artistic Expression through architecture, painting, sculpture, music, literature, and dance is universal, although what is considered art by one culture may not be so considered by another. Knowledge concerning these factors can be useful in therapy and rehabilitation.

Recreational and Leisure-Time Interests and Activities, as defined by each cultural group, are essential for health and must be considered in the nursing history and in medical diagnosis.

Religious and Magical Ideas and Practices exist in the form of various beliefs, taboos, ethical codes, rituals, mythology, philosophy, or the organized institution of the church, and serve to guide the behavior of a cultural group during health and illness.

Knowledge Basic to Survival and Expansion of the Group is always present. In civilized or "advanced" societies, the development of *science, systematized knowledge based on observation, study, and experimentation,* is basic to technological innovation and improving material living standards. In modern Western cultures, science is highly valued as a basis for health care. Medical science influences man biologically and socially.

Cultural Structuring of Basic Human Patterns includes rules for competition, conflict, cooperation, collaboration, and games. Also, the intimate habits of daily life, both personally and in groups, the manner in which one's house and body are perceived, and the many "taken-for-granted" activities between people are basically structured.

All the foregoing components and patterns influence and are influenced by climate, natural resources, geography, sanitation facilities, diet, group biological and genetic factors, and disease conditions and health practices.

COMPARISON OF CULTURES

Cultural Values in the United States

Several orientations and value systems may be simultaneously present in a given society or culture, but only one orientation dominates over a given period of time. Presently in the United States, the middle-class orientation and value system are dominant. This is further discussed in Chapter 12.

In the past (and to some degree still now), the Protestant ethic described by sociologist Max Weber was the prime influence on American culture, even for those Americans who were not Protestants. An *ethic is defined as an outlook or view made up of assumptions that are not often noticed and still less often questioned or tested.* These assumptions are blindly and passively accepted because they have been handed down from generation to generation and had their origins in an unimpeachable, but long forgotten, authority. With new knowledge, the assumptions are often found invalid, but assumptions about living undergo a slow process of change. The Protestant ethic encompasses a harsh, pessimistic view of man. It upholds the five following assumptions: (1) Man is basically imperfect and must struggle against his imperfection. (2) Man was placed on earth to struggle, and so struggle must be valued. Any sign of surrender or softness denotes weakness in the person and is bad. (3) Self-sacrifice and aspiring to good conduct are essential to overcome evil and gain personal salvation. (4) Emotions cannot be overtly expressed. Displaying anger is basically un-Christian. One should love one's neighbor; but expressing love openly is suspect, especially if related to sexuality, since sex is considered an animal pleasure and therefore a taboo topic. Even too intense an expression of nonsexual love can be a sign of weakness, and one must be strong and self-controlled in order to struggle. Anxiety must be avoided or denied, for it shows that the struggle is not going well. (5) The world is seen as useful to man and should provide for his material satisfaction, since his life is devoid of inner satisfaction. Thus the exploitation of land, even ruthlessly, is acceptable. Mastery of the environment is emphasized. Conservation of natural resources is secondary, since the resources of the world (which are supposedly inexhaustible) were put there for man's use [72].

Earlier in this century, Puritanical values and rigid Christian morality upheld the tenet of fear of God's judgment. A strong conscience was developed in fear of punishment and social disfavor. Society was stable because traditions were adhered to and proverbs were taken seriously. Hard work, plain living, self-control, responsibility, will power, honesty, and initiative were emphasized. Family and community roles were clearly defined: father was the patriarch; mother was subservient to him; and children were obedient to all. Education also emphasized discipline, order, and obedience to authority. People were tradition-bound and hard-working, and provided stability in society. Your understanding that many elderly and middle-aged persons still live by these values can help you better accept them and plan their care.

You need only look around at what Toffler calls our superindustrial society to realize that the Protestant ethic is losing its hold [69]. Yet parts of this ethic are being revived by some of the growing fundamentalist religious groups.

The American value system is worldly, in spite of its religious roots, since the most highly valued activities involve practical, secular pursuits rather than contemplation, devotion, or esthetic satisfaction. Thus the ideal society, originally the Kingdom of God on earth, has for many people been secularized into a good society with ideals of liberty, justice, general prosperity, and equality of opportunity [50].

Keniston describes how the issue of violence is to this generation in America what the issue of sex was to the Victorian world. Today's young adults have grown up with the ever-present possibility of instantaneous death or permanent maiming by thermonuclear, chemical, or biological warfare agents. The threat and fear of violence are therefore constant facts of life. Fear of violence has led to a fascination with violence that further surrounds people with its symptoms. American society is preoccupied with, almost mesmerized, by the violence of organized crime, urban rioting, and political assassinations. Violence on television and in the movies shows the potential for brutality and aggression in all [30].

People react differently to constant exposure to violence: they may tolerate it, develop disease symptoms, project their own aggression onto others, develop a neurotic preoccupation with it, or act violently themselves in order to discharge rage. We see examples of each of these reactions in our society in the form of physical, emotional, and social illness.

Persad discusses how concepts of aggression and dependency vary from culture to culture. In American culture, aggression is regarded as an innate force that has survival value and that requires appropriate channels for its expression; it is considered an integral part of social success. However, if aggression is not dealt with appropriately, the person becomes psychopathic. In some cultures, aggression is considered the result rather than the cause of psychopathy. Americans teach their children to be independent and emphasize the importance of the adolescent or young adult leaving home. Psychiatric therapy in the United States is often directed toward these goals. In traditional Oriental cultures, however, the young adult may be castigated for abruptly leaving home or striving for independence. Consideration for family elders is more important than one's desires to pursue personal goals. In American culture a well-developed ego is considered necessary for maturity. In Oriental cultures personal preoccupation with the ego is considered as absurd[53].

Three Cultures: Greek, Spanish-American, and Japanese

Tables 10-1 through 10-7 contrast Greek culture, Spanish-American culture in the southwestern United States, and Japanese culture. Discussion will center on the family unit, male and female relationships, childrearing, the group versus privacy, time orientation, work and use of leisure time, education, and attitudes regarding change. The following discussion then compares the attitudes of Americans regarding health and illness with the corresponding attitudes in each of these cultures[3, 4, 10, 19, 25, 38, 45, 50, 69]. Although neither a comprehensive study nor a stereotype of everyone in these cultures, these comparisons indicate that subtle as well as obvious differences, along with some similarities, exist among different groups' values and behavior. Understand that these cultural patterns will be followed by different persons in each culture to varying degrees, denied by some, and not identified, yet taken for granted by others. Chapters 12 and 13 will discuss some of these values in relation to American culture.

Attitudes Regarding Health and Illness

How health is identified, physically and emotionally, varies from culture to culture, as do ideas about the factors related to health and disease. American definitions are emphasized in Chapter 1.

Attitudes in the United States toward health are influenced considerably by society's emphasis on mastery of the environment as opposed to adjustment to it. Illness is seen as a challenge to be met by mobilizing resources: research, science, funds, institutions, and people. Americans tax themselves to finance health and welfare organizations, and persons giving time and effort to these organizations are given special status by the community. Since independence is

TABLE 10-1

A Comparison of Cultures: The Family Unit

COMPONENT	GREEK	SPANISH-AMERICAN	JAPANESE
Basis for Marriage	Social and family welfare. All of society patterned on family.	Family welfare central.	Value family and household lineage.
Type of Family System	Paternalistic. Extended family. Monogamy. Marriage bond strong.	Paternalistic. Extended. Monogamy. Marriage bond strong.	Traditional value on authority of father and elderly. Family strongly identified with father. Subordinate position of women and arranged marriage still accepted by older generation.
Family Size	Want many children.	Large so parents not alone in old age.	Family planning, including use of abortion to control size in modern family.
Pattern of Interaction	Authoritarian. Man head of house. Sex roles traditional male and female. Mother powerful in own way; credited with sustaining child with moral strength. Children subordinate. Oldest son responsible for family if husband not present. Child not focus of family activity. No special activities for child, even birthday a time to wish family long happiness with child rather than focus on child. Family together most of time with child learning to enjoy adult behavior and anticipate adulthood. Peer contacts through family.	Authoritarian. Man head of house. Sex roles traditional male and female. Child seldom center of activity or attention. Avoid admiration of child for fear of "evil eye." Child proud of home responsibilities. Age respected. Family loyalty strong.	Family revered as an institution, but interrelationships lacking companionship and warmth. Major decisions made by family. Subordination of individual to family interest. Traditional autocratic family system stronger in rural areas, with eldest son inheriting family property and hesitant to rebel against father. Young generation choosing own marriage partner, establishing own household, and daughter-in-law gaining freedom from mother-in-law's dominance. Increasing premarital and extramarital sexual affairs.

283

TABLE 10-2

A Comparison of Cultures: Childrearing Patterns

COMPONENT	GREEK	SPANISH-AMERICAN	JAPANESE
Process of Childbirth	Considered normal process, not to be feared.	Considered normal process. Husband little involved. Special practices surrounding process.	Considered normal process.
Philosophy of Childrearing	Effectiveness sought as parent not as a pal. Child raised to be strong, hard, firm, straight, since that is ideal personality. Wishes of elders put before child's wishes.	Effectiveness sought as parent, not as a pal. Child taught to do as parents do, to listen to parents' advice, learn from their experience, and not advance further than their parents.	Traditionally child to be dutiful and responsible. Young urban generations not bound as firmly by traditions.
Practices of Childrearing	Mother firm, not overprotective. Baby kept in straight position when carried or in bed. Follow rigid schedule, consistent.	Consistent, traditional, faith in own judgment.	Mother enveloping child in warmth during early years, but when child older, relationship more distant. Oldest son reared differently from other brothers, and brothers from sisters, so every child aware of his place.
Responsibility for Child Care	Primarily mother, but older children involved in daily activities, including care of younger siblings. Attitude of love and responsibility among siblings.	Husband ultimately responsible as head of household. Any family member, including siblings and cousins, responsible at times.	Mother primarily, but all of family involved.

TABLE 10-2 (cont.)

COMPONENT	GREEK	SPANISH-AMERICAN	JAPANESE
Discipline	Consistent. Obedience very important and taught to child at early age. Child praised when good and told when bad. Taught that it is important to be good and not shame family. Use group pressure to set limits on behavior.	Consistently correct child because his behavior is bothersome and warned not to act in a way to provoke father. Instill fear of consequences. Pride in self-control and fear of being shamed instilled in child. Seldom told he is "good" or "bad"	Firm, consistent, lack strong emotions. Emphasis on responsibility, duty, loyalty. Promote feeling of insecurity when do wrong.
Training of Child	Taught to value interdependence, cooperation. Sibling rivalry when new baby arrives but does not last long. Mother delighted with new baby but shares self equally with older child, including offer of free breast during feeding. Older child invited to share excitement about baby. Parents never clowning for child's amusement or giving many material things.	Taught to value interdependence, companionship. Little sibling jealousy. Freely show affection and attention.	Taught to value interdependence but responsible for own behavior. Taught to carry out obligation regardless of personal cost and to control behavior to avoid personal shame and disgrace of group. Develop strong sense of responsibility. Poor communication between generations because of differences in experiences, education, language comprehension, and values fostering problems in modern society.

285

TABLE 10-3

A Comparison of Cultures: Interaction with Others versus Privacy

COMPONENT	GREEK	SPANISH-AMERICAN	JAPANESE
Basic Values of Person and Behavior	Strong sense of self-esteem. Inner core of personality not to be exposed or shamed. Value equality, individuality. Aloneness not sought, but borne with fortitude. Pride in glorious past of Greece.	Anxiety about being alone and concern for people who are alone. Not considered proper to compete, push self forward in group through achievements. Better to submit than provoke anger in another. Violence atypical.	Strong sense of self-respect and important to be treated respectfully by others. Privacy not valued, apparently unwanted, and seen as loneliness.
Personal Possessions	Value in shared living and sharing possessions, especially with family and friends.	Sharing of possessions. One's own house nebulous; frequent unannounced visiting among family and friends.	Possessions not highly valued. Shared living space and possessions in family.
Status of Person	Valued for what he is rather than position or achievement. Family unit valued, not individual.	Valued for what he is, depends on family.	Belonging to right clique or faction important to status and future success. Try to join influential group at early age.
Interaction among Persons	Resented when treated impersonally, mechanically, or like a number on a chart. No word for "group," but born into group of family and friends. Extended family working together for benefit of each other. Units of cooperation retained from past, not created. Work to achieve common goal with those to whom he feels loyalty. Speech of much importance because it establishes interactions.	Much neighborhood socializing, especially among women to borrow, help, consult, discuss, or exchange gifts. Interchange of gifts and services frequent. Accepting as gracious as giving, and person not satisfied until he has returned a gift to show appreciation; return gift not necessarily same kind or form. Strangers not completely accepted unless related to established family by marriage.	Suppression of emotion in many situations. Most docile with strong urge to conform. Pleasant, polite, correct but aloof behavior to others in all classes. Restrained, formal, hierarchal relationships in family, company, and political party rather than horizontal, comradely behavior. Ceremonious, at ease, and apologetic to acquaintances and friends but less so with strangers. Man unappreciative of domineering woman.
Social Activities	Family basic social group. Circle of friends important.	Few formalized social groups. Family basic social group. Women thought of as one social group, men another. Remain close to own social group for job or	Fondness for crowds and physical proximity of people. Participation and spectator roles in social activities and sports enjoyed.

TABLE 10-4

A Comparison of Cultures: Time Orientation

COMPONENT	GREEK	SPANISH-AMERICAN	JAPANESE
Concept of Time	Present important but prepare for something in future that is sure part of life. No automatic faith in future. Distasteful to organize activities according to clock. Life regulated by body needs and rhythms, daily pattern of light and dark, and seasons.	Present important but validated by past. Expect future to be like present. Perform with distinction in present rather than emphasize efficiency, quantity. Life not regulated by clock but by body needs and rhythms, light and dark, seasons, religious holidays.	Time neither an absolute nor objective category but a process—the changing of nature with man as part of it. Planning for future valued. Present considered important, and past priceless.
Use of Time	Time used spontaneously. Elastic attitude toward time. "Tomorrow" thought of as tomorrow, next week, or never. Activities and appointments usually not starting on time, but person not hurried.	Time used spontaneously. Little value in planning ahead. "Right now" meaning now or later.	Appreciation of time. Calmness and time for daily ceremony highly valued. Ceremony carried out in spite of rush of work.

TABLE 10-5

A Comparison of Cultures: Work and Use of Leisure Time

COMPONENT	GREEK	SPANISH-AMERICAN	JAPANESE
Concept of Work	Work thought of as life, a joy and dignity, not drudgery. Work interrupted primarily for religious reasons, not as claim to idleness or leisure. Women as hard workers as men. Tenacious and resourceful at making the best of what they have and coping with difficulty. Person not to be hurried but works efficiently at own pace.	Work considered inevitable part of daily life. Not done just to keep busy or earn more money if present needs met. No moral corruption in being idle. Work at own pace and no specially defined working hours if possible. Everyone expected to cooperate and do his part. Work shared to decrease loneliness. Work roles of sexes and age groups distinct but each aware of tasks performed by the other. Able to take over work roles of other family members. Child a part in work of home and family and feels important. No special rewards.	Enjoyment of work more important than money earned. Strong ties between person, his job, and his company. Job mobility frowned upon. Independence in work traditionally valued but younger workers adjusting to Western concept of employment.
Concept of Leisure	Leisure an attitude, a dimension of all life and work. Not confined to certain time but a continual expression of internal freedom, at work or rest.	Leisure synonymous with free time. No emphasis on leisure for own sake. Intersperse work with rest, socialize during work. Free time spent visiting.	Some leisure time used in solitude. Much leisure time spent in traveling with peers. Freer expression of emotion in recreational pursuits.

TABLE 10-6
A Comparison of Cultures: Education

COMPONENT	GREEK	SPANISH-AMERICAN	JAPANESE
Value on Education	Highly prized, especially professional education. Educated person accorded much respect. Use of creative intellect and being cultured citizen valued, but can be achieved through life's experiences and work as well as by education.	Learns that which interests him. Absent from school if learning little or if something more interesting going on elsewhere. Not seen as only way to achieve.	Education highly valued, with emphasis on scientific information. Eager to learn. Believe in value of practical experience as well. Choice of college influences status in life. Much competition in education.
Educational Methods	Emphasize quickness, curiosity, cleverness, realism, reason. Education applied to matters of life.	No emphasis on excelling or competing for high grades or honors.	Educational reform by American occupation after World War II counter to traditional methods: replaced rote memorization with progressive methods, deemphasized moral training and unquestioning acceptance of authority, granted equal status to women, broadened opportunity for women.

TABLE 10-7

A Comparison of Cultures: Attitudes Regarding Change

COMPONENT	GREEK	SPANISH-AMERICAN	JAPANESE
Value of Change	Not valued for itself. Progress hoped for but not taken for granted. Change not necessarily bringing progress or improvement.	Change condemned simply because it is change. Little faith in progress or control over own destiny.	Physical world considered transient. Person appreciative but does not cling to things, thus change accepted.
Pace of Change	Deliberate.	Slow. Deliberate.	Able to adjust life style to rapid economic, industrial, and urban changes.
Effect of Change	No value on unlimited progress. Wants what is better than present but what is known and can be achieved. A plan to an American synonymous with a dream to a Greek. Adaptive to change. Utilizes material goods. Do not discard useful articles. Repair to maintain usefulness of object. Traditional Greek culture changing, becoming Westernized, affecting behavior of young.	Value system seen as constant. Feel many individuals not amenable to change by human endeavor. Adjust to environment. Utilize material goods to capacity. Generally remain near traditional home, maintaining stable relationships with people. Change in main culture affecting behavior of young, causing insecurity in elders.	Urgency of Western-like activity a new phenomenon. Breaking traditional patterns and solidarity, increased individualism, competition, and individual insecurity. Youth seeking new values to replace old dogmas. Parent generation generally revere authority of family and state—now rejected by younger generation.

highly valued, the weak are expected to help themselves as much as possible. The strong help the weak as long as the latter's problems are caused by events beyond their control; otherwise, the physically, socially, or emotionally weak, deformed, or unsightly are devalued.

A person is evaluated on his productivity or "doing good." Since the ability to be productive is dependent in part on health, individual health is highly valued. Health in the broadest sense is considered necessary for successful interaction with others, educational accomplishment, ability to work, leadership, childrearing, and capacity to use opportunities. Thus development of medical, nursing, and other health sciences and technology is considered important. The physical causation of illness is generally accepted. Only recently have the sociocultural causes of disease also been emphasized.

The importance of health has been accentuated by industrialization, urbanization, high-level technology, greater social controls, and mass communications, as well as by a high level of responsibility and stress placed upon the person. Americans at times react to the complexities of society by retreating into ill health, physically, emotionally, or socially. Levels of pathology that could be tolerated in preindustrial societies cannot be tolerated in complex modern life. Americans are more likely to interpret a person's difficulty in fulfilling social-role expectations as illness than would some other societies. Thus the person who is ill is less likely to be tolerated or kept in the family. When the person is ill, he is supposed to leave home, isolate himself from the family, and be cared for in a strange place, the hospital, by strange people who are authorities on illness. One's capacity for meeting social-role expectations is developed primarily through family socialization and education, but it is protected and restored through the health care system. The ill person is expected to want to return to his normal roles and to leave behind the feelings of alienation, regression, and passivity that are part of the deviance of illness. The impersonal agency of the hospital exerts pressures that discourage staying dependent and ill.

In Greece, health is important and desired, but it is not a preoccupation. One should not pamper the self. Straight living gives a healthy body, and so fortitude, hardness, and a simple standard of living are pursued. Excesses in living—in eating, drinking, or smoking—are avoided, and in general the level of public health is high.

Going to bed is a sign of weakness except for recognized disease. People do not go to a doctor unless there is something seriously wrong; but then they expect the doctor, who is a father figure, to have the answers for their problems. Home remedies and the services of an herbalist are tried first as treatment. Prayers are said and vows made. Illness is thought to arise from evil or magical sources that can be counteracted through magical practices. Entering the hospital is a last resort.

The organs of highest significance are the eyes, for they reflect the real person. Next in importance are the lips because of the words that come out of them.

A girl's hair and a man's mustache are important symbols of sexual identity and attractiveness. The genital organs are not freely talked about but are respected for their reproductive functions. The body is meant to be covered, and exposed only when necessary. Dress and ornamentation are essential to complete one's body image.

Childlessness is unfortunate, and until recently the woman was held responsible. The woman dislikes any examination or treatment of the reproductive organs and will accept gynecological problems rather than seek medical care for fear fertility will be affected. Special care is given to the woman during pregnancy, when special regulations about hygiene, rest, activity, and a happy environment are followed.

The handicapped are not easily accepted because of the emphasis on a whole, strong, firm body. To be crippled, blind, or lame means one is not a whole person and is dependent, unable to do anything for oneself.

Attitudes among Spanish Americans in the U.S. Southwest are quite unlike attitudes in mainstream America. The Spanish American considers himself to be a whole person; thus "better health" has no meaning. Good health is associated with the ability to work and fulfill normal roles, since one gains and maintains respect by meeting one's responsibilities. Criteria of health are a sturdy body, ability to maintain normal physical activity, and absence of pain. The person does not have to perfect his health; as long as his family is around, he is all right. Thus preventive measures are not highly valued. The person does seek to care for himself, however, through moderation in eating, drinking, work, recreation, and sleep, and by leading a good life.

The Spanish American believes that hardship and suffering are the destiny of man and that reward for being submissive to God's will and for doing good will come in the next life. Ill health is accepted as part of life and is thought to be caused by an unknown external event or object, such as natural forces of cold, heat, storms, water, or as the result of sinning—acting against God's will. For example, the Spanish American thinks that one cause of illness is bad air, especially night air, which enters through a cavity or opening in the body. Thus a raisin may be placed on the cord stump of the newborn, and surgery is avoided if possible; both practices help prevent air from entering the body. Avoiding drafts, keeping windows closed at night, keeping the head covered, and following certain postpartum practices have the same basis. Other causes of disease (according to Spanish-American beliefs) include overwork, poor food, excess worry or emotional strain, undue exposure to weather, uneven wetting of the body, taking a drink when overheated, and giving blood for transfusion. *Evil eye, mal ojo, is a cause of disease that results when a person looks admiringly at the child of another.* Usually children are not openly admired, but precautions against illness include patting the child on the head or a light slap. (Do you know people in other subcultures with similar beliefs? Such causes are commonly stated when illness occurs.) A common illness, in this culture, *susto,* with symptoms of agitation and depression, results from traumatic, frightening experiences and may result in death. Psychosocial forces causing disease are also seen in *empacho*, a gastrointestinal disease that results from eating food that is disliked, or from overeating, or from eating hot bread. Disease may also result from organs or parts of the body moving from the normal position. Little attention is paid to colds, minor aches, or common gastrointestinal disorders.

The role of the family is important in time of illness. The head of the house, the man, determines whether illness exists and what treatment is to be given. The person goes to bed when he is too ill to work or to move. Treatment from a lay healer is sought if family care does not help. The medical doctor is called only when the Spanish American is gravely ill; this is combined with visiting, so the patient does not get the rest and isolation advised by health workers in the majority culture. The sick person does not withdraw from the group; doing so would only make him feel worse. Acceptance of his present fate amounts to saying, "If the Lord intends for me to die, I'll die." The discomfort of the present is considered, but not in terms of future complications. Being ill brings no secondary advantage of care or coddling. Communicable diseases are hard to control, for resistance to isolation is based on the idea that family members, relatives, and familiar objects cannot contaminate or cause illness. Taking of home remedies, wearing special articles, and performing special ceremonies are accepted ways of getting and staying well. The person feels he will keep well by observing the ritual calendar, being brotherly, being a good Catholic and member of the community. If the health worker uses any procedure such as X-ray, that is considered to be the treatment, and hence the person should be cured.

Accidents are feared because they disrupt the wholeness of the person. In addition, the Spanish American fears surgery, the impersonality of the hospital and nurses, and any infringement on modesty. The hospital represents death and isolation from family or friends. The "professional" (Anglo) approach of the majority culture is regarded as showing indifference to needs and as causing anxiety and discomfort.

Attitudes in Japan toward health strongly reflect the belief in a body-mind-spirit interrelationship. Spiritual and temporal affairs in life are closely integrated; thus health practices and religion are closely intertwined, influenced considerably by the magicoreligious practices of Shinto, Japan's ancient religion. For example, bathing customs stem from Shinto purification rites, and baths are taken in the evening before eating not only for cleanliness but for ceremony and relaxation as well.

There is a strong emphasis on physical fitness, an intact body, physical strength, determination, and long life. Self-discipline in daily habits is highly valued, as are the mental, spiritual, and esthetic aspects of the person. These remain equally important to the sick person.

As a child, the person is taught to minimize his reactions to injury and illness. Hence to the Westerner the sick person may appear stoic. Part of the reserve in expressing emotion and pain is also influenced by childrearing and interaction practices, which emphasize correct behavior and suppression of emotion. However, the sick person, as much as the well, expects to be treated with respect. He resents being addressed informally by his first name, the dominating behavior in women, and people entering his hospital room without knocking. He is eager to cooperate with the medical care program, but wishes to be included in planning and decisions regarding care. The so-called professional approach of the average American health worker is likely to insult the average Japanese, although he may be too polite to say so.

By studying the life patterns of people in various cultures, (especially those of patients for whom you care), and by taking into account the factors discussed in the following chapters on religion and social class, you can better understand and handle varying levels of health, health problems, and attitudes toward care of different groups.

INFLUENCES OF CULTURE ON HEALTH

Because every culture is complex, it can be difficult to determine whether health and illness are the result of cultural or of other factors, such as physiological or psychological factors. However, there are numerous accounts of the presence or absence of certain diseases in certain cultural groups and reactions to illness that are culturally determined. [For further information, see references, 3, 28, 40, 43, 47, 51, 56, 61, 68, 76.] Cultural influences may include food availability, dietary taboos, methods of hygiene, and effects of climate—all factors related to culture. Several examples of the influences of culture on health and illness follow. Of necessity, the examples are limited.

Three cultures have been studied by Leaf in which many of the people live to be very old, often well over 100 years. These people live in Vilcabamba, Ecuador; in Hunza, located in Pakistani-controlled Kashmir; and in Abkhazia in the Caucasus Mountain region of the Soviet Union [34]. In each of these cultures the old people, even centenarians, share in a great deal of the hard labor and are physically active at levels that fatigue the average Westerner. Exercise appears to be a major factor in their longevity, in that constant physical activity improves cardiopulmonary functions so that the oxygen supply to the heart is superior to that of sedentary or urban people. A coronary attack (without overt symptoms) may have occurred when the person was 60 or 70 without having interfered with his activity or his life. The body apparently compensated without difficulty.

In each of these cultures, the aged are accorded high social status. They occupy a central and privileged position in the extended family. They live with close relatives, are given useful roles, continue daily to perform useful tasks, contribute to the economy of the community, and are sought for counsel and for their wisdom. Sense of family continuity is strong. Marriage and a regular, prolonged sex life seem important to longevity. Centenarians admit that a spouse who made them unhappy aged them, meaning they *felt* old in earlier life. Women who have borne children often live longer; some centenarian women have more than 20 children. The elderly are not shunted aside as in Western industrial societies, nor are they forced to retire, but remain independent and expect great longevity. Once they lose their useful roles in the community, however, they die quickly.

Cultural dietary habits may also influence these people's health and longevity. In Abkhazia, many of the elderly people ate primarily beans and other vegetables in early life, and while their present diet is more varied, they still do not overeat. In Vilcabamba and in Hunza, the diet is low in calories, protein, fat, and carbohydrate and would be considered deficient by Western standards.

The geographical and cultural isolation of the people in Hunza and Vilcabamba may have resulted in generations of people with an absence of genes that would contribute to disease. However, in Abkhazia there are centenarians from many different ethnic groups. One common factor for centenarians in all three cultures is that their parents were also long-lived.

The influence of other cultural folkways on health was studied by Graham[22]. Using groups with low and high incidence of illness, he studied the influence of race, social class, ethnic group, and religion on distribution of disease. His epidemiological findings suggest that Jewish women have less cancer of the cervix than non-Jewish women and that these results can be related to circumcision of the Jewish male or to abstinence from intercourse as prescribed by Jewish law for a certain period after the menses. Nuns also have low risk for cancer of the cervix. Lower-class and black women generally in the United States, with earlier sexual intercourse and early and more frequent childbirth, run a higher risk than the rest of the population in general and than Jews in particular. Prostitutes also have a higher incidence of cancer of the cervix, possibly because of multiple sex partners. Graham was influenced by the etiological theory proposed by Martin that the uncircumcised non-Jewish male is more likely to harbor a carciogenic virus, although only certain men carry it. Therefore, a woman who has sexual intercourse with a greater number of men during her life has a greater chance of being exposed to the virus and hence runs a greater risk of cervical cancer[44].

Culturally induced belief in magic can cause illness and death. The profound physiological consequences of intense fear, including inability to eat or drink, may be responsible. However, there may be no physiological changes except in the terminal moments. If the behavior of friends and relatives—what they say or do—strongly reinforces the person's conviction of his imminent death, the victim becomes resigned to his fate and soon meets it[40].

A culture's favored drink may have implications for health. For example, in a remote Mexican village, health workers found that the only available beverage was an alcoholic drink made from the juice of a local plant. A safe water supply was brought in, but the people did not fare well on it. The local drink was a rich source of essential vitamins and minerals not otherwise present in the local diet. Thus, although it may have appeared desirable to change a cultural pattern for certain health reasons, the unanticipated consequences proved detrimental to health in another way[20].

NURSING IMPLICATIONS

Importance of Cultural Concepts for Nursing

Knowledge of other cultures helps you examine your own cultural foundations, values, and beliefs, which in turn promotes increased self-understanding. But avoid *ethnocentricity, believing that your own ways of behavior are best for everyone*. For example, emphasizing daily bathing to a group who has a severely limited water supply is useless, since the water will be needed for survival. Recognize that your patterns of life and language are peculiar to your culture.

Learning about another's culture can promote feelings of respect and humility as well as enhance understanding of the person and his family—his needs, likes and dislikes, behavior, attitudes, care and treatment approaches, and sociocultural causes of disease. Cultural differences should be anticipated not only in foreigners and first-generation immigrants, but also in persons even further removed in time from their native country and in persons from other regions within your country. The person's behavior during illness is influenced by cultural definitions of how he should act and of the meaning of illness. Understanding this and seeking reasons for behavior avoid stereotyping and labeling the person as uncooperative and resistant just because his behavior is different. As you consider alternate reasons for behavior, care can be individualized. People from different cultural backgrounds classify health problems differently and have certain expectations about how they should be helped. If cultural differences are ignored, your ability to help the patient and his ability to progress toward his own culturally defined health status may be hampered. You should be able to translate your knowledge of the health care system into terms that match the conceptions of your patients. Several authors have written of their successful experiences in adapting care to certain cultural groups without compromising service. In fact, care is usually enhanced because of acceptance and compliance by the group to the desired health practices. [See references 2, 5, 13, 15, 27, 36, 37, 47, 54, 58, 60, 63.]

Relations between the patient and his family may at times seem offensive or disharmonious to you. Differentiate carefully between patterns of behavior that are culturally induced and expected and those that are unhealthy for the persons involved.

Learn about the significant religious practices and the everyday patterns of hygiene, eating, sleeping, elimination, and various rituals that are a part of the person's culture. Interference with normal living patterns or practices adds to the stress of being ill. You will encounter and need to adapt patient care to the following customs: drinking tea instead of coffee with meals, eating the main meal at midday instead of in the evening, refusing to undress before a strange person, avoiding use of the bedpan because someone else must handle its contents, maintaining special religious or ethnic customs, refusing to bathe daily, refusing a pelvic exam by a male doctor, moaning loudly when in pain, and showing unreserved demonstrations of grief when a loved one dies.

The changing society may cause families to have a variety of problems. Be a supportive listener, validate realistic ideas, prepare the family to adapt to a new or changing environment, and be aware of community agencies or resources that can provide additional help. When a patient has no family nearby and seems alone and friendless, you may provide significant support.

Respecting the person's need for privacy or to have others continually around is essential. Understand that some patients or families will not be expressive emotionally or verbally. Respect this pattern, recognizing that nonverbal behavior is also significant. Be aware, too, that word meanings may vary considerably from culture to culture, so that the person may have difficulty understanding you and vice versa.

A patient with a strict time orientation must take his medicines and receive his treatments on time or he will feel neglected. You are expected to give prompt and efficient, but compassionate, service to the patient and family. Time orientation also affects making appointments for the clinic and plans for medication routine or return to work after discharge, and influences the person's ideas about how quickly he should get well. The person with little future-time orientation has difficulty planning a future clinic appointment or a long-range medication schedule. He cannot predict now how he will feel at a later date, and he thinks that clinic visits or medicines are unnecessary if he feels all right at the moment.

For some patients, the hurrying behavior of the nurse is distressing; it conveys a lack of concern and lack of time to give adequate care. In turn, the patient expresses guilt feelings when he has to ask for help. Although you may look very efficient when you are scurrying, you are likely to miss many observations, cues, and hidden meanings in what the patient says.

Examine your own attitude about busyness and leisure in order to help others consider leisure as a part of life. The disabled patient, whose inability to work carries a stigma, must develop a positive attitude about leisure and may seek your help.

Develop a personal philosophy that promotes a feeling of stability in your life so that you in turn can assist the patient and family to explore feelings and to formulate a philosophy for coping with change. Toffler speaks about ways in which the person can learn to cope with rapid change. One important way is to develop some ritual or pattern in your personal life that you can practice regardless of where you are and thus maintain some sense of continuity and stability[69].

Promoting Health in Other Cultures through Education

One of the ways to have a lasting effect upon the health practices of a different cultural group is through health teaching that includes a philosophy of prevention. Present-day China as compared with China during the 1940s is an example of how public health standards can be effectively raised through an emphasis on prevention[63]. Increasingly your role includes health education, as discussed in Chapter 5. Outsiders cannot make decisions for others, but people should be given sufficient knowledge concerning alternate behavior so that they can make intelligent choices themselves.

Various pressures interfere with attempts at health teaching[9, 12, 51]. Behind poor health habits lie more than ignorance, economic pressure, or selfish desires. Motivation plays a great part in continuing certain practices, even though the person has been taught differently by you. Motivation, moreover, is influenced by the person's culture, his status and role in that culture, and social pressures for conformity. Starting programs of prevention can be difficult when people place a low value on health, cannot recognize cause-and-effect relationships in disease, lack future-time orientation, or are confused about the existence of preventive measures in their culture. Thus preventive programs or innovations in health care must be shaped to fit the cultural and health profiles of the population[22]. Long-range prevention goals stand a better chance of implementation if they are combined with measures to meet immediate needs. A mother is more likely to heed your advice about how to prevent further illness in her sick child if you give the child immediate attention.

Be ever mindful of how people view you. If they cannot understand you, if you threaten their values, or if they view you as an untouchable professional, you will not cross the cultural barrier.

REFERENCES

1. Abercombie, Thomas, "Japan's Historic Heartland," *National Geographic*, 137: No. 3 (1970), 295-339.
2. Aichlmayr, Rita, "Cultural Understanding: A Key To Acceptance," *Nursing Outlook*, 17: No. 7 (1969), 20-23.
3. Baca, Josephine, "Some Health Beliefs of the Spanish Speaking," *American Journal of Nursing*, 69: No. 10 (1969), 2172-76.
4. Beland, Irene, *Clinical Nursing: Pathophysiological and Psychosocial Approaches* (2nd ed.). London: Collier-MacMillan Ltd., The MacMillan Company, 1970, chapter 7.
5. Berry, E., "HOPE Docks in Guinea," *American Journal of Nursing*, 66: No. 10 (1966), 2238-42.

6. Biesanz, John, and Mavis Biesanz, *Modern Society* (3rd ed.). Englewood Cliffs, N.J.: Prentice-Hall, Inc., 1964.

7. Bossard, J., and E. Boll, *The Sociology of Child Development* (4th ed.). New York: Harper & Row, Publishers, 1966.

8. Brinton, D., "Health Center Milieu: Interaction of Nurses and Low Income Families," *Nursing Research*, 21: No. 1 (1972), 46-52.

9. Brockington, Fraser, "Health Education as a Cultural Philosophy," *International Journal of Nursing Studies*, 1: No. 1 (1964), 17-25.

10. Brown, Esther, *Newer Dimensions of Patient Care, Part III: Patients As People*. New York: Russell Sage Foundation, 1964.

11. Campbell, Teresa, and Betty Chung, "Health Care of the Chinese in America," *Nursing Outlook*, 21: No. 4 (1973), 245-49.

12. Cassel, John, "The Social and Cultural Implications of Food and Food Habits." Paper presented at Joint Session of Dental Health, Food and Nutrition, Public Health Education, and Public Health Nursing Sections of the American Public Health Association at the 84th Annual Meeting, Atlantic City, N.J., 1956.

13. Cunningham, M., H. Sanders, and P. Weatherly, "We Went to Mississippi," *American Journal of Nursing*, 67: No. 4 (1967), 801-4.

14. Davis, W., Allison Havighurst, and R. Havighurst, *Father of the Man*. Boston: Houghton Mifflin Company, 1947.

15. Devitt, H., "Nursing in a Vietnam Village," *Nursing Outlook*, 14: No. 12 (1966), 46-49.

16. Dilliard, J., "Negro Children's Dialect in the Inner City," *Florida FL Reporter*, Fall 1967, n.p.

17. _____, "Non-Standard Negro Dialects: Convergence or Divergence?" *Florida FL Reporter*, Fall 1968, pp. 9-12.

18. Dimancescu, Dan, "Kayak Odyssey from the Inland Sea to Tokyo," *National Geographic*, 132: No. 3 (1967), 295-336.

19. Eliot, Alexander, *Greece*, Life World Library. New York: Time, Inc., 1963.

20. Fuerst, Elinor, and LuVerne Wolff, *Fundamentals of Nursing* (4th ed.). Philadelphia: J. B. Lippincott Company, 1969.

21. Garn, S. M., "Cultural Factors Affecting Study of Human Biology," in *Man in Adaptation: The Biosocial Background*, ed. Y. A. Cohen. Chicago: Aldine Publishing Company, 1968.

22. Graham, Saxon, "Cancer, Culture, and Social Structure," in *Patients, Physicians, and Illness* (2nd ed.), ed. E. Gartly Jaco. New York: The Free Press, 1972, pp. 31-39.

23. _____, "Studies of Behavior Change to Enhance Public Health," *American Journal of Public Health*, 63: No. 4 (1973), 327-34.

24. Guralnik, David, ed., *Webster's New World Dictionary of the American Language* (2nd. college ed.). New York: World Publishing Company, 1972.

25. Hanson, Robert, and Lyle Saunders, *Nurse-Patient Communication: A Manual for Public Health Nurses in Northern New Mexico.* Washington, D.C.: United States Department of Health, Education, and Welfare, 1964.

26. Hartley, William, "The Old Ways Linger: Chinese Herb Doctors Still Treat Taiwanese," *Wall Street Journal,* October 10, 1969, p. 9.

27. Jacobson, Phyllis, "The Y. Family," *American Journal of Nursing,* 69: No. 9 (1969), 1951-52.

28. Jewell, D., "A Case of a 'Psychotic' Navajo Indian Male," in *Social Interaction and Patient Care,* eds. J. Skipper and R. Leonard. Philadelphia: J. B. Lippincott Company, 1965, pp. 184-95.

29. Johnson, Nichols, "Keep Your Eye on TV," *AAUW Journal,* 66: No. 5 (1973), 13-15.

30. Keniston, Kenneth, *The Young Radicals.* New York: Harcourt, Brace & World, Inc., 1968.

31. King, Imogene, *Towards a Theory for Nursing.* New York: John Wiley & Sons, Inc., 1971.

32. Kluckhorn, C., et al., "Values and Value Orientations in the Theory of Action," in *Toward a General Theory of Action,* eds. T. Parson and E. Shils. Cambridge, Mass.: Harvard University Press, 1951.

33. Koos, Earl, *The Health of Regionville.* New York: Columbia University Press, 1951.

34. Leaf, Alexander, M.D., "Every Day Is a Gift When You Are over 100," *National Geographic,* 143: No. 1 (1973), 93-119.

35. Leininger, M., "The Culture Concept and Its Relevance to Nursing," *Journal of Nursing Education,* 6 No. 2 (1967), 27-37.

36. Leonard, Sister Margaret Ann, and Sister Carol Ann Joyce, "Two Worlds United," *American Journal of Nursing,* 71: No. 6 (1971), 1152-55.

37. Loughlin, B., "Pregnancy in the Navajo Culture," *Nursing Outlook,* 13: No. 3 (1965), 55-58.

38. Lynn, F., "An American Nurse Visits Two Mental Hospitals in Greece," *Nursing Outlook,* 14: No. 12 (1966), 50-53.

39. McCabe, Gracia, "Cultural Influences on Patient Behavior," *American Journal of Nursing,* 60: No. 8 (1960), 1101-4.

40. Maclachlan, J., "Cultural Factors in Health and Disease," in *Patients, Physicians, and Illness: Behavioral Science and Medicine,* ed. E. Gartly Jaco. Glencoe, Ill.: Free Press of Glencoe, 1958, pp. 95-105.

41. Malmstrom, Jean, "Dialects—Updated," *Florida FL Reporter,* Spring/Summer 1969.

42. Mandell, Arnold, and Mary Mandell, "What Can Nursing Learn from the Behavioral Sciences?" *American Journal of Nursing,* 63: No. 6 (1963), 104-7.

43. Mangin, William, "Mental Health and Migration to Cities: A Peruvian Case," *Annals of the New York Academy of Science,* 84 (1960), 911-17.

44. Martin, C., "Marital and Coital Factors in Cervical Cancer," *American Journal of Public Health*, 58: No. 5 (1967), 803-14.

45. Mead, Margaret, *Cultural Patterns and Technical Change*. New York: The New American Library, Mentor Books, 1955.

46. ____, *Culture and Commitment: A Study of the Generation Gap*. Garden City, N.Y.: Natural History Press/Doubleday & Company, Inc., 1970.

47. Murphy, Patricia, "Tuberculosis Control in San Francisco's Chinatown," *American Journal of Nursing*, 70: No. 5 (1970), 1044-46.

48. Ogburn, William, and M. Nimkoff, *Sociology* (2nd ed.). Boston: Houghton Mifflin Company, 1950.

49. Parson, Talcott, *Essays in Sociological Theory* (rev. ed.). London: Collier-MacMillan Ltd., 1964, pp. 275-97.

50. ____, "Definitions of Health and Illness in the Light of American Values and Social Structure," in *Patients, Physicians, and Illness* (2nd ed.), ed. E. Gartly Jaco. New York: The Free Press, 1972, pp. 118-27.

51. Paul, Benjamin, "Anthropological Perspectives on Medicine and Public Health," *Annals of the American Academy of Political and Social Science*, 346: No. 3 (1963), 34-43.

52. Paynich, M., "Cultural Barriers to Nurse Communication," *American Journal of Nursing*, 64: No. 2 (1964), 87-90.

53. Persad, Emmanuel, "Some Cultural Factors in Psychiatric Training," *Canadian Mental Health*, 19: Nos. 3-4 (1971), 11-15.

54. Peters, J., "On The Patient's Terms," *American Journal of Nursing*, 65: No. 2 (1965), 130-31.

55. Richardson, Stephens, N. Goodman, A. Hostorf, and S. Dornbusch, "Cultural Uniformity in Reaction to Physical Disabilities," *American Sociological Review*, 26: No. 2 (1961), 241-47.

56. Rubel, Arthur, "Concepts of Disease in Mexican-American Culture," *American Anthropologist*, 62 (1960), 795-814.

57. Russell, B., and L. Lofstrom, "Health Clinic for the Alienated," *American Journal of Nursing*, 71: No. 1 (1971), 80-83.

58. Saba, V., "A Nurse Goes to Saudi Arabia," *Nursing Outlook*, 14: No. 5 (1966), 58-61.

59. Saunders, Lyle, *Cultural Differences and Medical Care*. New York: Russell Sage Foundation, 1954.

60. Schneider, V., "Letter from Lambarene," *American Journal of Nursing*, 65: No. 10 (1965), 128-30.

61. Scotch, Norman, "A Preliminary Report on the Relation of Sociocultural Factors to Hypertension Among the Zulu," *Annals of the New York Academy of Science*, 84 (1960), 1000-1009.

62. Shor, Franc, "Japan: The Exquisite Enigma," *National Geographic*, 118: No. 6 (1969), 733-77.

63. Stallsmith, J., "Treat or Tribulation?" *American Journal of Nursing*, 66: No. 8 (1966), 1782-83.

64. Stanley, Margaret, "China: Then and Now," *American Journal of Nursing*, 72: No. 12 (1972), 2213-18.

65. Stewart, W., "Sociolinguistic Factors in the History of American Negro Dialects," *Florida FL Reporter*, Spring 1967, n.p.

66. _____, "Continuity and Change in American Negro Dialects," *Florida FL Reporter*, Spring, 1968, n.p.

67. Suchman, Edward, "Social Patterns of Illness and Medical Care," in *Patients, Physicians, and Illness* (2nd ed.), ed. E. Gartly Jaco. New York: The Free Press, 1972, pp. 262-79.

68. Tao-Kim-Hai, A., "Orientals Are Stoic," in *Social Interaction and Patient Care*, eds. J. Skipper and R. Leonard. Philadelphia: J. B. Lippincott Company, 1965, pp. 142-55.

69. Toffler, Alvin, *Future Shock*. New York: Bantam Books, 1970.

70. Tyler, E. B., *Primitive Culture* (7th ed.). New York: Brentano's, 1924.

71. von Bertalanffy, Ludwig, *General System Theory*. New York: George Braziller, 1968.

72. Weber, Max, *The Protestant Ethic and the Spirit of Capitalism*, trans. Talcott Parsons. New York: Charles Scribner's Sons, 1930; students' edition, 1958.

73. Weiss, M. Olga, "Cultural Shock," *Nursing Outlook*, 19: No. 1 (1971), 40-43.

74. Whiting, B., ed., *Six Cultures: Studies of Child Rearing*. New York: Jurley and Sons, 1968.

75. Young, Kimball, *Social Psychology* (2nd ed.). New York: F. S. Crofts and Company, 1944.

76. Zborowski, Mark, "Cultural Components in Response to Pain," in *Sociological Studies of Health and Sickness*, ed. Dorrian Apple. New York: McGraw-Hill Book Company, 1960, pp. 118-33.

CHAPTER 11

Religious Influences
on the Person

Study of this chapter will enable you to:

1 Contrast the major tenets of Hinduism, Buddhism, Shintoism, Confucianism, Taoism, Islam, Judaism, and Christianity.

2 Compare the major tenets of the various branches of Christianity: Roman Catholicism, Eastern Orthodoxy, various Protestant denominations, and other Christian sects.

3 Discuss how religious beliefs influence life style and health status in each of the above religious groups.

4 Identify your religious beliefs, or lack of them, and explore how they will influence your nursing practice.

5 Discuss your role in meeting the spiritual needs of a patient and family.

6 Describe specific nursing measures that can be used to meet the needs of persons with different religious backgrounds.

7 Work with a patient who has religious beliefs different from your own or refer him to an appropriate resource.

Until an illness occurs, the person may give no thought to the meaning of his life or spiritual beliefs. But when he feels vulnerable and fearful of the future, he seeks solace. Religion can provide that solace.

A patient sneezes. You say, "God bless you." Why? Perhaps unconsciously you are coordinating the medical-physical with the religious-spiritual. But you may feel afraid to work professionally with the combination.

The attitude that medical science is superior to religion has affected us all. Yet religion is there as it always has been. Each culture has had some organization or priesthood to sustain the important rituals and myths of its people. Primitive man combined the roles of physician, psychiatrist, and priest. The Indian medicine man and the African witch doctor combine magic with religion; with their herbs, psychosuggestion, and appeals to the gods, they realize that man is a psychophysical-spiritual being[35].

In the midst of our specialized world, you must attempt again to bring the three areas together. Segmenting the person has not worked. You now have an opportunity and an obligation to study the religions of your patients. And those are world religions, not your personal or country's basic religion. Mass media, rapid transportation, and cultural exchange have made void the provincial approach.

Religion is defined on various levels: *a belief in a supernatural or divine force that has power over the universe and commands worship and obedience; a system of beliefs; a comprehensive code of ethics or philosophy; the conscious pursuit of any object the person holds as supreme*[8].

This definition, however, does not portray the constancy and at times the fervency that can underlie religious belief. In every human there seems to be a quality that defies definition, that strives for inspiration, reverence, and awe. Religious symbols have developed as a result of this striving. They, too, cannot be fully understood because they represent the infinite, but learning some of their significance can advance your understanding[33].

In this chapter, nine personalities are presented. Each has a fictitious name and represents not a single person but rather a composite of knowledge gained from the authors' interviewing, reading, and personal experience.

MAJOR WORLD RELIGIONS

Hinduism

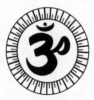

Rama tells us that nothing is typically Hindu and that anyone who puts religion in neat packages will have difficulty comprehending his outlook. Rama is named after Ramakrishma, the greatest Hindu saint of the nineteenth century. The history of Rama's religion goes back to approximately 1500 B.C., when the **Vedas—** *divine revelations*—were written. His main religious texts are the **Upanishads,** *or scriptures,* and the **Bhagavad-Gita,** *a summary of the former with additions. The most expressive and universal word of God is* **Om,** *or* **Aum**—providing the most important auditory and visual symbol in Rama's religion.*

Rama speaks of some of the worship popular in India today: of the family and local deities; of the trinity—**Brahma,** *the creator*; **Vishnu,** *the preserver and god of love*; and **Shiva,** *the destroyer.*

Rama tells of his own shrine in his home where, in the presence of various pictures of **incarnations** *(human forms of God)*, and with incense burning, he meditates. He also thinks of Buddha, Muhammed, and Jesus as incarnations and sometimes reads from the scriptures inspired by their teachings, although they represent other major religions.

In spite of this vast array of deities and the recognition that all religions are valid, Rama believes in one universal concept—*Brahman, the Divine Intelligence, the Supreme Reality.* Rama believes all paths lead to the understanding that this "reality" exists as part of all physical beings, especially humans. Rama's entire spiritual quest is directed toward uniting his *inner and real self,* the **atman**, with the concept of Brahman. So although Rama has gone through several stages of desire—for pleasure, power, wealth, fame, and humanitarianism—the last stage, his desire for freedom, for touching the infinite, is his main goal.

Rama is interested in health and illness only as it guides him to this goal. He feels that the human love for the body is a cause for illness. He says, for example, that we overeat and get a stomachache. He views the pain as a warning, in this case to stop overeating. He does not oppose any medical treatment if absolutely necessary, but he feels that medicine can sometimes dull the pain and then the person overeats again, thus perpetuating the cause of the problem. Medical or psychiatric help Rama says, is at best transitory. The cause of the pain must be rooted out.

So that he does not dwell on physical concerns, Rama strives for moderation in his eating pattern as well as in other bodily functions. He considers only the atman as real and eternal, the body as unreal and finite. The body is a temple, a vehicle, no more. He tries to take care of it so that it will not scream at him because of his overindulgence or underindulgence. Rama is a vegetarian. He feels that meat and intoxicants would excite his senses too much. However, the Hindu diet pattern is flexible; definite rules are not set. If Rama is sick, he tries to bear his illness with resignation, knowing its temporary nature. He believes that the prayer of supplication for bodily cure is the lowest form of prayer, while the highest form is devotion to God. To him death and rebirth are nearly synonymous, as the atman never changes and always remains pure. He compares

*See the symbol at the beginning of this section. A transliteration of the script is *a, u, m.* It is written in English as *Om,* or *Aum. Om, God,* and *Brahman* are synonymous and mean a *consciousness* or *awareness* rather than a personified being.

the atman to the ocean: as ocean water can be put into various containers without changing its nature, so can the atman be put into various physical and human containers without changing its nature.

Rama says that as a devotee of God he is following a *training course* called *yoga*. As a preliminary, however, he must establish certain moral qualifications. He must strive for self-control, self-discipline, cleanliness, and contentment. He must avoid injury, deceitfulness, and stealing. His overwhelming desire to reach God can be implemented through one or a combination of the four yoga paths. These are (1) *inana yoga* through *reading and absorbing knowledge;* (2) *bhakti yoga* through the *devotion of emotion and love*; (3) *karma yoga* through *work dedicated to God*; and (4) *raja yoga* through *psychological experiments on oneself*. Rama combines the first three by reading and memorizing portions of the ancient scriptures, by meditating daily at his shrine, and by dedicating the results of his professional work to God.

For Rama, religion is not something that can be picked up and put down according to a schedule or one's mood. It is a constant and all-pervading part of his life and the life of his country. India's literature and art are witness to this.

If you give nursing care to a person with Rama's background, consider how his religious beliefs will influence your approach. For example, be accepting if he seems to minimize his bodily ills. Keep in mind his view of the body as only a vehicle to carry the atman and his belief that the desire for bodily cure is a low form of prayer. Yoga training, emphasizing self-control and devotion to God through reading and meditation, may cause him to seek help from his inner resources and the literature of Hinduism rather than from medication or consultation with staff. Your provision of an atmosphere conducive to this practice will be appreciated.

Buddhism and Shintoism

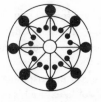

Umeko Sato is a member of the *Buddhist sect, Soka Gakkai.* Recently this sect has become a powerful new religion in Japan, with a government party, a university, and a grand temple representing it. Based on the *Lotus Sutra, part of the Buddhist scriptures*, its doctrine advocates the three values of happiness: profit, goodness, and beauty. Sato is attracted by the practicality of the teachings, the mottoes that she can live by, the emphasis on small group study, and present world benefits, especially healing.

Although Sato's beliefs at some points seem in direct contrast to the original Buddhist teachings, she is happy to explain the rich multireligious tradition that her family has had for generations. She emphasizes that she is affected by the Confucian emphasis on the family unit; by Christianity's healing emphasis; by Shintoism, the state religion of Japan until 1945; and by Buddhism, which originated about 600 B.C. in India with a Hindu named *Siddhartha Gautama*.

Gautama, shortly after a historic enlightenment experience during which he became the Buddha, preached a sermon to his followers and drew on the earth a wheel representing the continuous round of life and death and rebirth. Later eight spokes were added to illustrate the sermon and to provide the most explicit visual symbol of Buddhism* today. Sato repeats Buddha's four noble truths: (1) man's life is disjointed or out of balance, especially in birth, old age, illness, and death; (2) the cause of this imbalance is man's ignorance of his own true nature; (3) removal of this ignorance is attained by reaching *Nirvana, the divine state of release, the ultimate reality, the perfect knowledge* via (4) the eightfold path.

The eight spokes of the wheel represent the eightfold path used to reach Nirvana. Sato says that followers subscribe to right knowledge, right intentions, right speech, right conduct, right means of livelihood, right effort, right mindfulness, and concentration. From these concepts has arisen a moral code that, among other things, prohibits intoxicants, lying, and killing of any kind (which explains why Buddhists are often vegetarians). She further explains that the Mahayana branch of Buddhism took hold in Japan as opposed to the Theravada branch. The *Theravada branch emphasizes an intellectual approach through wisdom, man working by himself through meditation and without ritual.* The *Mahayana branch emphasizes involvement with mankind, ritual, petitionary prayer, and concern for one's brother.* Sato feels that the Mahayana branch provides the happier philosophy of the two, and she tells of the ritual of celebration on Gautama's birthday. But most Japanese believe in *Amitabha Buddha, a god rather than a historical figure,* who in replacing the austere image of Gautama is a glorious redeemer, one of infinite light. Also, the people worship *Kwannon, a goddess of compassion.*

Sato explains that she cannot omit mention of the one austere movement within the Mahayana branch, the *Zen* sect. Taking their example from Gautama's extended contemplation of a flower, Zen followers care not much for discourse, books, or other symbolic interpretations and explanations of reality. Hours and years are devoted to meditation, contemplation of word puzzles, and consultation with a Zen master. In seeking absolute honesty and truthfulness through

*See the symbol at the beginning of this section.

simple acts such as drinking tea or gardening, the Zen student hopes to experience enlightenment.

Sato next turns to her former state religion, *Shintoism*. While Buddhism produced a solemnizing effect on her country, Shintoism had an affirmative and joyous effect. Emperor, ancestor, ancient hero, and nature worship form its core. Those who follow Shintoism, she says, feel an intense loyalty and devotion to every lake, tree, and blossom in Japan as well as to the ancestral spirits abiding there. They also have a great concern for cleanliness, a carryover from early ideas surrounding dread of pollution in the dead.

Sato says that her parents have two god shelves in their home. One contains wooden tablets inscribed with the name of the household's patron deity and a symbolic form of the goddess of rice, as well as other texts and objects of family significance. Here, each day, her family perform simple rites such as offering a prayer or a food gift. In a family crisis, perhaps an illness, the family conducts more elaborate rites such as lighting tapers or offering rice brandy. The other god shelf, in another room, is the Buddha shelf, and if a family member dies, a Buddhist priest, the spiritual leader, performs specified rituals there.

Sato strongly emphasizes that if illness or impending death causes a family member to be hospitalized, another well family member will stay at the hospital to bathe, cook for, and give emotional support to the patient. Sato feels that recovery is largely dependent on this family tie.

So although Sato has grasped a new religious path for herself, her respect for tradition remains.

In giving care to a person with Umeko Sato's background, be aware of the varied religious influences on her life. Her sect's emphasis on the here and now rather than on the long road to Nirvana may cause her to value physical health highly so that she can benefit from the joys and beauty of this life. She may readily voice impatience with her body's dysfunction. You can also respond to her great concern for cleanliness, her desire to have family nearby, and her need for family rites that are offered for the sick member.

Confucianism and Taoism

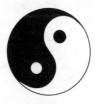

Wong Huieng is a young teacher in Taiwan simultaneously influenced by *Taoism*,* *the romantic and mystical*, and **Confucianism**, *the practical and pragmatic*. To provide insights into these Chinese modes of thinking, although

*Pronounced "dowism."

it is more representative of Taoism, Wong Huieng uses the *yin-yang symbol.* *
The symbol is a circle, representing *Tao* or *the absolute*, in which two tear shapes
fit perfectly into one another, each containing a small dot from the other. Generally, yang is light or red, and yin is dark. Ancient Chinese tradition says that
everything exists in these two interacting forces. Each represents a group of qualities. Yang is positive or masculine—dry, hot, active, moving, and light. Yin is
feminine or negative—wet, cold, passive, restful and empty. For example, fire is
almost pure yang, and water almost pure yin—but not quite. The combination of
yin and yang constitutes all the dualisms a person can imagine: day/night, sum-
mer/winter, beauty/ugliness, illness/health, life/death. Both qualities are necessary
for life in the universe; they are complementary and, if in harmony, good. Yang
and yin energy forces are embodied in the body parts and affect food preferences
and eating habits as well.

Huieng translates this symbol into a relaxed philosophy of life: "If I am
sick, I will get better. Life is like going up and down a mountain; sometimes I
feel good and sometimes I feel bad. That's the way it is." Though educated, she
is not interested in climbing up the job ladder, accumulating wealth, or conquer-
ing nature. Her goal is to help provide money to build an orphanage in a natural
wooded setting.

Huieng thinks of death as a natural part of life, as the peace that comes
when the body is worn out. She admits, however, that when her father died,
human grief took hold of her. Before his death her mother went to the Taoist
temple priest and got some incense that was to help cast the sickness from his
body. After death, they kept his body in the house for the required time, 49
days. The priest executed a special ceremony every seven days. Her mother
could cry only one hour daily, 2:00 until 3:00 in the morning. Now her
mother talks through the priest to her father's ghost. Although Huieng re-
gards this practice as superstitious and thinks that painting a picture of a lake
and mountains is a more fitting way to erase her grief, she looks at the little
yellow bag, containing a blessing from the priest, hanging around her neck, and
finds it comforting if not intellectually acceptable.

Now Huieng turns to her practical side and talks about *Confucius, the
first saint of the nation.* Although *Lao-tzu, the founder of Taoism,* is a semi-
legendary figure said to have vanished after he wrote the *bible of Taoism, Tao-
te-ching,* Confucius has a well-documented existence.

Confucius, born in 551 B.C., wrote little. His disciples wrote the *Analects,
short proverbs embodying his teachings*. He is revered as a teacher, not as a god.
Huieng does not ask him to bless her but tries to emulate him and his teachings,
which she has heard since birth. The temple in his memory is a place for studying, not for praying. And on his birthday, a national holiday, people pay respect
to their teachers in his memory.

Five important terms in Confucius' teaching are *Jen, a striving for good-*

*See the symbol used at the beginning of this section.

ness within; **Chun-sui,** *establishing a gentlemanly/womanly approach with others;* **Li,** *knowing how relationships should be conducted and having respect for age;* **Te,** *leading by virtuous character rather than by force;* and **Wen,** *pursuing the arts as an adjunct to moral character.* Huieng stresses that in *Li* are the directives for family relationships. So strongly did Confucius feel about the family that he gave directives on proper attitudes between father and son, elder brother and junior brother, husband and wife. Also Huieng feels she can't harm her body because it was given to her by her parents. Immediate family to her include grandparents, uncles, aunts, and cousins. Her language has more words for relationships between relatives than the English language does.

Huieng feels, as she cares for her body, she cares for her family, the country, and the universe. Essentially, to her, all men are brothers.

Important in your understanding of a person with Wong Huieng's background is the dualism that exists in her thinking. Acceptance of her particular version of mysticism and practicality, and of the yin and yang forces that she sees operating within herself, will help in building a foundation of personalized care.

She may have more respect for older rather than younger staff members. She may respond well to teaching. And she may have a strong desire to attain and maintain wellness. All these factors are directly related to her religious teaching; you can use them to enhance care.

Islam

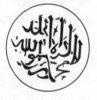

Omar Ali is **Muslim,** *a member of Islam, the youngest of the major world religions.* This faith, with its Arabic coloring and tenacious monotheistic tradition, serves as a bridge between Eastern and Western religions. "There is no God but Allah; Muhammed is His Prophet"* provides the key to Omar's beliefs. He must say this but once in his life as a requirement, but will repeat it many times as an affirmation.

Omar is an Egyptian physician whose religious tradition was revealed through Muhammed, born approximately A.D. 571 in Mecca, then a trading point between India and Syria on the Arabian peninsula. Hating polytheism and influenced by Judaism and Christianity, Muhammed wrote *God's relevation to*

---

*These words are a translation of the sacred calligraphy in the symbol shown at the beginning of this section. The prophet's name is sometimes spelled *Muhammad.*

him in the **Quran**,* *scriptures* that to Omar confirm the truths of the Jewish-Christian Bible. Omar believes in the biblical prophets, but he calls Muhammed the greatest—the Seal of Prophets.

Through the *Quran* and the **Hadith**, *the traditions,* Omar has specific guidelines for his thinking, devotional life, and social obligations. Basically he believes himself to be a unique individual with an eternal soul. He believes in a heaven and hell, and while on earth he wants to walk the straight path.

To keep on this path, Omar prays five times a day: generally upon rising, at midday, in the afternoon, in the early evening, and before retiring. Articles needed are water and a prayer rug. Because the *Quran* emphasizes cleanliness of body, Omar performs a ritual washing before each prayer. Then, facing Mecca, he goes through a series of prescribed bodily motions and repeats various passages in praise and supplication.

Omar also observes **Ramadan**, *a fast month,*† during which time he eats or drinks nothing from sunrise to sunset; after sunset he takes nourishment only in moderation. He explains *fasting (abstinence from eating)* as a *discipline aiding him to understand those with little food.* At the end of Ramadan, he enters a festive period with feelings of good will and gift exchanges.

Omar has made one pilgrimage to Mecca, another requirement for all well and financially able Muslims. He feels the experience created a great sense of brotherhood, as all the pilgrims wore similar modest clothing, exchanged news of followers in various lands, and renewed their mutual faith. The *twelfth day of the Pilgrimage month is the* **Feast of Sacrifice,** when all Muslim families kill a lamb in honor of Abraham's offering of his son to God.

In line with the *Quran's* teaching, Omar does not eat pork (including items such as bologna, that might contain partial pork products), does not gamble, and does not drink intoxicants. He worships no images or pictures of Muhammed, as the prophet is not deified. He gives a portion of his money to the poor, since Islam advocates a responsibility to society.

Omar outlines the ideas of his religion as it applies to his profession. He feels that he can make a significant contribution to health care, but that essentially what happens is God's will. Submission to God is the very meaning of Islam.

Muslim patients are excused from religious rules, but many will still want to follow them as closely as possible. Even though a patient might be in a body cast and can't get out of bed, he may want to go through his prayers symbolically. He might also recite the first chapters of the *Quran*, centered on praise to Allah, which are often used in times of crises. Family is a great comfort in illness, and praying with a group is strengthening, but the Muslim has no priest. His relation-

---

*Sometimes spelled *Koran.*

†Coming during the ninth month of the Muslim year, always at a different time each year by the Western calendar, and sometimes spelled *Ramazan.*

ship is directly with God. Some patients may seem completely resigned to death, while others, hoping it is God's will that they live, cooperate vigorously with the medical program. After death a body must be washed and the hands folded in prayer. Knowledge of these attitudes and traditions can greatly enhance your care.

Judaism

Seth Lieberman, strongly influenced by the social-concern emphasis in Judaism, is a psychiatrist. He can't remember when his religious instruction began— it was always there. He went through the motions and felt the emotion of the Sabbath eve with its candles and cup of sanctification long before he could comprehend his father's explanations. Book learning followed, however, and he came to understand the fervency with which his people study and live the law as given in the *Torah, the first five books of the Bible;* and in the *Talmud, a commentary and enlargement of the Torah.* His *spiritual leader is the rabbi.* His spiritual symbol is the *menorah.* *

Although raised in an *Orthodox* home, Seth and his family are now *Reform.* And he mentions another group, the *Conservatives. The Orthodox believe God gave the law;* it was written exactly as He gave it; it should be followed precisely. *Reform Jews believe the law was written by inspired men* at various times and therefore is subject to reinterpretation. Seth says he follows the traditions because they are traditions rather than because God demands it. *Conservatives are in the middle,* taking some practices from both groups. Overriding any differences in interpretation of ritual and tradition is the fundamental concept expressed in the prayer, "Hear, O Israel, the Lord our God, the Lord is One." Not only is He one, He loves His creation, wants His people to live justly, and wants to bless their food, drink, and celebration. Judaism's double theme might be expressed as, "Enjoy life now, and share it with God." Understandably then, Seth's religious emphasis isn't on an afterlife, although some Jewish people believe in one. And although Jews have had a history of suffering, the inherent value of suffering or illness isn't stressed. Through their observance of the Law, the belief of their historical role as God's chosen people, and their hope for better days, Jews have survived seemingly insurmountable persecution.

---

*See the symbol at beginning of this section. The seven-branched candelabrum stands for the creation of the universe in seven days; the center light symbolizes the Sabbath; and the candlelight symbolizes the presence of God in the Temple.

Seth works with physically, emotionally, and spiritually depressed persons. He feels that often the spiritual depression is unnoticed, misunderstood, or ignored by professional workers. He cites instances where mental attitudes have brightened as he shared a common bond of Judaism with a client. He offers guidelines for working with a Jewish person in a hospital or nursing home. Although Jewish law can be suspended when a person is ill, he will be most comfortable following as many practices as possible.

Every Jew observes the *Sabbath, a time for spiritual refreshment, from sundown on Friday to shortly after sundown on Saturday.* During this period Orthodox Jews may refuse freshly cooked food, medicine, treatment, surgery, and use of radio, television, and writing equipment lest the direction of their thinking be diverted on this special day. An Orthodox male may want to wear *a yarmulke or skullcap* continuously; use a *prayerbook called Siddur*; and use *phylacteries, leather strips with boxes containing scriptures,* at weekday morning prayer. Also the ultra-Orthodox male may refuse to use a razor because of the Levitical ban on shaving.

Jewish dietary laws have been considered by some scholars as health measures: to enjoy life is to eat properly and in moderation. The Orthodox, however, obey them because God so commanded. Food is called *treyfe* (or treyfah) if it is *unfit,* and *kosher* if it is *ritually correct.* Foods forbidden are pig, horse, shrimp, lobster, crab, oyster, and fowl that are birds of prey. Meats approved are from those animals that are ruminants and have divided hooves. Fish approved must have both fins and scales. Also, the kosher animals must be healthy and slaughtered in a prescribed manner. Because of the Biblical passage stating not to soak a young goat in its mother's milk, Jews do not eat meat products and milk products together. Neither are the utensils used to cook these products ever intermixed, nor the dishes from which to eat these products.

Guidelines for a satisfactory diet for the Orthodox are: (1) Serve milk products first, meat second. Meat can be eaten a few minutes after milk, but milk cannot be taken for six hours after meat. (2) If a person completely refuses meat because of incorrect slaughter, encourage a vegetarian diet with protein supplements such as fish and eggs, considered neutral unless prepared with milk or meat shortening. (3) Get frozen kosher products marked (*U*) or *pareve.* (4) Heat and serve food in the original container and use paper utensils.

Two holy days of paramount importance are *Rosh Hashanah* and *Yom Kippur. Rosh Hashanah, the Jewish New Year,* is a time to meet with the family, give thanks to God for good health, and renew traditions. Ten days later is *Yom Kippur, the day of atonement,* a time for asking forgiveness of family members for wrongs done. On Yom Kippur Jews fast for 24 hours, a symbolic act of self-denial, mourning, and petition. *Tisha Bab, the day of lamentation,* recalling the destruction of both Temples of Jerusalem, is another 24-hour fast period. *Pesach* or *Passover* (eight days for Orthodox and Conservative, seven days for Reform) *celebrates the ancient Jews' deliverance from Egyptian bondage. Matzo, an unleavened bread,* replaces leavened bread during this period.

While family, friends, and rabbi may visit the ill, especially on or near holidays, they will also come at other times. Visiting the sick is a religious duty. And although to many Jews death is final except for living on in the memories of others, guidelines exist for this time. A dying person should not be left alone; his soul should leave in the presence of people. And if he should die on the Sabbath, he cannot be moved, except by a non-Jew, until sundown.

So from circumcision of the male infant on the eighth day after birth to his deathbed, and from the days of the original menorah in the sanctuary in the wilderness until the present day, the followers of Judaism reenact their traditions. Since many of these traditions remain an intrinsic part of the Jew as he strives to maintain or regain wellness, the above guidelines offer a foundation for knowledgeable care.

Christianity

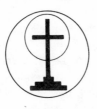

Beth Meyer, a *Roman Catholic*, Demetrius Callas, an *Eastern Orthodox*, and Jean Taylor, a *Protestant*, are Christian American nurses representing the three major branches of Christianity. Although Christianity divided into Eastern Orthodox and Roman Catholic in A.D. 1054, and the Protestant Reformation provided a third division in the sixteenth century, these nurses share some basic beliefs, most importantly that Jesus Christ as described in the Bible is God's son. Jesus, born in Palestine, changed "B.C." to "A.D." The details of His 33 years are few, but His deeds and words recorded in the Bible's New Testament show quiet authority, loving humility, and an ability to perform miracles and to visit easily with people in varied social positions.

The main symbol of Christianity is the cross,* but it signifies more than a wooden structure on which Jesus was crucified. It also symbolizes the finished redemption—Christ rising from the dead and ascending to the Father in order to rule with Him and continuously pervade the personal lives of His followers.

Christians observe *Christmas as Christ's birthday; Lent as a season of penitence and self-examination preceding Good Friday, Christ's crucifixion day;* and *Easter, His Resurrection day.*

*See the symbol at the beginning of this section.

Beth, Demetrius, and Jean rely on the New Testament as a guideline for their lives. They believe that Jesus was fully God and fully man at the same time, that their original sin (which they accept as a basic part of themselves) can be forgiven, and that they are acceptable to God because of Jesus Christ's life and death. They believe God is three persons—the Father, the Son, and the Holy Spirit (Holy Ghost), the latter providing a spirit of love and truth.

Beth, Demetrius, and Jean differ in some worship practices and theology, but all highly regard their individuality as children of God and hope for life with God after death. They feel responsible for their own *souls, the spiritual portions of themselves,* and for aiding the spiritual needs of their patients.

Roman Catholicism, according to Beth, is a religion based on the dignity of man as a social, intellectual, and spiritual being, made in the image of God. She traces the teaching authority of the church through the scriptures: God sent his Son to establish the Church. Jesus chose apostles to preach, teach, and guide. He appointed Saint Peter as the Church's head to preserve unity and to have authority over the apostles. The mission given by Jesus to Saint Peter and the apostles is the same that continues to the present through the pope and his bishops.

Beth follows the seven *sacraments* as *grace-giving rites* that help her follow Jesus' example and strive for a life above the mundane in faith, love, and service. The sacraments that occur once in life are baptism, confirmation, and holy matrimony or dedication of life to God through taking holy orders.

Through baptism the new soul is incorporated into the life of Christ and shares His divinity. Any infant in danger of death should be baptized, even an aborted fetus. If a priest is not available, you can perform the sacrament by pouring water on the forehead and saying, "I baptize thee in the name of the Father, of the Son, and of the Holy Ghost." Adults are also baptized when they join the church. *Confirmation is another strengthening step,* taken when a child begins to reason and be responsible for a more mature religion. *Marriage acknowledges the love and lifelong commitment between a man and a woman.* Strict laws uphold the sanctity of the union; it is not to be dissolved by a human power, as in divorce. *Holy orders ordain deacons, priests, bishops, and some monks.*

The sacraments that are repeated are *confession* (penance), the *Eucharist,* and *anointing of the sick.* Although required to confess only once a year, Beth feels that *confession, a recitation of her sins to God in the presence of her spiritual leader, the priest,* with the determination not to commit the sin again, should be practiced as needed. The *Mass, the religious service whose central portion is the Eucharist, in which bread and wine are miraculously transformed into the body and blood of Christ and are then partaken of,* is the sustaining power of Beth's religion. Each Sunday in her liturgical celebration, she communes with God; sheds the routine, dullness, or disappointments of each day; reexamines and refuels her life so the Holy Spirit can lead her.

Beth is glad that the anointing of the sick is being modified and broadened. Formerly known as extreme unction or last rites, this sacrament was reserved for those near death. Now *anointing of the sick, symbolic of Christ's healing love and the concern of the Christian community,* can provide spiritual strength to those less gravely ill. Some priests are talking to groups of patients, along with family and health workers, to explain the newer interpretation of this sacrament. Group anointing may follow. And instead of anointing the five senses with olive oil and reciting a separate prayer each time, the priest might anoint only the forehead and recite one prayer.

Beth is convinced that her religious practice contributes to her health. She feels that the body and mind work together and that a mind rid of guilt, grievances, and mundaneness is a mind that has a positive effect on the body. She believes, however, that suffering is an integral part of life and can be a means toward achieving growth. She says that no Catholic looking at a *crucifix, a representation of Christ suffering on the cross,* can miss the implication of how He suffered for each man's redemption.

While in the hospital, a Roman Catholic may want to attend Mass or receive the Eucharist at bedside. (Fasting one hour before the sacrament is traditional unless physical illness prevents.) Other symbols that might be comforting are the miraculous medal; holy water; a lighted candle; a statue of the Blessed Virgin Mary, Mother of Jesus; a rosary; a relic; or a prayer book.

The Greek Orthodox Faith is discussed by Demetrius. The Eastern Orthodox church, the main denomination, is divided into groups by nationality. Each group has the *Divine Liturgy, the Eucharistic service,* in the native language and sometimes in English also. While similar in many respects to the Roman Catholic, the Eastern Orthodox have no pope. The seven sacraments are followed with slight variations. Baptism is by triple immersion: the priest places the infant in a basin of water and pours water on his forehead three times. He then immediately confirms the infant by anointing him with holy oil. If death is imminent for a hospitalized infant and the parents or priest cannot be reached, you can baptize by placing a small amount of water on the forehead three times. Even a symbolic baptism is acceptable, but only a living being should receive the sacrament. Adults who join the Church are also baptized and confirmed.

The *unction of the sick* has never been practiced as a last rite by the Eastern Orthodox; *it is a blessing for the sick.* Confession at least once a year is a prerequisite to participation in the Eucharist, which is taken at least four times a year: at Christmas, at Easter, on the Feast Day of Saint Peter and Saint Paul (June 30), and on the day celebrating the Sleeping of the Virgin Mary (August 15).

Fasting from the last meal in the evening until after *Communion, another term for the Eucharist,* is the general rule. Other fast periods include each

Wednesday, representing the seizure of Jesus; each Friday, representing His death; and two 40-day periods, the first before Christmas and the second before Easter. Fasting to Demetrius means avoiding meat, dairy products, and olive oil. Its purpose is for spiritual betterment, to avoid producing extra energy in the body and, instead, thinking of the spirit. Fasting is not necessary when ill. Religion should not harm one's health.

Demetrius retains the Eastern influence in his thinking. He envisions his soul as blending in with the spiritual cosmos and his actions as affecting the rest of creation. He is mystically inclined and feels insights can be gained directly from God. He tells of sharing such an experience with a patient, Mrs. A., also Greek Orthodox.

Mrs. A. had experienced nine surgeries to build up deteriorating bones caused by rheumatoid arthritis. She faced another surgery. On the positive side, the surgery promised hope for walking; on the negative, it was a new and risky procedure. Possibly she would not walk; possibly she would not live. Demetrius saw Mrs. A. when he started working at 3:30 P.M. She was depressed, fearful, and crying. Later, at 6:30 P.M., he saw a changed person—fearless and calm, ready for surgery. She explained that she had seen Jesus in a vision, and that He had said, "Go ahead with the surgery. You'll have positive results. But call your priest and take Communion first." Demetrius called the priest, who gave her Communion. She went into surgery the next day with supreme confidence. She now walks.

In addition to Communion, other helpful symbols are prayer books, lighted candles, and holy water. Especially helpful to the Orthodox are *icons, pictures of Jesus, Mary, or a revered saint*. Saints can intercede between God and man. One of the most loved is **Saint Nicholas**, *a third-century teacher and father figure* who gave his wealth to the poor and became an archbishop. He is honored on Saint Nicholas Day, December 6, and prayed to continuously for guidance and protection.

Every Sunday morning Demetrius participates in an hour-long liturgy. Sitting in an ornate sanctuary with figures and symbols on the windows, walls, and ceiling, facing the tabernacle containing the holy gifts and scripture, Demetrius finds renewal. He recites, "I believe in one God, the Father Almighty, Maker of Heaven and Earth, and of all things visible and invisible. And in one Lord Jesus Christ, the only begotten Son of God."

Protestantism is divided into many denominations and sects. Jean Taylor is a member of the *Church of God* (Anderson, Indiana). She identifies the church by its headquarters because there are some 200 independent church groups in the United States using the phrase "Church of God" in their title. Her group evolved late in the nineteenth century as members of various churches felt organization and ritual were taking precedence over direction from God. They banded together in a drive toward Christian unity, toward a recognition that any people who followed Christ's teachings were members of a universal Church of God and could worship freely together.

This example speaks of one of the chief characteristics of Protestantism: the insistence that God has not given any one person or group of persons sole authority to interpret His truth to others. Protestants employ a freedom of spiritual searching and reinterpretation. Thus new groups form as certain persons and their followers come to believe that they see God's teaching in a new and better light. Jean feels that reading the Bible for historical knowledge and guidance, having a minister to teach and counsel her, and relying on certain worship forms are all important aids. But discerning God's will for her life individually and following that will is her ultimate religious goal.

Jean defines her corporate worship as free liturgical, with an emphasis on congregational singing, verbal prayer, and scripture reading. A sermon by the **minister, *the spiritual leader,*** may take half of the worship period. As with many Protestant groups, two sacraments or ordinances are observed: (1) baptism (in this case **believer's** or **mature baptism** *by total immersion into water*) and (2) Communion. To Protestants, the bread and wine used in Communion are symbolic of Christ's body and blood rather than the actual elements. One additonal ordinance practiced in Jean's church and among some other groups is **footwashing**, *symbolic of Jesus washing His disciples' feet.* These ordinances are practiced with varied frequencies.

The spectrum of beliefs and practices makes defining Protestants, even within a single denomination or sect, nearly impossible. Some Protestant groups, retaining their initial emphasis on individual freedom, have allowed no written creed but expect members to follow an unwritten code of behavior. Jean does suggest some guidelines, however. She lists some of the main Protestant bodies in the United States, beginning with the most formal liturgically and sacramentally, the *Protestant Episcopal* and *Lutheran* churches. The in-betweens are the *Presbyterians, United Church of Christ, United Methodists,* and *Disciples of Christ (Christian Church).* The liturgically freest and least sacramental are the *Baptists* and *Pentecostals.*

Among these groups, some of the opposing doctrines and practices are as follows: living in sin versus living above sin; predestination versus free will; infant versus believer's baptism; and loose organization versus tightly knit organization. Some uphold **fundamental precepts**, *holding to the Scriptures as infallible,* while others uphold **liberal precepts**, *using the Scriptures as a guide, with various interpretations for current living.*

With this infinite variety, Jean feels that learning the individual beliefs of her Protestant patients is essential. For example, when and if a patient wants Communion; if an infant should be baptized; and what will be most helpful spiritually to the patient—these are learned by careful listening. Generally, Jean feels that prayer, a scriptural motto such as "I can do all things through Christ who gives me strength," or a line from a hymn can give strength to a Protestant. Some patients will also want anointing with oil as a symbolic aid to healing.

Practices or Beliefs Unique to Certain Christian Groups should be part of the knowledge of every health worker.

Seventh-Day Adventists rely on Old Testament laws more than do other Christian churches. As in Jewish tradition, the Sabbath is from sundown Friday to sundown Saturday. And as the Orthodox Jew, the Seventh-Day Adventist may refuse medical treatment and the use of secular items such as television during this period and prefer to read spiritual literature. Diet is also restricted. Pork, fish without both scales and fins, and tea and coffee are prohibited. Some Seventh-Day Adventists are *lacto-ovo-vegetarians: they eat milk and eggs but no meat.* Tobacco, alcoholic beverages, and narcotics are also avoided. Health reform is high on their list of priorities, and they sponsor health institutes, cooking schools, and food-producing organizations. Much of their inspiration comes from Ellen G. White, a nineteenth-century prophetess who gave advice on diet and food.

The Church of Jesus Christ of Latter-Day Saints (Mormons) takes much of its inspiration from the **Book of Mormon**, *translated from golden tablets found by the prophet Joseph Smith.* The Mormons believe that this book and two others supplement the Bible. Every Mormon is an official missionary. There is no official congregational leader, but a *seventy* and a **high priest** *represent successive steps upward in commitment and authority.*

Specific Mormon beliefs are that the dead can hear the Gospel and can be baptized by proxy. Marriage in the temple seals the relationship for time and eternity. After a special ceremony in the temple, worthy members receive a white garment. This garment, worn under the clothes, has priesthood marks at the navel and at the right knee and is considered a safeguard against danger. The church believes in a whole-man approach and provides education, recreation, and financial aid for its members. A health and conduct code called "Word of Wisdom" prohibits tobacco, alcohol, and hot drinks (interpreted as tea and coffee) and recommends eating, though sparingly and with thankfulness, herbs, fruit, meat, fowl, and grain, especially wheat.

While the two groups discussed above—the Seventh-Day Adventists and the Mormons—generally accept and promote modern medical practices, the next two groups hold views that conflict with the medical field. The first group, *Jehovah's Witnesses*, refuse to accept blood transfusions. Their refusal is based on the Levitical commandment, given by God to Moses, declaring that no one in the House of David should eat blood or he would be cut off from his people, and on a New Testament reference (in Acts) prohibiting the tasting of blood. Every Jehovah's Witness is a minister. Members meet in halls rather than in traditional-style churches, and they produce massive amounts of literature explaining their faith.

The second group, *Church of Christ, Scientist (Christian Scientists)*, turn wholly to spiritual means for healing. They refuse not only blood transfusions, but also intravenous fluid and medication. Occasionally they allow an orthopedist to set a bone if no medication is used. In addition to the Bible, Christian Scientists use as their guide Mary Baker Eddy's *Science and Health with Key to the Scriptures,* originally published in 1875. The title of this work indicates an approach to wholeness, and those who follow its precepts think of God as Divine Mind, of spirit as real and eternal, of matter as unreal illusion. Sin, sickness, and death are unrealities or erring belief. Christian Scientists do not ignore their erring belief, however, as they have established nursing homes and sanitoriums, the latter recognized in the United States under the federal Medicare program and in insurance regulations. These facilities are operated by trained Christian Science nurses who give first-aid measures and spiritual assistance. The nurse supports the work of the *practitioner who devotes his full time to the public practice of Christian Science healing.* Healing is not thought of as miraculous, but as the application of natural spiritual law. A Christian Scientist who is in a medical hospital has undoubtedly tried Christian Science healing first, and may have been put there by a non-Scientist relative, or may be at variance with his beliefs.

Two more groups of special interest because of their positive personal and health emphasis are the *Unity School of Christianity* and the *Friends (Quakers).* While most Roman Catholics acknowledge the earthly spiritual authority of the pope, and most Protestants regard the Bible as their ultimate authority, the Friends' authority resides in his own direct experience of God within himself. A Friend obeys the *light within. Sometimes called the inner light or the divine principle, this spiritual quality causes the Friend to esteem himself and listen to inner direction.* All Friends are spiritual equals. Without a minister and without any symbols or religious decor, unprogrammed corporate worship consists of silent meditation with each person seeking divine guidance. Toward the end of the meeting, people are free to share their inspiration. The meeting closes with handshaking. Always interested in world peace, Friends have been instrumental in establishing organizations that work toward human brotherhood and economic and social improvements resulting in better health. Friends have staffed hospitals, driven ambulances, and served in medical corps, among numerous other volunteer services.

The *Unity School of Christianity* advocates the view that health is natural, sickness unnatural. While followers think illness is real, they think it can be overcome by concentrating on spiritual goals. Late in the nineteenth century, Charles and Myrtle Fillmore started this group after studying, among other religions, Christian Science, Quakerism, and Hinduism. Thus it blends several established concepts in a new direction. Today Unity Village in Missouri has a publication center that publishes several inspirational periodicals, is beautifully landscaped and open for guests to share in the beauty, and houses its real force, Silent Unity. *Silent Unity consists of staff who are available on a 24-hour basis to answer telephone calls, telegrams, and letters from people seeking spiritual help.* They offer prayer and counseling to all faiths with no charge.

Another facet of Christianity in America is *neo-Pentecostalism.* This is not a group but a trend or phenomenon that has gained support from some Roman Catholics, Presbyterians, and Lutherans, as well as from those churches traditionally closer to the Pentecostal spirit. ***Pentecostalism*** *connotes revivalism, ultrafundamentalism, and the manifest working of the Holy Spirit, often causing people to talk in unknown tongues, to shout, dance, and fall into trances.* However, with the trend in America away from formal organized worship, with changing concepts of family structure, including experiments in communal living, and with increasing mobility and the arrival of the drug culture, many youth are searching for some security in neo-Pentecostalism. They "get high on Jesus," a substitute for the ecstasy of drugs without the dangerous aftereffects.

This chapter so far has concentrated on worship of God, the divine spirit, with an emphasis on traditional teaching. Devil worship is also a form of religion for some. And others live by ethical standards, considering themselves either ***agnostic,*** *incapable of knowing whether God exists, or* ***atheistic,*** *believing that God does not exist.*

NURSING IMPLICATIONS

You can use the foregoing—basic beliefs, dietary laws, and ideas of illness, health, body, spirit, mysticism, pragmatism, pain, death, cleanliness, and family ties—as a *beginning*. Even more basic than understanding these concepts is for you to respect your patient and perform your job adequately. No one will respect your spiritual aid if you do not appear competent and thoughtful in your work. You are not expected to be a professional spiritual leader, for which lengthy training and experience would be required. You can, however, aid patients. You are the transition, the key person between the patient and spiritual help. Even if you feel inadequate, you can make an intelligent referral.

For too long there has been no communication between the nurse and the chaplain. You can fill that gap. When you are determining medical background such as drug or food allergies, you could also ask about religious dietary laws, special rituals, or restrictions that might be just as important a part of the patient's history. Recording and helping the patient follow his beliefs could speed his recovery. Later, when you care for the patient, you will have to watch for religious needs that may be expressed through nonreligious language. You must let the patient know what options are open for spiritual help. If you hide behind busyness and procedures, you may lose a valuable opportunity to aid in health restoration.

Case Study

The following case presents a classic picture of a man with spiritual needs.

Jason Smith is a 40-year-old middle-class white bank president. He lives in a small town with his wife and four children. He also deals in real estate, works with civic and Roman Catholic church groups, and is developing an advertising company. He seems constantly busy. He discusses business over lunch, and competes with friends when playing golf or tennis.

One evening he started vomiting and defecating blood and learned, after being hospitalized locally, that he had a bleeding duodenal ulcer. He was then taken in an ambulance to a metropolitan hospital 200 miles away, where a specialist successfully performed a partial gastrectomy, surgical removal of part of the stomach.

For the first time in his life, Jason was stopped. He was away from family and friends, and was confined. Good and bad memories flooded his mind. He began to evaluate his activities, his emphasis on material gain and competition, how his children were growing so fast, how his religious activities were superficial, and how, without skilled surgery, he might have died.

At first he tried being jovial with the staff in order to strike out these new and troubling thoughts. But he couldn't sleep well. He was dreaming about death in wild combinations with his past life. He began to mention these dreams along with questions about how the surgery would affect his life span, diet, and activities. He mentioned a friend who seemed severely limited from a similar surgery. He also said he was worried about the problems his teenagers were beginning to face and about his own ability to guide them properly.

The staff members never forced Jason to express more than he wished, but answered the questions that were medically based and asked him if he would like to see the chaplain, since his own priest was not available. Jason agreed. An appointed nurse then informed the chaplain of Jason's physical, emotional, and spiritual history to date. In the course of several sessions the chaplain helped Jason work through a revised philosophy of life that put more emphasis on spiritual values, family life, and healthy use of leisure.

Assessment

While you can learn a great deal by picking out points in case studies, you must remember that they provide only a basis. You will have to accept each patient at his religious level. For example, the sacraments have quite a different meaning to Jason than to a child. To a 10-year-old, the meaning of baptism might be carrying an ugly little baby on a pillow to the front of the church, pouring water on its head, and trying to believe that the baby emerges as a beautiful child of God. A teenager caught up in sorting out various facets of his learned idealism and trying to fit them into more realistic daily patterns may temporarily discard his religious teaching. He may reject the guidance of a spiritual leader because he associates the latter with his parents' beliefs; yet he is nevertheless searching and needs guidance. An elderly person suffering the grief of a recently lost mate may repeatedly question how a God of love could allow this loss. Some physiologically mature people are not religiously mature; they may expect magic from God. In all people, personality and temperament affect how they live out their religious experience. A particular Hindu and a given Roman Catholic may

be more in agreement religiously than two Lutherans. You can't make generalizations about a religion from knowing a single follower.

Furthermore, realize that people can use the same religious terms differently: *saved, sanctified, fell out, slain by the spirit,* and *deathbed conversion* all
connote religious experiences, but you should listen carefully and may have to
ask questions to accurately determine the individual person's meaning.

Your greater understanding of social-class and cultural differences gleaned
from other chapters should help you comprehend some of the religious differences. For instance, a poor Protestant American who has grown up with the
barest survival materials, who has no economic power, no money for recreation,
no hope for significant gain, and no positive attitude about this life may center
his whole being in the church. It provides as best it can for his emotional, recreational, and spiritual needs. When he sings about heaven in terms of having beautiful clothes, a crown, and a mansion, he is singing with a much different meaning than the wealthy Protestant American who is really more concerned about
mansions *here* than *over there.*

In a wider sense, an Egyptian Christian and an American Christian, although voicing the same basic beliefs, will differ in their approaches to religion.
The Egyptian, influenced by the Islamic attitudes of his country, might say,
"No matter what happens, it's God's will. I can do no more about it." The
American Christian may be more influenced by the individual drive to guide his
life, a philosophy so prevalent in his culture. Another cultural difference will
center on the influence of the family with an ill member. The Egyptian, accustomed to having family and friends surrounding him nearly constantly, will
expect a continuation of such activity during illness. He will seek spiritual and
emotional support from their presence. The American, more mobile and used to
the American hospital system of limiting visitors in number and time, will be
better able to detach himself from the emotional and religious support given by
the presence of his family.

Religion influences attitudes and behavior regarding: (1) work—whether
you work to expiate sin or simply because it's there to do; (2) money—whether
you save money to deny yourself something, do installment buying, or buy
health insurance, or whether you consider money the root of all evil; (3) political
behavior—ideas about the sanctity of the Constitution, effects of communism,
importance of world problems, spending abroad versus that for national defense,
school or residential desegregation, welfare aid, and union membership; (4) family—kinds of interaction within the family, honoring of parents or spouse;
(5) childrearing—interest in the child's present and future, attitudes regarding
punishment or rewards for behavior, values of strict obedience as contrasted with
independent thinking, or how many children should be borne; (6) right and
wrong—what is sin, how wrong is gambling, drinking, birth control, divorce,
smoking, and abortion[4].

Consider how essentially the same situation can be diversely interpreted
by two teenagers of different faiths. One, a fundamentalist Protestant, may

spend an evening dancing and playing cards and suffer crushing guilt because she participated in sinful acts. The other, a Jewish teenager, may participate in the same activities and consider it a religiously based function. Your knowledge of and sensitivity to such differences are important, for essentially similar kinds of decisions—right and wrong as religiously defined—will be made about autopsy, cremation, and organ transplants. [See reference 12 for additional information.] Furthermore, although religious bodies may hand down statements on these issues, often the individual person will alter his group's stand as he incorporates his own circumstances into the decision.

Ideally, religion provides strength, an inner calm and faith with which to work through life's problems. But you must be prepared to see the negative aspect. To some, religion seems to add guilt, depression, and confusion. Some may blame God for making them ill, for letting them suffer, or for not healing them in a prescribed manner. One Protestant felt she had made a contract with God: if she lived the best Christian life she could, He would keep her relatively well and free from tragedy. When an incurable disease was diagnosed, she said, "What did I do to deserve this?" Another Protestant, during her illness, took the opposite view of her similar contract with God. She said, "I wasn't living as well as I should and God knocked me down to let me know I was backsliding."

Healing, too, has varied meanings. Some will demand that God provide a quick and miraculous recovery, while others will expect the process to occur through the work of the health team. Still others combine God's touch, the health workers' skill, and their own emotional and physical cooperation. Some will even consider death as the final form of healing.

Sometimes you will have to deal with your own negative reactions. Your medical background and knowledge will cause you to be dismayed at some religious practices. For instance, how will you react as you watch a postoperative Jehovah's Witness patient die because she has refused blood? How will you react to a Christian Scientist patient who, in your opinion, should have sought medical help a month ago to avoid present complications? Here is one response given by a Christian Science nurse: "People can be ruined psychologically by going against a long held belief. They may live and get better physically, but will suffer depression, guilt, and failure in not holding to their standard." In essence, they prefer to die. Should you dictate otherwise? You may need to think through and discuss such situations with a spiritual leader.

Intervention

With all these aspects to consider, a team approach that includes the patient, family, health workers, and chaplain or other spiritual leader seems imperative. Because Americans want weekends away from the job, the weekend hospital staff often has double responsibility. Furthermore, weekends are when most people attend corporate worship. Preparing the patient for chapel service, or seeing that the Sabbath ritual is carried out, puts a special responsibility on you, the nurse.

If a patient is confined to his room, you can simply prepare a worship center or shirine by arranging his flowers, prayer book, relics, or whatever other objects have spiritual meaning to him.

You should keep one or more calendars of various religious holidays. The Eastern Orthodox Easter usually does not coincide with the Roman Catholic and Protestant Easter. Jewish holidays usually do not fall on the same dates of the Western calendar in successive years. Remember also that holidays are family days, and that ill people separated from the family at such times may be especially depressed.

Maintaining a list of available spiritual leaders, knowing when to call them, and knowing how to prepare for their arrival are other important responsibilities. If a patient can't bring himself to make the request, consult with the family. One woman said, "If my sister sees a priest, she will be sure she is dying." Once a health worker took the initiative to call an Eastern Orthodox priest who unfortunately represented the wrong nationality; the patient's main source of comfort was to have come from discussion and prayers in his own native language. Sometimes the family need reassurance and guidance from the chaplain. You can suggest this option.

As you prepare the patient and the setting for the spiritual leader, help create an atmosphere that reflects more than sterile procedure. Emphasis has previously been given to privacy by drawing curtains and shutting doors. While acceptable to some, this approach may produce a negative response in others. Perhaps more emphasis should be given to cheerful surroundings: sunshine, flowers, lighted candles, openness, and participation by family and staff in at least an introductory way. Perhaps the patient and spiritual leader could meet outdoors in an adjoining garden. The Shintoist and Taoist would especially benefit from the esthetic exposure. If the patient is a child on a prolonged hospitalization, a special area might be designated for religious instruction.

You should brief the spiritual leader on any points that might give him special insight, and be sure the patient is ready to receive him. Prepare any special arrangements, such as having a clean, cloth-covered tray for Communion. Guard against interruption by health workers from other departments who may be unaware of the visit. Finally, incorporate the results of the visit into the patient's record.

While many will benefit from the sacraments, the prayers, Scripture reading, and counseling given by the spiritual leader, others will want to rely on their own direct communication with God. The Zen Buddhist, Hindu, Muslim, and Friend might be in the latter category. All may wish reading material, however. Most will bring their sacred book with them, but if they express a desire for more literature, offer to get it. Some hospitals furnish daily and weekly meditations as well as copies of the King James Version of the Bible. Or you might suggest the Bible paraphrased in modern language by Kenneth Taylor called *The Living Bible* (Tyndale House, 1971). The same edition is available as *The Children's Living Bible* (Tyndale House, 1972) with appropriate illustrations. *The Way* (Tyndale House, 1972) has the same wording as *The Living Bible* with guidelines and illustrations for youth. A positive interfaith magazine is *Guideposts* (Guideposts Associates, Inc.), and a novel with religious insights is *Christy* (Avon Books, 1968) by Catherine Marshall.

If you feel comfortable doing so, there will be times when you can say a prayer, read a Scripture, or provide a statement of faith helpful to the patient. And if spiritual leaders aren't available, you could organize a group of health workers willing to counsel with or make referrals for patients of their own faiths.

Although a hospital setting has been used as a point of reference throughout this chapter, you can improvise in your setting—nursing home, school, industry, clinic, home, or other health center—in order to provide adequate spiritual assistance.

REFERENCES

1. Abbott, Walter M., and Joseph Galleger, eds., *The Documents of Vatican II*. New York: The America Press, 1966, pp. 37-39, 158, 363.
2. Allport, Gordon, *The Individual and His Religion*. New York: The Macmillan Company, 1961, pp. 24-27.
3. Berkowitz, Philip, and Nancy Berkowitz, "The Jewish Patient in the Hospital," *American Journal of Nursing*, 67: No. 11 (1967), 2335-37.
4. Bossard, J., and E. Boll, *The Sociology of Child Development* (4th ed.). New York: Harper & Row, Publishers, 1966.
5. Brown, Robert, *The Spirit of Protestantism*. New York: Oxford University Press, 1961.
6. Campbell, Teresa, and Betty Chang, "Health Care of the Chinese in America," *Nursing Outlook*, 21: No. 4 (1973), 245-49.
7. Glustrom, Simon, *When Your Child Asks: A Handbook for Jewish Parents*. New York: Block Publishing Company, 1959.
8. Guralnik, David, ed., *Webster's New World Dictionary of the American Language* (2nd. college ed.). New York: World Publishing Company, 1972.
9. Hackney, E. J., personal letter on Zen Buddhism. January 19, 1973.
10. Hudson, Virginia, *O Ye Jigs and Juleps*. New York: MacFadden-Bartell Corporation, 1964.
11. Kepler, Milton, "The Religious Factor in Pediatric Care," *Clinical Pediatrics*, 9: No. 3 (1970), 128-30.
12. ____, "Human Values in Medicine: Some Helping Organizations," *Journal of the American Medical Association*, 15: No. 3 (1973), 305-7.

13. Kertzer, Rabbi Morris, *What Is a Jew?* (rev. ed.). New York: The Macmillan Company, 1969.
14. Long, Luman, ed., *The World Almanac and Book of Facts, 1971*. New York: Newspaper Enterprise Association, 1971, pp. 327-28.
15. Luce, Henry R., ed., *The World's Great Religions*. New York: Time, Inc., 1957.
16. *Manual on Hospital Chaplaincy*. Chicago: American Hospital Association, 1970, pp. 55-66.
17. Marty, Martin, "Religion in America, 1972," *P.T.A.*, December 1972, pp. 15-19.
18. Mastrantonis, George, ed., "St. Nicholas: The Popular Wonder Worker," *Ologos*. St. Louis: Ologos, n.d.
19. Mead, Frank, *Handbook of Denominations in the United States* (4th ed.). Nashville, Tenn.: Abingdon Press, 1965.
20. Morris, Karen, and J. Foerster, "Team Work: Nurse and Chaplain," *American Journal of Nursing*, 72: No. 12 (1972), 2197-99.
21. Naimann, H., "Nursing in Jewish Law," *American Journal of Nursing*, 70: No. 11 (1970), 2378-79.
22. Noss, John, *Man's Religions* (rev. ed.). New York: The Macmillan Company, 1956, pp. 399-427.
23. Petersen, Mark, *A Word of Wisdom*. Salt Lake City: Church of Jesus Christ of Latter-Day Saints, n.d.
24. Piepgras, Ruth, "The Other Dimension: Spiritual Help," *American Journal of Nursing*, 68: No. 12 (1968), 2610-13.
25. Porath, Thomas, "Humanizing the Sacrament of the Sick," *Hospital Progress*, 53: No. 7 (1972), 45-47.
26. Rosten, Leo, ed., *Religions in America* (rev. ed.). New York: Simon and Schuster, 1963.
27. *Saint Louis Globe Democrat*, January 19, 1973, sec. A, p. 8, "Pope Paul Eases the Rules for Anointing of the Sick."
28. Satprakashananda, Swami, ed., *The Use of Symbols in Religion*. St. Louis: The Vedanta Society, 1970.
29. Saunders, E. Dale, *Buddhism in Japan*. Philadelphia: University of Philadelphia Press, 1964, pp. 265-86.
30. "Second Thoughts About Man: Searching Again for the Sacred," *Time*, April 9, 1973, pp. 90-93.
31. Shibata, Chizuo, "The New Religions and the Christian Church," *Japan Christian Quarterly*, Summer 1971, pp. 173-80.
32. Smith, Huston, *The Religions of Man*. New York: Harper & Row, Publishers, Inc., 1965.
33.ʼ Smith, Wilfred, *The Faith of Other Men*. New York: The American Library of World Literature, Inc., 1963.
34. *Unity School of Christianity*. Unity Village, Mo.: Unity School of Christianity, n.d.

35.   Walker, H. B., "Why Medicine Needs Religion," *International Surgery*, 56: No. 8 (1971), 37B-40B.

36.   Wasson, Elgin, personal letter and paper from Christian Science Committee on Publication for Missouri, January 8, 1973.

37.   Westberg, Granger, *Nurse, Pastor, and Patient*. Philadelphia: Fortress Press, 1955.

38.   Wood, Verna, personal letter on Religious Society of Friends, January 29, 1973.

PERSONAL INTERVIEWS

39.   Andrews, Constantine, pastor, St. Nicholas Greek Orthodox Church, St. Louis, January 26, 1973.

40.   Bregman, Alan, rabbi, Temple Israel, St. Louis, January 27, 1973.

41.   Crump, Ronald, pastor, Rock Hill Church of God, St. Louis, January 30, 1973.

42.   Danker, William, professor of world mission, Concordia Seminary, St. Louis, January 26, 1973.

43.   Dickes, Hans, a seventy in the Church of Jesus Christ of Latter-Day Saints, St. Louis, January 20, 1973.

44.   Gowing, Peter, regional professor, South East Asia, Graduate School of Theology, Singapore, January 10, 1973.

45.   Griswell, John, pastor, Seventh Day Adventist Central Church, St. Louis, January 31, 1973.

46.   Guirguis, Youssef, and Laila Guirguis, Egyptian Christians, January 13, 1973.

47.   Katsarus, Georgia, Greek Orthodox, January 19, 1973.

48.   Khalifa, Saeed, Soheir Eltoumi, E. Z. Eltoumi, Mohamed Ahmed, and Fatma Ahmed, Egyptian Muslims, January 13, 1973.

49.   Kimelman, Dr. Nathan, Mrs. Nathan Kimelman, Dr. Harry G. Mellman, and Jane Tarlow, American Jews, January 29 and February 2, 1973.

50.   Liao, Nancy, graduate, National Taiwan University, Tapei, Taiwan, January 15, 1973.

51.   Lonnemann, Anne, Roman Catholic, January 8, 1973.

52.   Luehrman, Ernest, chaplain, Deaconess Hospital, St. Louis, January 17, 1973.

53.   Purvis, Doreen, administrator, Peace Haven Nursing Home, St. Louis, and trained Christian Science nurse, January 9, 1973.

54.   Rupani, Navinchandra L., Hindu spiritual teacher, Collinsville, Ill., January 28, 1973.

55.   Satprakashananda, Swami, leader, Vedanta Society, St. Louis, January 7, 1973.

56.   Zentner, Reid, pastoral counselor, January 2, 1973.

CHAPTER 12

Social-Class Life Styles and Their Influences on the Person

Study of this chapter will help you to:

1 Define *social class* and describe the specific social-class levels in the United States.

2 Describe the main concepts of social organization as they relate to social class.

3 Discuss and contrast the main characteristics of the upper-, middle-, and lower-class life styles.

4 Differentiate between the life styles and values of persons in the upper and lower divisions of each social class.

5 Identify characteristics of your life style and the influence of these upon you as a health care worker.

6 Compare class-related attitudes toward health and health care, determining how these attitudes will affect your nursing practice.

7 Discuss the value of understanding social-class life styles and related nursing implications.

8 Assess and care for a person and family from a social class different from your own, individualizing care in a nonjudgmental manner.

There are no classless societies, and the United States is no exception. In this chapter some of the differences among the social classes in the United States are discussed, along with social-class attitudes toward health and the health care system and related nursing implications.

CONCEPTS OF SOCIAL ORGANIZATION

Social class is defined as a group of people who share similar life styles because of similarities in occupation, wealth, education, recreation, interests, beliefs, attitudes, and values, and who regard themselves as belonging to one group.
Social class has been one criterion used to describe heterogenous populations. People at different levels of income and wealth often represent correspondingly different backgrounds and different levels of education. Additionally, they create for themselves different life styles, adopt different values and goals, and maintain different types of relationships[14]. This knowledge is valuable in understanding patients.

Social classes are formed because in any society some functions are more important than others. Since not all members of society are equally capable of performing these functions, certain abilities, time, and self-sacrifice are required for training to perform the special functions. Privileges and special rewards are offered to induce the capable to undertake such training, and with these privileges and rewards come later prestige and social superiority within the group. Thus different jobs have different prestige values in different cultures or countries, and prestige and material rewards may maintain the power of a person (or group) even after his (or its) role in society has diminished in importance[8].

At birth the person is given a place in society according to the social status of his parents. Families are generally aware of their own status and that of others in their community. Others may be seen as "our kind of people," or "those who live across the tracks," or "those who live on millionaire row." A community may be comprised predominately of one class or it may consist of several, depending on its location in the city, suburb, rural area, or section of the United States[10].

A description of a society in terms of classes and their relationship reveals *class structure. Open class structuring exists in a society that permits ease of movement from one social class to another. When mobility is difficult or impossible, the society possesses a* **caste system**[2]. Even open class systems develop castelike characteristics, since people try to preserve class advantages for their offspring.

In the United States, however, some controls limit the preferential advantages of children in higher status groups: these include adequate income distributed among a large number of middle-class people, inheritance taxes, and free access to education. Nevertheless, the class into which each person is born affects in some way his position in life.

Determining Social Class

Class is more than an arbitrary placement along a line. It is a reality that provides us with an awareness that people live, eat, play, mate, dress, work, and think at similar and contrasting levels. The Index of Status Characteristics (I.S.C.) was developed to objectively determine the social class of a given family[30]. Its ratings are based on data derived from studying families in various locations throughout the United States. The specific characteristics examined were occupation, source of income, housing arrangement, and living location, with occupation rated as the most important item to consider. According to this index, people may fit into more than one category.

Another study utilized occupation as a characteristic but also included other factors: possessions, interaction, class consciousness, and value orientation[2]. Any one of the factors mentioned is not sufficient alone to determine one's social class or to explain the American class structure. Some characteristics may loom larger than others in the minds of people and thus strongly influence placement within a class.

Although most persons can be objectively placed with a certain class, they are still accorded a status classification by others around them, and they may see themselves at yet a different status level, based on race, sex, religion, ancestry, ethnic origin, or wealth in material goods[2]. What seems natural and logical in determining status for some may be rejected by others.

Class levels alone do not shape values and personalities. There is similarity between those who share like cultural and social backgrounds, but each individual person is unique. People differ in inherited capacities, temperament, and, most important, in the interpersonal experiences that have made them the distinct person they are[13].

Description of Classes

Three classes have long been recognized in the United States: upper, middle, and lower—which translate to mean the rich, the in-between, and the poor. The high social mobility of Americans blurs the boundary lines, but trends are still discernible. Today the number and proportion of families in the middle class are increasing rapidly, along with higher levels of income and education. One in every four or five families, usually in the upper-lower or lower-middle class, has an upward mobility of one class during its lifetime.

Warner divided each class into upper and lower levels, making six social classes[30]. The brief descriptions of the characteristics of each of these six classes, as noted next, and the more extensive discussions that follow will help you better understand the persons you care for. The purpose is not to label, stereotype, or imply that one class is more valuable than another, but to help you realize that important class differences, sometimes unexpected ones, do exist. Realize that while the descriptions in this chapter include data that have been found generally applicable to persons in certain classes, a given person sometimes possesses characteristics of more than one status.

By understanding the *life style* of the person for whom you care, you will be better able to assess his needs and to adapt your care to meet those needs. In addition, you must be aware of how your patients or clients see you, for your upbringing, partially influenced by class values, affects how you view other people and their health and illness patterns.

*The **upper-upper class** is referred to as the "old aristocracy."* These are long-established families who live in the most exclusive sections of the community, usually in homes built by their ancestors. Inherited wealth, rather than income, usually determines their status. These families often take pride in tracing their heritage back several generations. They stress gracious living, supervise their inherited wealth, and generally associate with one another in exclusive clubs. Children are sent to private schools that cater to members of their own class.

*The **lower-upper class** is composed of people who have recently acquired their wealth* and who therefore are not completely accepted socially by the upper-upper class. They belong to the less exclusive but "good" clubs and live as much as possible like the upper-upper class.

*The **upper-middle class** in general is composed of professional persons*, including university professors, scientists, dentists, and those holding responsible managerial positions in business, industry, and government. *This class of people has been referred to as the "backbone of the community."* They live in the better, though not exclusive, sections of the community.

*The **Lower-middle-class** people live in respectable sections of town in comfortable homes.* They strive to give their children a good education and some advantages they may have lacked in their youth. Honesty, fair dealing, and decency are important values to them. They work hard in so-called white-collar jobs as schoolteachers, shopkeepers, clerks, secretaries, bookkeepers, and salespeople. Skilled workmen and successful farmers are sometimes in this class, depending on their values.

*The **upper-lower class**, along with the lower-middle class, constitute the level of "the common man."* The upper-lower class may live in rented houses or apartments not far from deteriorating areas of the community. The father is usually a blue-collar worker earning his income in a factory, mine, mill, or in a civil service capacity. Many times the wife and older children work to help meet all the needs of the family. *These people work hard and strive to maintain a respectable, independent life.*

*The **lower-lower class** live in deteriorated or slumlike dwellings in a day-to-day existence, as there is not enough money to meet their needs.* Their income is derived from wages earned by the father, and usually the mother, at unskilled jobs that alternate with unemployment compensation. The children usually enter the labor force at an early age, dropping out of school to do so.

The following descriptions of the social classes are based on the traditional upper-middle-lower classification, with particular distinctions being made within the classes as necessary.

UPPER-CLASS LIFE STYLE

Lineage and Status

Belonging to the upper class is based on the high status a family has within a community, either through inheritance or acquired privileges, or both.

Established Upper-Class Families. **Lineage**, or *ancestry*, is a crucial factor in established upper-class families. More emphasis is placed on one's ancestors and relatives than on personal attainments[14]. Background becomes especially important when marriage is considered, since it is the institution that allows for maintenance and continuation of the family group. Closing ranks in the family is seen when a member proposes to marry someone not of "the aristocracy." The erring member, more frequently a male than a female, is then coerced, through pressure from many relatives, to recognize that admitting an outsider would be a grave error: family and class codes would be violated; and the expected trust or promised position would pass to someone else.

The high degree of solidarity between relatives and among intraclass marriages provides for maximum stability in the established upper class. The nuclear family (parents and offspring) maintains a separate household, but sees itself as belonging to the larger kin group, which includes all descendants in addition to the added members accepted by marriage.

The upper-class wife may oversee several homes, plan entertainment, hire and supervise the help (an increasingly difficult task), and involve herself in community organizations and charity work. These duties, in addition to teaching the children the role they will play in society, are expected[32]. If finances decrease, she may also have to maintain a front (go through the usual routines even though circumstances have changed).

The New-Upper-Class Families have the wealth of established families but not the lineage. The extended family group does not have as much relevance, and therefore they cannot exert as much influence on a recalcitrant member. Consequently, members of the new-upper class have broken ties many times with kin during their upward mobility, behavior not acceptable to the aristocracy. The newly rich are more independent and rely primarily on the nuclear family; because of mobility and family instability, they may become insecure and exhibit more signs and social pathology, including divorce and alcoholism.

To the ire and discredit of the aristocracy, many people equate this behavior with being upper class[14].

   The Lower-Upper-Class Families. Usually the economic status of the new or lower-upper class has been achieved within a relatively short period (possibly one generation). The family wastes no time accumulating the status possessions—a large house with swimming pool and tennis courts, expensive clothes and furniture, and membership in less exclusive clubs. Nevertheless, the lack of a two- or three-generation upper-class family tree means that lower-upper-class families are not accorded the local status of established families.

   The new-upper-class family must also translate its wealth into socially approved behavior that supposedly matches its position. For example, a family applies to join an exclusive private yacht club and is refused. They find out that they have not made their "money talk" for the right people: they donated money to charity, but not to the charity supported by the yacht club! They make amends by donating to the favored charity and are promptly accepted by the club.

Income Levels

Recently West estimated that there are about 100,000 millionaires in the United States. Another 200 persons are worth 100 times that amount. Still a third small group of 12 measure their wealth up to $2 billion[32]. Some in the aristocracy live on their inheritance for generations. They handle their money in various ways. Some invest in municipal bonds or real estate. Others give their resources and their time to public service, as shown by the Rockefeller and Ford foundations. Many people benefit from the interchange of money, such as cities and research centers. However, these investments also result in a substantial monetary gain for the investor, who may spend 12-14 hours a day maintaining the family business or engaging in professional obligations.

Education

A high social class generally indicates more extensive formal education. Children in the upper class attend private primary and secondary schools or attend public schools with a high rating in the educational system, generally located in their own community. Higher education is expected of most upper-class youth, usually at the best universities and colleges. Learning several languages, worldwide travels with a tutor in attendance, indoctrination to the arts, and development of a gracious style of living are part of the normal educational process.

Dating Patterns of Youth

Upper-class youth nearly always attend social events with persons from their class, although males (more so than females) are noted for dating outside their class. During the high-school years, relationships usually do not lead to a marriage commitment. Supposedly, future aspirations of attendance at exclusive colleges are jeopardized by getting involved with another at the high-school level. While in college, upper-class youth continue to associate with those in their own class.

A study done on a Virginia college campus in 1965 showed that members of high-ranked fraternities (those whose members had fathers in high-ranked occupations) confined their serious dating to girls from high-ranked sororities (similarly defined). In this situation, a continuity of class, leading from home to campus activity, in dating pattern, can be seen[23].

Attitudes toward Sexual Behavior

Reiss believes that no sharp social-class differences exist in the acceptance of premarital sex, and that permissiveness exists at every level and is becoming more acceptable in the upper third of the social strata[23].

In addition to being concerned about his offspring's personal welfare, the upper-class parent is concerned with the family name and thus fears the social damage that would result if a son or daughter engaged freely in premarital sex and became a source of gossip or an unintentional parent. But this attitude can also be found in parents from other social classes[23].

MIDDLE-CLASS LIFE STYLE

The American Way

Eighty-five percent of American children are growing up in financially stable families. Tomorrow's citizens, including those not presently middle-class, are receiving an early indoctrination to middle-class ways and values through the mass media and the educational system. This growth reflects the social and economic progress of the country as well as individual personal growth. Being middle-class is synonymous with the "American way." The middle class has helped to build the system, has proven the system to be operative in an urban-industrialized society, and in turn has been shaped and reinforced by the system[10]. This premise reinforces the commonly held belief that the middle-class way is the way of success.

The names of middle-class occupations imply some of the vast achievements and responsibilities of the middle class. Members of this class aid in economic progress, scientific advancements, medical research, and accomplishments in outer space. They construct, maintain (through financial contributions), and staff hospitals, schools, churches, and a variety of other service organizations and institutions. They also contribute to the growth of others and themselves through contributions to the theater, museums, art galleries, libraries, and the concert hall.

Despite all their contributions, middle class members are not exempt from the weaknesses of man. Middle-class persons engage in their share of crimes, including those crimes more typical of the upper class, such as blackmail, fraud, and extortion. Many of these people have struggled to become middle-class and have to keep striving to maintain their status. Consequently, they often resort to methods of making more money outside their regular occupations, usually legally, but sometimes illegally.

Upper-Middle Class

Stability is the key word in upper-middle-class families. The nuclear unit, often composed of husband, wife, and two or three children, is generally a closely knit group who work hard, are happy, and enjoy life.

Because people in this class generally possess a well-integrated personality and display confidence in their abilities, they are able to make concrete plans and carry them through. Because of their abstract thinking ability, they can make decisions concerning the future and are usually optimistic that they have acted wisely and that planning will bring results. They plan for emergencies through insurance coverage, savings plans, or investments. Also, the wife in an upper-middle-class family usually has some educational preparation, training, or perhaps some working experience and is considered a valuable source of economic security. Her capabilities can be utilized in a time of crisis.

The main goals for the upper-middle-class parents revolve around success and satisfaction in a business or comparable occupation, higher education for their children, and provision for themselves after retirement[14].

Education is a primary goal; the norm for formal education is 14 to 16 years[28]. Youth receive support and encouragement for their educational endeavors. They talk freely about school and become involved in school-related activities. Because the home environment is suited for these achievements, the majority of high-school graduates in this class automatically enter college, which is recognized as a way of completing one's personal development. Educational institutions in the United States have expanded enormously to help fulfill this goal.

Dating, Courtship, and Marriage are usually within the same class, although upper-middle-class girls also date boys from the upper class. Middle-class teenagers may limit their premarital sexual experiences because of future goals to which they are committed; family expectations, stability, interest, and participation of parents with their youth; and religious ties. However, their sexual practices are not sharply contrasted to those of other social classes[10].

Marriage is generally with a person of similar background, religious belief, or educational experience. Often they are young adults before entering marriage, having completed their education or any other commitments first. Separation, divorce, and desertion are infrequent, although these are generally increasing in our society for some of the reasons discussed in Chapters 10 and 13. Group support from friends and kin groups seems to strongly influence prevention of divorce, and such support seems stronger emotionally and economically in the middle classes[1].

If marriages are unhappy, the partners may be so intent on maintaining their status that they willingly maintain a facade of stability. Furthermore, people in this class generally accept professional help and may seek guidance of a marriage counselor.

In childrearing, parents are generally concerned with the development of respectable, obedient behavior in children, although emphasis on discipline is less strict than in lower-class families. A feature frequently seen in middle-class childrearing is overpermissiveness. Parent attitudes are more oriented toward psychological growth and development of children and less geared toward maintaining discipline than lower-class parents tend to be[15].

Lower-Middle Class

There are no notable differences between the lower-middle class and the upper-middle class in terms of nuclear unit stability. As in the lower-upper class, a large number of lower-middle-class persons have achieved their positions mainly through their own efforts. A large number of these adults began as working-class people whose ability, hard work, and support from the family aided their upward mobility.

Problems of the lower-middle-class family revolve around economic stability and education for children[14]. Most see the need for college education and want it for their children even if it means their making sacrifices. These people want their children to have opportunities that they (the parents) lacked as youth. Parents have achieved upward mobility and want their children to achieve one more step—the upper-middle class. They know that higher education is the tool to help achieve this goal. Ironically, this willingness to sacrifice for their children's rise could be what fosters a later generation gap: the children attain upper-middle-class characteristics, while the parents do not. On the other hand, those children who remain appreciative of their parents' admiration and sacrifice will continue to bridge the gap[23].

LOWER-CLASS LIFE STYLE

Upper-Lower Class

The amount and types of skills possessed are the basis for subdividing the lower or "working class." In the upper level of this class are the skilled workers: those employed in industry; in building or road construction; in mining, extracting, and producing basic materials; in plumbing, masonry, baking; and in operating small self-owned farms. The problems resulting from technology have expanded the labor union movement, which can claim many, but not all, blue-collar workers as members. As a result of union efforts, working hours and conditions have improved, along with social welfare benefits such as insurance plans and workmen's compensation. Working-class wages are now equal to or greater than those of many lower-middle-class workers. Thus the economic criterion is no longer the main difference between this level and the middle class[6].

Nevertheless, class differences in the *life themes* seem to prevail. The distinction appears to center around the different values of the two groups[2]. The blue-collar worker feels he has reached the highest level possible for him and he is pleased. But clerks and salesmen in the lower-middle class, the white-collar group, feel differently, especially if their income is similar to that of the blue-collar worker. These white-collar men are at the bottom of their ladder, while the blue-collar men are at the top of theirs.

Education that the lower-class youth receives is related to amount of parental education and parents' occupation. Data from a short-term study revealed that only 37 percent of high-school graduates from working-class families went to college. Various factors could explain why. The child may receive little parental help or encouragement. Also environmental conditions at home, such as noise or overcrowding, could be deterrents to study. Or the child could feel rejected by his teacher, who often comes from a middle-class background[10]. Nevertheless, some youth from this group are continuing with college education. Upward mobility is attributable partially to education, and the greatest amount of upward mobility begins at the lower-middle-class and upper-lower-class levels.

Courtship, Marriage, and Childrearing Patterns are characteristic in certain respects. Early dating and marriage are common among working-class youth. They have fewer social pressures and therefore less achievement drive. They are often anxious to leave crowded home conditions. They have few reasons to postpone marriage, sexual activity, and pregnancy. However, their maintenance of a successful marriage can be hindered by limited education, lack of a trade or skill, and the consequent economically insecure position of the family[10, 23].

All of these stressful factors influence childrearing, which is adult-centered, authoritarian, and based on reward and punishment. Children are supposed to behave like miniature adults as much as possible. Girls seven and eight years of age assist their mothers, and likewise boys assist their fathers. Children are reared to meet the dictates of the family's need[3]. Lower-class parents are apparently as concerned with developing respectable, obedient behavior as their middle-class counterparts[15].

Lower-Lower Class

At the lowest end of the economic scale are the people who exist below the poverty level. Within the affluence of the United States there are many poor people (13 percent of the population in 1967). The greatest number of these are unskilled, chronically ill, and either under 18 or over 64. They are usually living in a family with more than four children, which is often headed by a woman, and they are frequently nonwhites[7, 10]. The War on Poverty began in 1964 with the passage of the Economic Opportunity Act, which was concerned with providing everyone with the opportunity for education, training, work, and the opportunity to live in decency and dignity. Alleviating the lot of the impoverished has assumed a major place among national priorities. However, most poor people cannot be helped by simply expanding the economy, for there are factors beyond economic ones preventing them from getting or keeping better-paying work: age, family responsibilities, poor health, lack of ability, or the barriers of discrimination.

Life's Theme as Seen by the Poor is unpatterned, unpredictable, and beyond personal control. Their constant struggle with inadequate and crowded living conditions, reduced access to education and consequently to jobs requiring any skill, and limited recreation are some of the causes of these feelings. There are four themes characteristic of lower-class attitudes and behavior: (1) fatalism, (2) orientation to the present, (3) authoritarianism, and (4) concreteness[15].

A feeling of powerlessness is the source of their *fatalistic* attitude. Because they cannot predict or avoid events, they feel a sense of resignation. If anything gives them a reason to feel any optimism, it is ascribed to chance—a lucky break. Since they cannot rely or build on positive past experiences, they *focus on the present*. If all their resources must be spent for daily survival, how can they think about the future? They exist for today and allow the future to take care of itself.

The *authoritarian* theme stems from their belief that physical strength is the source of authority. To them, the strong survive; toughness and aggressiveness are thus valued traits. This attitude is a result of frequent simplification of their life experiences. They have learned to accept and prefer cut-and-dried solutions to their difficulties, as long-range solutions too often bring few results, resulting in even less ability to do future planning. This authoritarian theme transfers to childrearing patterns, which support severe punishment for deviance and disobedience as opposed to any type of reasoning.

Concreteness is the fourth theme in life. These families usually deemphasize verbal communication and instead value tangible rather than intellectual matters. They have no use for abstract reasoning abilities, but rather want the products of action. Immediate results are considered most important.

Values and Aspirations of the Poor in the United States, including aspirations for their children, are the same as for the middle class—a good education, career, and happiness. Findings show that 65 percent of lower-class parents desire a college education for their children[15]. However, their aspirations are vague, for they have no realistic means of future planning.

The poor are not satisfied with their housing or living conditions. The term **ghetto** has been applied to their *substandard housing, environment of* *violence and crime, and poor neighborhood conditions, usually located in large cities.* They desire nice homes, fine furniture, and other objects characterized as "American necessities." To the disdain of many middle-class people, television sets are frequently seen in their apartments. Materialism sometimes wins out over other needs and supports their present-time emphasis since they usually see no way out of their present living situation.

They value safety, economic and emotional security, religious beliefs, some ascribed status and respect, and families of typical middle-class size—two or three children.

Because of the sharp difference in their life style from the other five classes, their moral codes may also be different. They value stable marriages to an extent, but do not reject other forms of intimate partnerships. Common-law marriages are acceptable, as are out-of-wedlock children. There is some sense of achievement in parents who support children born out of wedlock.

Family Structure is distinguished by a female-based family and a transient, marginal male, one who does not live steadily with the female and does not contribute fully to the family economy. Or the family circle may comprise only females.

This type of family has been described as "broken," "incomplete," "fatherless"—or as "the grandmother family." These terms imply harsh, negative value judgments about the poor. A relatively new and value-free term, *matrifocal, or mother-centered, is used in reference to a strong mother-child bond found in most lower-class households*[22]. The matrifocal family does not conform to the middle-class idea of a stable nuclear unit. The mother and her children usually socialize with her female kin and friends, while the male, if present, seeks excitement or thrills with others outside the home. If marriage is present, it is not expected to provide the same interest or intimacy as expected in middle-class marriages.

Economic insecurity is probably the main factor contributing to the continuation of the matrifocal family. The transient, marginal male, with his limited education and his inability to succeed in the working world, depends on wage labor. Thus he is subject to low-paying seasonal employment alternating with relief. Unskilled labor is no longer in demand as it was in past years. Anyway, such jobs offer little prestige or opportunity for learning and almost no chance for advancement. The female has more job opportunities in restaurants, hospitals, factories, private homes, and discount stores[22]. All these factors contribute to low self-esteem and motivation in the male and further marginal behavior.

Matrifocality is the end product of poverty and deprivation, not its source. It should be appreciated as a survival pattern for the family rather than as a pathology. Matrifocality is not a disease, but a social adaptation.

CLASS-RELATED DIFFERENCES
IN HEALTH ATTITUDES

Suchman has found that certain sociocultural background factors, particularly the *social group, those with whom one most closely associates,* predispose the person toward accepting or rejecting formal, scientific medical care. Illness is an experience that occurs frequently in the life of everyone and that also involves well people significant to the sick person. Significant group norms and expectations have evolved that influence attitudes and behavior related to health and illness. The more homogeneous and cohesive the group, the more likely is the person to react to illness and medical care according to group norms, which may mean rejecting the formal, impersonal, official medical care system. Social-group organization can be broken down into ethnic, friendship, and family groups. *Cosmopolitan social groups have an outlook that is progressive, individualistic, open, and accepting of impersonal, scientific medical practices. Parochial sociocultural groups are tradition-bound, authoritarian, emotionally expressive, closed, and less likely to accept modern medical practices*[26].

Persons who belong to cultural groups that are ethnically exclusive, to friendship groups that are cohesive, and to family groups oriented toward tradition and authority have less knowledge of disease and a higher suspicion or skepticism of formal medical care. They have a greater dependency, in illness, on nonmedical workers. A parochial group has a subjective, informal health orientation rather than a scientific, objective, professional, and independent approach to illness and medical care characteristic of the cosmopolitan group. The person with nonscientific, closed ideas about medicine is more likely to seek diagnosis and help from his lay peers, to use folk remedies and self-medications, and to delay sound treatment. He reacts more strongly to painful symptoms and is concerned with immediate relief rather than long-term cure or prevention. Such a person feels uncertain about modern medical practices, uneasy in a group practice setting, is poorly informed about health care services, and has difficulty adapting to hospital routines. He is likely to resist and to avoid utilizing modern medical care programs and resources.

Generally, members of the lower class have a parochial social structure and less scientific ideas about health care than the upper class, who tend to be more open to professional, scientific care and to make greater use of modern medical services. However, there are parochial, closed groups within the upper class who are not particularly scientific in their definition of health and illness, who are also more likely to use lay help and home remedies than formal medical care.

Women are generally more parochial and more easily influenced by the group than are men in areas other than health, but they are better informed about disease and less skeptical of the medical care system than are men, perhaps because they are responsible for family health. Thus they learn more about disease and place more faith in doctors.

Regardless of sex or social class, epidemiological research shows that more illness exists among the old than the young, including chronic disease, medically attended conditions, and mental disability (with the exception of more mental disability among young upper-class males than old upper-class males). Women report more chronic conditions, medically attended conditions, and mental disability than men within each age and social-class group. This finding may be related to women's greater willingness to seek care, which makes them available to be included in a statistically counted group. Men may have equal health problems but are not counted in medical statistics because they less frequently seek treatment. Groups with parochial, traditional characteristics report more illness than cosmopolitan, open groups.

What effect does experience with illness and medical care have on one's medical orientation? The more one is exposed to illness and medical care, the more likely the person is to have a scientific health orientation, regardless of social class or social-group structure. The upper-class person and the older person are more likely than the lower-class and the younger person to make use of private physicians. Thus social status and age affect where an ill person seeks medical care. The person with a parochial viewpoint is also more likely than the cosmopolitan, scientific person to seek care from a private physician, probably because of the former's need for a more informal, personal relationship. The scientific person is more willing to utilize the impersonal sources of medical care, such as clinics, group practice, and specialists in medicine.

Many persons in the upper and middle classes buy health insurance and use preventive services. They get periodical medical check-ups, receive immunizations, eat a balanced diet, and seek dental care and eye examinations. In addition, they consult a physician for specific symptoms such as a fever or rash.

Modern medicine is increasingly scientific, formal, complex, impersonal, objective, specialized, and focused on disease rather than on the patient. This trend will cause increasing conflict with the traditional, parochial, closed persons who seek a personal, layman's, nonscientific approach to medical care. Consequently, many groups in the United States, as well as in the underdeveloped areas of the world, continue to resist modern medical programs. Unless health care programs are adapted to the type of social group to be served, the people in that group will not be likely to utilize or cooperate with the health team.

Health care must become more personalized, focusing on the patient and family as a unit, adapting to local customs when reaching out to the community, and eliminating long waiting lines at public clinics. The public must be educated about medical services and the importance of seeking care rather than given reams of factual, anxiety-provoking data about etiology, signs, and symptoms. Medicine must forego the traditional, controlling approach to people, for some people react negatively, even to the point of self-neglect, to such an approach[26].

NURSING IMPLICATIONS

The nursing implications from Chapter 10 can be applied to the material in this chapter as well. Knowing the significant differences among classes and the predictable knowledge and attitudes about health and health care gives you more information to work with.

All people have some prejudice; it emerges in such expressions as, "Those upper-crust people always...," or, "Those welfare people never... ." Examine your thinking for unconscious prejudice, understand your own class background, and distinguish your values from those held by the persons you care for. Try to withhold value judgments that interfere with your relationship with the patient and with objective care. There are too many unknown factors in people's lives to set up stereotyped categories. For example, a family may be in the middle class or upper class in terms of income, education, and goals, and yet live in an upper-lower-class neighborhood because they refuse to emphasize material wealth. A farmer according to our criteria may be labeled upper-lower-class and yet regard himself very much a part of the middle class. A person who lives in an economically depressed section of the United States and is poor may have an adequate public education, a middle-class value system, and upper-class graciousness.

If you feel you are stooping to help lower-class people, you may be labeled a "do-gooder" and be ineffective. Recognize the behavior of the lower class not as pathological but as adaptive for their needs. Realize, too, that not only the poor need your help. The upper-class person may need a great deal of help with care, health teaching, or counseling. Having money does not necessarily mean one is knowledgeable about preventive health measures, nutrition, and disease processes. Persons of all classes deserve competent care, clear explanations, and a helpful attitude.

Knowledge about social classes may help explain repeated broken clinic appointments resulting from fear of rejection or lack of transportation rather than from indifference toward the health program or laziness. Take time to talk with the person and you will learn of his fears, problems, aspirations, concern for health and family, and his human warmth.

For example, a woman in labor who is a product of a parochial background with reliance on lay medical help and suspicious of the impersonal hospital and professional-looking nurses, asks to have a knife placed under the bed to help "cut labor pains." While you implement scientific health care, you can be more prepared to act on this belief that psychologically helps the patient.

The misinterpretation of behavior typical of a social class does not always go in one direction, from upper to lower. For example, if you are a nurse with a working-class background, you may be overwhelmed by the 50-year-old corporation president, admitted for coronary disease, who is a member of the newly rich class. He seems obsessed with learning when he can resume his professional duties, exactly how many hours he can work daily, and his chances for a recurrence. An understanding of his class position, along with his possible motives, values, and status (which he feels must be maintained), will enable you to work with his seeming obsession rather than simply label him an "impossible patient."

Try to accept people as they are, regardless of social class. Allow them the freedom to be themselves. Picture the world from the eyes of others—those you care for. In this way you can maintain your own personal standards without being shocked by theirs.

REFERENCES

1. Ackerman, Charles, "Affiliations: Structural Determinants of Differential Divorce Rates," *American Journal of Sociology*, 75 (July 1969), 13-21.

2. Bell, Earl H., *Social Foundations of Human Behavior*. New York: Harper & Row, Publishers, 1961.

3. Bossard, James H., and Eleanor Stoker Boll, *The Sociology of Child Development* (4th ed.). New York: Harper & Row, Publishers, 1966, pp. 235-67.

4. Bower, Fay Louise, *The Process of Planning Nursing Care, A Theoretic Model*. St. Louis: The C. V. Mosby Company, 1972, pp. 1-7.

5. Brinton, Diana M., "Health Center Milieu: Interaction of Nurses and Low-Income Families," *Nursing Research*, 21: No. 1 (1972), 46-51.

6. Brown, Esther L., *Newer Dimensions of Patient Care: Patients as People, Part 3*. New York: Russell Sage Foundation, 1964, pp. 87-132.

7. Bullough, Bonnie, and Vern L. Bullough, *Poverty, Ethnic Identity, and Health Care*. New York: Appleton-Century-Crofts, Educational Division, Meredith Corporation, 1972.

8. Davis, Allison, and R. Havighurst, *Father of the Man*. Boston: Houghton Mifflin Company, 1947.

9. Davis, Kingsley, "Sexual Behavior," in *Contemporary Social Problems*, eds. Robert K. Merton and Robert A. Nesbit. New York: Harcourt, Brace & World, Inc., 1966, pp. 322-72.

10. Duvall, Evelyn, *Family Development* (4th ed.). Philadelphia: J. B. Lippincott Company, 1971, pp. 28-55.

11. Freeman, Ruth B., *Community Health Nursing Practice*. Philadelphia: W. B. Saunders Company, 1970, pp. 206-22.

12. Harrington, Michael, *The Other America*. Baltimore, Md.: Penguin Books, Inc., 1962.

13. Hodges, Harold M., *Social Stratification*. Cambridge, Mass.: Schankman Publishing Company, 1964.

14. Hollingshead, August B., "Class Differences in Family Stability," in *Sourcebook in Marriage and the Family* (3rd ed.), ed. Marvin B. Sussman. Boston: Houghton Mifflin Company, 1968, pp. 153-59.

15. Irelan, Lola M., *Low Income Life Styles*. Washington, D.C.: United States Department of Health, Education, and Welfare, 1966.

16. "Issue on Poverty and Health Care," *Nursing Outlook*, 17: No. 19 (1969), 33-75.

17. Jourard, Sidney M., *The Transparent Self* (rev. ed.). New York: Van Nostrand Reinhold Company, 1971, pp. 177-207.

18. Knutson, Andie L., *The Individual, Society, and Health Behavior*. New York: Russell Sage Foundation, 1965, pp. 98-110.

19. LaFargue, Jane P., "Role of Prejudice in Rejection of Health Care," *Nursing Research*, 21: No. 1 (1972), 53-58.

20. McGrath, Eileen M., "Guidelines for New Community Nurses," *Nursing Outlook*, 19: No. 7 (1971), 478-80.

21. Norman, John C., "Medicine in the Ghetto," *New England Journal of Medicine*, 281: No. 23 (1969), 1271-75.

22. O'Crawford, Charles, *Health and the Family: A Medical-Sociological Analysis*. New York: The Macmillan Company, 1971.

23. Reiss, Ira L., *The Family System in America*. New York: Holt, Rinehart & Winston, Inc., 1971.

24. Schulz, David, *The Changing Family*. Englewood Cliffs, N.J.: Prentice-Hall, Inc., 1972.

25. Standeven, M., "What the Poor Dislike About Community Health Nurses," *Nursing Outlook*, 17: No. 9 (1969), 72-75.

26. Suchman, Edward, "Social Patterns of Illness and Medical Care," in *Patients, Physicians, and Illness*, ed. E. Gartly Jaco. New York: The Free Press, 1972, pp. 262-79.

27. "Syndrome of Poverty," *American Journal of Nursing*, 66: No. 8 (1966), 1750-62.

28. Tinkham, Catherine W., and Eleanor F. Voorhies, *Community Health Nursing: Evolution and Process*. New York: Appleton-Century-Crofts, Educational Division, Meredith Corporation, 1972, pp. 1-102.

29. Warner, W. Lloyd, and Paul S. Lunt, *The Social Life of a Modern Community*. New Haven: Yale University Press, 1941.

30. _____, and Mildred H. Warner, *What You Should Know About Social Class*. Chicago: Science Research Associates, 1953, pp. 22, 25.

31. Watts, W. "Social Class, Ethnic Background, and Patient Care," *Nursing Forum*, 6: No. 2 (1967), 155-62.

32. West, Ruth, "The Care and Feeding of the Very Rich," *McCalls*, 96: No. 11 (1969), 57, 109-10, 112.

CHAPTER 13

The Family —
Basic Unit for
the Developing Person

Study of this chapter will enable you to:

1 Define *family* and view the family in historical perspective.

2 List the developmental tasks of the family.

3 Describe the roles and functions of the family and the relationship of these to the development and health of its members.

4 List the eight-stage cycle of family life and the developmental tasks for the establishment and expectancy phases.

5 Discuss your role in helping the family achieve its developmental tasks for the establishment and expectancy phases.

6 Relate the impact of feelings about the self and childhood experiences upon later family interaction patterns.

7 List and describe the variables affecting the relationship between parent and child and general family life style.

8 Identify ways in which your family life has influenced your present attitudes about family.

9 Discuss the influence of twentieth-century changes upon the family life and childrearing practices.

10 Predict how changing trends in family life may affect the development and health of its members.

11 Explore your role in promoting physical and emotional health of a family, and assess community services that might assist you.

12 Assess and work with a family to enhance its welfare while simultaneously giving health care to one of its members.

"It's an uncanny feeling—to suddenly know that I am answering my son's question with the same words—even the same tone—as my father used with me 30 years ago."

"Even though I have a happy, successful marriage, two loving children, a nice home, and a profession in which I feel competent, I constantly fight a feeling of inferiority. A contributing factor must be that my parents never encouraged or complimented me. When I took a test, they emphasized the 2 wrong, not the 98 right."

"I always admired my aunt. If my cousin, her son, had told her he wanted to build a bridge to the moon, she would have furnished the nails."

These three men are speaking of aspects of a social and biological phenomenon that is often taken for granted: the family. So strongly can this basic unit affect the developing person that he may live successfully or unsuccessfully because of its influence.

Between society and the individual person, the family exists as a primary social group. Most people share the experiences of very early years almost exclusively with the members of a family. Many experts agree that the family is a basic unit of growth, experience, and adaptation; for the purposes of this text, it is also a basic unit of health or illness.

There are countless ways of examining or analyzing the family. Entire texts have been devoted to some of the topics briefly considered here. This chapter is not an exhaustive study of families or family life. Instead, it is an overview of the various forms, stages, and functions of contemporary American families and of how nursing can use this knowledge. Although various aspects of the family are separately discussed, keep in mind that family purposes, stages of development, developmental tasks, and patterns of interaction are all closely interrelated, all influenced by historical foundations, and all continually evolving into new forms.

DEFINITIONS

According to the Federal Bureau of the Census, a *family is a group of two or more persons related by marriage, blood, or adoption who reside together*. Cavan extends the definition: the family *provides a unit that maintains a common culture, derived from the general culture, in which members learn and practice expected social roles*[9].

Messer, in turn, defines the family as *an organization or social institution with continuity (past, present, and future), in which there are certain behaviors in common that affect each other: sharing of goals and identity, mutual concern for physical and emotional needs, and patterns of response that do not require the person to be constantly on guard*[26].

Aside from the natural family, many other units assume characteristics of a family. The employer may be seen as a "father" to his employees. The nurse may be perceived as "mother" to the patients. The behavior of ancestors may be so important to a family that they are in a sense part of the family, living strongly in the memory of present family members and serving as a guide for behavior. For example, an alcoholic ancestor may remind the present family members not to drink.

In the light of changing social attitudes toward living arrangements involving new "family units," researchers suggest that the definition of *family* may have to be changed to accommodate the increasing variety of nonprocreational forms of families. Such units may be sibling families, homosexual marriages, and other forms of friendship families. Indeed, the future may bring with it an increase in social ties and household arrangements where procreation is not a factor. This may necessitate stretching the definition of *family* even farther[21].

HISTORICAL PERSPECTIVE

Although there are many theories about the origin of the family, all are speculative. The only safe assumption is that it is a very old practice for a man and woman, or several men and women, to live together in order to rear their children. Family life exists not only in Homo sapiens. For example, similarities to human family behavior and roles exist in the anthropoid apes—such as mate selection, rearing of offspring by both mates, the male role of protector, and the female role of nurturer. The great difference is that throughout the ape species, family life remains much the same; whereas, with man, family life varies greatly from place to place because of culture.

The ancient family was *patriarchal: the man had complete control over his family*. The large patriarchal family is still characteristic of a majority of the human race today. The development of the crafts in medieval times made the large patriarchal family inefficient. Specialists were needed away from the home base; thus the extended family became a smaller unit. But the man of the house still ruled with absolute authority, and children, considered chattels, were at his mercy. With the Industrial Revolution came new independence for young people. In the United States, for example, a young man no longer had to depend on the family for survival but could go out to obtain a factory job or free land, thereby gaining the right to set up his own household. The extension of democratic principles, with emphasis on individual freedom, contributed to the breakdown of the extended patriarchal family and to the emergence of the democratic, *nuclear-type family, the mother-father-child group*[26].

PURPOSES OF THE FAMILY

Family bonds seem to be a fusion of four universal aspects: biological, social, psychological, and economic. Biologically, the traditional family serves to perpetuate the species by providing for the union of male and female to produce offspring. Socially, the family assures their nurture and training within a given society. The family's biological functions can best be fulfilled in an appropriate social organization. Psychologically, family members depend on one another for the satisfaction of their respective emotional needs. Economically, they depend on each other for provision of their material needs. All aspects are regarded as necessary for the survival of society and are closely interrelated.

Within the framework of these universal aspects emerge the concepts of family functions, roles, and tasks. Definitions of these terms may seem very similar, and may be used almost interchangeably.

A *function is a normal or characteristic action expected or required of someone in a given situation. A* **role** *is a set of prescribed behaviors reflecting goals, values, and sentiments operating in a given situation, created, defined, and modified as a consequence of interaction between two or more people*[19]. *A* **task** *is a function, but with work or labor overtones assigned to or demanded of* the person. A *family developmental task is a growth responsibility that arises at a certain stage in the life of a family, successful achievement of which leads to satisfaction and success with later tasks. However, failure leads to unhappiness in the family, disapproval by society, and difficulty with later family developmental tasks and functions*[12].

Duvall lists eight basic tasks for American families:

1. Providing physical necessities—food, shelter, clothes, health care.
2. Allocation of resources—money, space, material goods.
3. Division of labor.
4. Socialization of family members.
5. Reproduction, recruitment into the family, and release of new members for society.
6. Maintenance of order through effective communication and patterns of interaction.
7. Placement of members into the larger society—church, school, politics.

8. Maintenance of motivation and morale[12].

Whatever the term used—task, role, or function—each of these eight behaviors is essential for the survival, growth, adaptation, and continuity of the family in any society. These behaviors also promote the continuing development of family members through the life cycle[12, 27].

Roles of the Family

The family apportions roles in a way similar to society at large[26]. In society there are specialists who enforce laws, teach, practice medicine, and fight fires. In the family there are also such performance roles: breadwinner, homemaker, handyman (or handywoman), political advisor, chauffeur, and gardener. There are also emotional roles: leader, nurturer, protector, healer, arbitrator, jester, rebel, and "sexpot." The fewer people there are to fulfill these roles, as in the nuclear family, the more demands there are that will be placed on one person. If a member leaves home, someone else takes up his role. Any member of the family can satisfactorily fulfill any of the roles in either category unless he or she is uncomfortable in that role. The man who is sure of his masculinity will have no emotional problems diapering a baby or cooking a meal. The woman who is sure of her femininity will have no trouble gardening or taking the car for repair.

The emotional response of a person to the role he fulfills should be considered. Someone may perform his job competently and yet dread doing it. The man may be a carpenter because his father taught him the trade, although he wants to be a music teacher. Changes in performance roles also necessitate emotional changes—for example, in the man who takes over duties in caring for the household when his wife becomes incapacitated.

The child learns about emotional response to roles in the family as he imitates the adults. The child experiments with various roles in play, and eventually will find one in which he is emotionally comfortable. The more pressure put on the child by the parents to respond in a particular way, the more likely he is to learn only one role and be uncomfortable in others, as evidenced by the athletic champion who may be a social misfit. He becomes less adaptive socially and even within his own family as a result.

Exercising a capacity for a variety of roles, either in actuality or in fantasy, is healthy. The healthy family is the one in which there is opportunity to shift roles intermittently with ease[26]. Through these roles family functions are fulfilled.

Functions of the Family

Ackerman states that all the functions of the family can be reduced to two basic ones: (1) insuring the physical survival of the species, and (2) transmitting the culture, thereby insuring man's essential humanness. The union of mother and father, of parent and child, forms the bonds of identity that are the matrix for the development of this humanness[1].

Physical Functions of the family are met through the parents providing food, clothing, and shelter; protection against danger; provision for bodily repairs after fatigue or illness; and through reproduction. In "primitive" societies, these physical needs are the dominant concern. In Western societies, many families take them for granted[26].

Affectional Functions are equally important. Although many traditional family functions—such as education, job training, and medical care—are being absorbed by other agencies, meeting emotional needs is still one of the family's major functions. The family is the primary unit in which the child tests his emotional reactions. Learning how to reach and maintain emotional equilibrium within the family enables him to repeat the pattern in later life situations. The child who feels loved is likely to contract fewer physical illnesses, to learn more quickly, and generally to have an easier time growing up and adapting to society[26].

Social Functions of the modern family include providing social togetherness, fostering self-esteem and a personal identity tied to family identity, providing opportunities for observing and learning social and sexual roles, accepting responsibility for behavior, and supporting individual creativity and initiative. The family actually begins the indoctrination of the infant into society when it gives him a name and, hence, a social position or status in relation to his immediate and kinship-group families. Simultaneously, each family begins to transmit its own version of the cultural heritage to the child. Because the culture is too vast and comprehensive to be transmitted to the child in its entirety and all at once, the family selects from the surroundings what is to be transmitted. In addition, the family interprets and evaluates what is transmitted. Through this process, the child learns to share his family's values[1, 26, 31].

Socialization thus is a primary task of the parents, since the parents teach the child about himself, his body, peers, family, community, and age-appropriate roles as well as language, perceptions, social values, and ethics. The family also teaches about the different standards of responsibility society demands from various social groups. For example, the professional person, such as a physician, nurse, or lawyer, those in whom people confide and to whom they entrust their lives and fortunes, are held more accountable than the farmer or day laborer. There is also a difference in the type of contact society has with a particular group: for example, the postman or milkman does not enter the home, but the exterminator has the freedom to enter a home and look into every corner.

The parent generation educates by literal instruction and by serving as models[26]. Thus the child's *personality, a product of all the influences that have and are impinging on him,* is greatly influenced by the parents[25]. The types and importance of family interactions in carrying out these functions in each life era are further discussed by Murray and Zentner[27].

STAGES OF FAMILY DEVELOPMENT

The concept of natural life history or cyclic family stages has been observed and analyzed by many students of family development[6, 12, 20, 34]. Like an individual person, a family also has a developmental history marked by predictable crises and preoccupations and interspersed with periods of relative calm. In this connection, the analogy of the family to a cell with a semipermeable membrane is especially appropriate[1]. Both exhibit the qualities of a living process and of a functional unity. Both demonstrate a selective interchange between the enclosed members and the outside world. These external and internal influences may result in an adverse or a favorable environment in which the cell (the family) must continue to exist and function.

Because family life is on a continuum, the cyclic concept is useful in predicting what stage the family is in at a given time and what they can expect in the future. Parents must develop and mature just as their children develop and mature. Parents have different responsibilities and functions in these successive life stages[12, 27]. A newly married couple form the core of the traditional family. With the coming of the first child and with successive children, a significant reorganization of family life occurs. The children grow, usually marry, and establish homes of their own. The aging parents are a solitary couple once again. In its simplest form, a family with children has a life cycle in two stages: the expanding and the contracting family.

Developmental Tasks

In the United States, marriage typically establishes a new family unit. The readiness for and customs of marriage in American society are discussed in relation to young adulthood by Murray and Zentner[27].

Establishment Phase. The *establishment phase of the family life cycle, a developmental crisis, begins with the marriage of the couple and continues until the couple become aware that they are expectant parents, or until certain developmental tasks are accomplished if they decide not to have children.* These developmental tasks of the married couple have their origin in the personal aspirations of the man and woman, in the cultural expectations of their given society, and in the partners' physiological drives for sexual fulfillment. The complexities of these developmental tasks provide some difficulties in adjusting to life as a married pair. Allowing for some variations in families, classes, and cultures, Duvall describes the developmental tasks in the establishment phase of the family as follows:

1. Establishing a home of their own, making a bodily and psychological departure from the parental home.
2. Working out acceptable patterns of daily living.

3. Formulating a workable philosophy of life as a couple, including systems of intellectual and emotional communication, and religious or moral codes.
4. Establishing a mutually satisfying sexual relationship.
5. Reworking relationships with relatives, friends, associates, and community.
6. Planning for the possibility and responsibility of children, or deciding against having children.
7. Devising a system of financial responsibility[12].

Expectant Phase. The **expectant phase** *begins with the awareness that the wife is pregnant and continues until the first child is born*. This phase is short in length but long in adjustments, crises, and responsibilities in becoming parents. All future family interaction is affected by the couple's attitude toward parenthood and their attitude toward children. Along with the exacting responsibilities, parenthood brings many changes in life style and new social roles[12].

Thus, pregnancy is a developmental or maturational crisis since the usual patterns of living and adaptation are no longer appropriate. Developmental crises are normal, but they may be disturbing and frightening because each life stage is a new experience. So it is with the first pregnancy. The changing identities and roles of both husband and wife can be sources of anxiety and concern[11]. For the woman there are new and extensive physical and psychological stimuli. The man must cope with the changes his wife is undergoing by "mothering" her through these difficulties as well as dealing with his own feelings about becoming a father and assuming a father's responsibilities.

Revisions in the family budget are frequently one of the first problems the expectant couple have to face, especially if the wife leaves employment, as the couple are facing today's high cost of hospital, obstetric, and pediatric care. In the United States, the estimated costs of prenatal care, delivery, furnishings and clothing for baby, and his care in the first year of life range from $1,500 to $2,000, depending on vicinity of residence.

Pregnancy frequently changes the pattern of sexual relations. These changes may be based on physician's restrictions or on the couple's own wishes. Studies reveal that pregnancy has an unpredictable effect on sexual desire in women: some find desire enhanced; others notice it is distinctly curbed, and even have an unexplained aversion to the husband. If sexual desire is different from what is usual and sexual activity is refused, misunderstandings frequently ensue. The couple should understand that these idiosyncrasies are temporary and need not affect their future sexual relationship[16]. You and the physician are resource persons with whom the couple can explore their feelings and attitudes toward sex, pregnancy, and parenthood.

You and the physician should also direct the expectant parents toward learning the specifics of pregnancy, labor and delivery, and child care. Many such educational programs are provided through Visiting Nurse Associations, local and state public health agencies, and private associations such as the Maternity

Center Association. In addition, there is a growing trend in the United States for maternity and general hospitals to provide classes for expectant parents. The goals of these classes are to increase knowledge related to physiology of pregnancy and labor, general hygiene, nutrition in pregnancy and lactation, and baby care and to increase understanding of ways to promote and maintain optimum health through the practice of good health habits in daily living. These programs enhance and broaden the services provided by the physician or clinic. The concept of family-centered care, which is becoming increasingly prevalent in health services today, could have no more appropriate application than to the expectant phase [16].

The couple will need to decide whether or not they plan to use the regular health care system for delivery or to have the baby at home. More couples are opting for the latter choice to avoid the depersonalization typical of a hospital delivery. Edwards describes the nurse's role in helping the couple prepare for a home delivery [13].

If you work in the hospital, you can influence policy and regulations to allow flexibility in maternal-child care. Presence of the father during labor and delivery, rooming-in, flexible visiting hours, and in-service education classes that give ancillary personnel a better understanding of the crisis of pregnancy will minimize the depersonalization.

Parenthood Phase. LeMaster's well-known study on the crisis of parenthood assumes that one of the reasons the transition to parenthood is so difficult is that the first child forces the pair relationship into a more complicated triangular system. The husband may find it difficult to accept the baby ranking first in claims upon his wife [22]. You and the physician, as resource persons, should be aware that couples may have an attitude toward parenthood distinct from that toward children. They may accept the concept of parenthood, yet reject their particular child because of the latter's sex, appearance, or threatening helplessness. Or the couple may reject the idea of parenthood, as in the case of unplanned conception, yet unite in genuine love and acceptance of their new baby. Often the parents repeat in their childrearing practices the treatment they received from their own parents. Understanding this is significant, for the basis for child abuse can be traced to how the parents were themselves reared. However, parental practices are modified by their experience with their children, by their perception of people, by the emotional satisfaction they gain from life, and by reworking their philosophy of life.

Much of a child's early development is a reflection of the mother's capacities, which are in turn related to her self-esteem, relationship with her husband, and feelings about her current life situation. A high rating in each of these three positive factors is correlated with enthusiasm and great warmth in childcaring [25].

Toffler notes that raising children successfully requires skills that are by no means universal. Yet our society allows virtually anyone, almost regardless of mental or moral qualifications to raise young human beings, so long as these humans are biological offspring. Despite the increasing complexity of the tasks involved, parenthood remains the greatest single preserve of the amateur[35]. To offset the amateur approach, family-life education is a part of the health curriculum in some schools. As a school nurse, you can initiate courses about family-life attitudes, usual problems in starting a family, and tasks in childrearing.

The developmental tasks of a couple with their first child are demanding. The woman is now wife-mother and the man husband-father, and blending these roles and adjusting to new expectations take time. Duvall lists the following tasks demanded of new parents, which even the single parent must perform to some degree. Essentially these tasks are those listed previously for the establishment phase, with alterations that account for adjusting to, and taking care of, a new baby:

1. Expanding and refining the communication system so that there is mutual recognition of the involvement and emotional ties with the newcomer and acceptance of sharing one's mate.
2. Adjusting to round-the-clock baby care, thereby reworking patterns of responsibility and accountability.
3. Meeting the increased costs of living as a childrearing family.
4. Gradually adapting housing arrangements to accommodate a growing child.
5. Reestablishing mutually satisfying sexual relationships.
6. Refashioning relationships within the larger family-relative circle.
7. Adjusting to community and social life as a childrearing family.
8. Planning for future pregnancies or postponing plans until another child is desired, or deciding to have no more children.
9. Reworking a suitable philosophy of family life in the childrearing stage[12].

These tasks are reworked with the birth of each additional child, although the outcomes may vary.

The three phases of family life discussed earlier—establishment phase, expectant phase, and parenthood phase—are only a small segment of life's developmental stages, each with specific tasks, that a person passes through from birth to death. The companion text, *Nursing Assessment and Health Promotion through the Life Span,* explores all stages and accompanying tasks[27].

FAMILY INTERACTION

Family interaction is a unique form of social interaction based on a set of intimate and continuing relationships. It is the sum total of all the family roles being played within a family at a given time[12]. Families function and carry out their tasks and life styles through this process.

Family therapists, psychiatrists, and nurses are giving increased attention to the emotional balance in family *dyads or paired role positions* such as husband and wife or mother and child. They have noted that a shift in the balance of one member of the pair (or of one pair) will alter the balance of the other member (or pair). The birth of a child is the classic example[22].

Interaction of the husband and wife, or of the adult members living under one roof, is basic to the mental, and sometimes physical, health of the adults as well as to the eventual health of the children. There are two factors that strongly influence this interaction: (1) the sense of self-esteem or self-love of each family member, and (2) the different socialization processes for boys and girls[36].

Importance of Self-Esteem

The most important life task for each person—to feel a sense of self-esteem, to love himself and have a positive self-image—evolves through interaction with his parents from the time of birth onward and will in turn affect how he interacts in later life with others, including with spouse and offspring.

The adult in the family who does not feel self-acceptance and self-respect is not likely to be a loving spouse or parent. His behavior will betray his feelings about himself and others because he will perceive no automatic acceptance and little love from others in the family. Since his perception of an event is his reality, such a person in turn reacts in ways designed to defend himself from the rejection that he *thinks* he will receive; he may criticize, get angry, brag, demand perfection from others, or withdraw. In this way he builds himself up, his emotional reasoning being: "I may not be much, but others are worse." Behavior of this kind is corrosive to any relationship, but particularly one as initimate as exists in the family. Because of his overt behavior, those intimate with him are not likely to appreciate or respond to his basic needs for love, acceptance, and respect. Indeed, the common responses to such behavior are counterattack or withdrawal, which in turn perpetuate the other's negative behavior. To remain open and giving in such situations is difficult for the mate; but this may be the only way to elevate the other's self-esteem. Perhaps only then can he reciprocate loving behavior. You can help family members realize the importance of respecting and loving one another and help them work through problems stemming from the low self-esteem of a family member[36].

Influence of Childhood Socialization

The second crucial influence on interaction between adults in the family is the difference in socialization processes for boys and for girls. These differences are so embedded in the American social matrix that until recently they had gone nearly unnoticed. There is a different social source for self-love in boys and girls. The girl is loved simply because she exists and can attract, as is evidenced by the admiration pretty little girls receive. The girl is also taught to be subtle, for such behavior is part of her attraction. The boy is loved for what he can do and become; he must prove himself. Boys, particularly from school age on, are given less recognition than girls for good looks and much recognition for what they can do. A boy learns to be direct, to brush aside distractions (sometimes including a woman's voice since most disciplining will come from the mother and from female schoolteachers and can be perceived as nagging after awhile), and to get to the essence of things[36] .

These concepts of what is appropriate boy and girl behavior are taught early and continue to affect heterosexual interactions throughout life. For example, in traditional courtship, the boy is expected to be in charge, to be dominant, to prove himself; the girl is expected to attract, to be passive. In marriage, however, these expectations cause problems, for the man is proving himself largely through his work, so this aspect of his earlier courtship behavior is now less visible to his wife. If the woman does not understand the dynamics of his behavior, she is likely to feel rejected and unloved, thinking she can no longer attract him. If the wife is also working, the husband may think of her as a competitor and work harder to keep his self-esteem. His physical self, including his involvement in lovemaking, is very much intertwined with his social, professional, and financial self, and failure in one is likely to cause feelings of failure in the total self, affecting his sense of masculinity, sexuality, and personhood[36] .

All of these factors are compounded by the shift in balance between the man and woman found in modern marriage. The husband often labors under the illusion that he enjoys the rights and responsibilities inherent in a patriarchal family system. Yet he must recognize the qualifications and drive for independence, the basic humanness, of his wife. You can help the couple to recognize the effect of their early socialization on their behavior and expectations, to work through misunderstandings, and to strive for healthy socialization of their children.

Variables Affecting Interaction between the Child and Adult

Long before the child learns to speak, sensory, emotional, and intellectual exchanges are made between the child and other family members. Through such exchanges, and later with words, the child receives and tests instructions on how to consider the rights of others and how to respond to authority. He also learns how to use language as a symbol, how to carry out certain routines necessary for health, how to compete, and what goals to seek. The games and toys purchased for and played with the child, the books selected and read, and the television programs allowed can provide key learning techniques.

The child's spontaneity can evoke in the adult fresh ways of looking at life long buried under habit and routine. The child says, "It's too loud, but my earlids won't stay down"; or, "I want one of those little red olives with the green around"; or, "Give me that eraser with the handle." The child can also recreate for the adult the difficulty of the learning process: "Is it today, tomorrow, or yesterday? You said when I woke up it would be tomorrow, but now you call it 'today.' ''

Family interaction for the child and adult is also affected by the ordinal position and sex of the children, as well as by the presence of an only child or of multiple births such as twins.

The Ordinal Position of the Child is important to his development[23, 26]. The first-born, who is an only child until the second one comes along, may enjoy some advantages in achievement of intellectual superiority and perspective about life, including a greater sense of responsibility. He has more contact with adults and is the sole recipient of attention for a time. The younger children benefit from the parents' experience with childraising and from having older siblings to imitate. The middle child is apt to get caught between the jealousy of the older child and the envy of the younger, who may form a coalition against him.

The Only Child may feel more loneliness, and may seem older and more serious than his peers who have siblings. He lacks the opportunities siblings could provide. Thus he usually does not share feelings and experiences with someone close, or cope with jealousy and envy from rivals in the home, or learn intimately about ways of the opposite- or same-sexed peers. He learns less about compromising with peers, sharing adult attention, and erecting strong defenses against the feelings displaced on him by adults and peers.

Children are the logical targets for fulfilling many of the parents' frustrated ambitions and needs. In a large family, these yearnings and aspirations can be parceled out among a number of children; but when there is only one child, this child can sense his parents' manipulation and expectations. Thus the only child tends to be a peacemaker if he and his parents are the only household members. He is inadvertently brought into his parents' conflicts and forced to help maintain harmony and preserve equilibrium in the household.

In a family with only one child, there are few people to fulfill the many roles of a family; thus more is demanded of each member. The only child may be forced prematurely to assume roles for which he is ill equipped. He may become deft at performing adult tasks and roles, but his confidence in his capacity to do so may be uncertain.

The only child sometimes has special problems when he becomes a parent, seeing in his child a longed-for brother or sister. The danger in the situation is that the child is also a rival for the spouse's attention. When the child becomes an adolescent, he may then pose a threat to his parent's own adult roles, and the parent may unconsciously become overly competitive.

Certainly the only child can develop into a wholesome, well-adjusted person. The qualities of being more serious, assertive, responsible, independent, able to entertain himself and find satisfaction in his own pursuits frequently develop because of the demands placed on him. These demands can enhance his abilities to be a mature, capable adult. The greater opportunities available for adult contact, beginning at home, develop his creativity, language skills, and intellectual potential. First-born and only children such as Isaac Newton, Franklin Roosevelt, Emile Zola, Herbert Spencer, Rainer Maria Rilke, and some of the American astronauts rank high on the roster of outstanding leaders, artists, and scientists. As you counsel parents who plan for or have only one child, emphasize the need for peer activity and the danger of too much early responsibility and pressure.

The Adopted Child may suffer some problems of the only child. In addition, he may have to work through feelings about rejection and abandonment by his biological parents versus being wanted and loved by his adoptive parents. The child should be told he is adopted as early as he can comprehend the idea generally. Usually by the preschool years he can incorporate the idea that he is truly a wanted child.

Multiple Births, such as twins, have considerable impact on family interaction. If ovulation has been inhibited with contraceptive pills, multiple births are more likely when a family is started, after stopping use of this method[17]. The needs and tasks of these parents will be different from the parents who have a single birth. Your helpful suggestions and support can influence how well the parents cope with their responsibility.

Since multiple births are often premature, the first four or five months are very demanding on the parents regarding both amount of energy and time spent in child care; this means the parents have less energy and time for each other or for other children. The mother should have help for several months if possible—from the husband, a relative, friend, or neighbor. Financial worries and concern about space and providing for material needs also may intrude on normal husband-wife relationships; or on relationships with older children.

Although books discourage the mother of twins from breast-feeding or using alternate breast-and-bottle-feeding, the mother may be able to successfully breast-feed both twins, by alternating breast- with bottle-feedings. The babies will not necessarily be poor breast-feeders with this arrangement.

You can suggest shortcuts in, or realities about, care that will not be detrimental to twin babies and that will give the parents more time to enjoy them. For example, a diaper service is well worth the investment, as 1000 may be used in a month's time. The parents should not be made to feel guilty if they are not as conscientious with two babies as they would be with one. For example, the babies can lie in wet diapers a little longer, and each can be given a total bath every other day instead of daily. Heating bottles before feeding is not necessary. The parents should try to avoid getting so wrapped up in meeting the babies' physical needs that resentment, anger, or excessive fatigue creep in. Multiple offspring should be fun as well as work.

Encourage the parents of twins (or multiple offspring) to perceive the babies as individuals and to consider the long-term consequences of giving them similar-sounding names, dressing them alike, having doubles of everything, and expecting them to behave alike. Tell parents about the national organization, Mothers of Twins, whose local branch can be a place to share feelings and ideas and gain practical suggestions.

Multiple-birth children are likely to be closer than ordinary siblings. They soon learn about the extra attention their birth status brings them and may take advantage of the situation. Interaction between them is often complementary; for example, one twin may be dominant and the other submissive. Each learns from reinforcement of his experiences about the advantages of the particular role he chooses.

The Sex of the Child also influences his or her development within the family [23]. In most cultures a higher value is placed on male children than on female children. For example, there are some cultures where only a boy's birth is welcomed or celebrated, and the family's status is partially measured by the number of sons. Or in a family with several girls and no boys, another baby girl may come as a disappointment. The girl may discover this attitude in later years from overhearing adult conversations, and she may try to compensate for her sex and gain parental affection and esteem by engaging in tomboy behavior and later assuming masculine roles.

If a boy arrives in a family hoping for a girl, he may receive pressure to be feminine. He may even be dressed and socialized in a feminine manner. If the boy arrives after a family has two or three girls, he will receive much attention but also the jealousy of his sisters. He will grow up with three or four "mothering" figures (some may be unkind) and in a family more attuned to feminine than to masculine behavior. Developing a masculine identity may be more difficult for him, particularly if there is no male nearby with whom to relate. In spite of being pampered, he will be expected by his family to be manly. The boy may feel envious of his sisters' position and their freedom from such great expectations.

The girl who arrives in a family with a number of boys may also receive considerable attention, but may have to become tomboyish in order to compete with her brothers and receive their esteem. Feminine identity may be difficult for her. You can help parents understand how their attitude toward their own sexuality and their evaluation of boys and girls influence their relationship with their children. Emphasize the importance of encouraging the child's unique identity to develop.

FAMILY LIFE STYLES
AND CHILDREARING PRACTICES

There is no single type of contemporary American family, but the life styles of many American families correspond to the factors discussed in this section, including family structure, family cultural pattern, the impact of the twentieth century, and the changing trends in the family. These factors, in addition to those already discussed, influence family interaction, and so an understanding of them will assist you in family care.

Family Structure

Childrearing and family relationships are influenced primarily by family structure. The biological and reproductive unit most commonly found in the United States is the mother-father-child group. Ordinarily the parents are married, have established a residence of their own, are viewed (along with their children) as an integral social unit, and live in an intimate, monogamous relationship. Emphasis in American marriage is on pursuit of love in a romanticized way and on the individual happiness, rather than on family bonds, as in many other cultures.

In many situations, however, a child may grow up in a family that differs from the typical one just described. An aunt, uncle, or grandparent may be a continuing member of the household unit; one or the other parent may be absent because of death, divorce, illegitimacy, military service, or occupation involving travel.

In many countries, the United States included, a person is also a member of a larger kinship group to which the term *family* is applied. These kinship-group families may develop around the male or female line, and are respectively referred to as *patrilinear* (such as the Hindu family) or *matrilinear* (such as the Hopi Indian family)[24]. In the United States, once a couple is married, kinship ties are generally recognized on both sides of the family and are called *bilateral*. Recognition of bilateral lines leads to the concept of the family as a social unit rather than as just a biological phenomenon, and means more people will have contact with, and influence on, the child.

Family Size

The size of a family is related to distinctive patterns of family life and child development. Most children in the United States are members of a small family system—that is, one with three children or less.

Common features observable in the small family system are that (1) emphasis is on planning (the number and the frequency of births, the objectives of childrearing, and educational possibilities); (2) parenthood is intensive rather than extensive (great concern is evidenced from pregnancy through every phase of childrearing for each child); (3) group actions are usually more democratic; and (4) greater freedom is allowed individual members. The child or children in the small family usually enjoy advantages beyond those available to children in large families of corresponding economic and social level, including that of receiving more individual attention. On the other hand, these children may retain emotional dependence on their parents, grow up with extreme pressure for performance, and retain an exaggerated notion of self-importance.

The large family, generally thought of as one with six or more children, is as a rule not a planned family. Parenthood is generally extensive rather than intensive, not because of less love or concern but simply because parents must divide their attention more ways. In the large family, emphasis is on the group rather than on the individual member. Conformity and cooperation are valued above self-expression. Discipline in the form of numerous and stringent rules is frequently stressed, and there is a high degree of organization in the activities of daily living[18].

Family Cultural Pattern

*The ways of living and thinking that constitute the intimate aspects of family group life are the **family cultural pattern**[8]*. The family transmits the cultural pattern of its own ethnic background and class to the child, together with the parents' attitudes toward other classes.

Within the national cultural pattern of the United States, significant variations have been found in family cultural patterns and social systems[8]. For example, in Millstadt, Illinois, the German farm family provides a distinctive social system with cultural features distinct from its Italian neighbors across the River in Saint Louis. The Maine Yankee and the North Carolina rebel barely speak the same language. Thus how families rear their children will depend on ethnic group and class, region, nation, and historical period.

Influence of Twentieth-Century Changes

The shift in this century from an agrarian to a complex technological society has produced dramatic changes for the American family. A greater proportion of children now survive childhood than did in 1900, and a higher proportion of mothers survive childbirth. Marriage on the average occurs at an earlier age than in former generations. Fewer children are born to most parents and are spaced closer together. Middle-aged couples now have more time together after their children are grown and leave home. And because of an increased life expectancy, families now have more living relatives than formerly, especially elderly relatives[12].

There are other trends related to living in a complex industrial society. Families live primarily in urban areas. More women work outside the home. Family members are becoming better educated. Family incomes are increasing, and acquisition of personal housing and equipment comes earlier in the marriage. Greater individual freedom exists.

In recent decades, the emphasis on the family-kinship group has been replaced by the acceptance of the nuclear family. The mother-child unit is more widely publicized as existing among poor urban blacks, but even there it is not a dominant pattern[38]. Because Americans are so mobile and are increasingly living in smaller homes or in apartments, many ties with kin other than the immediate family are loosened, or at least are geographically extended. Sometimes close friends become "the family." Yet many Americans strengthen kinship ties through letters, telephone calls, and holiday and vacation visits. Religious influences affect family ties. Jews, with their many family traditions, are generally more embedded in a network of relatives than are white Protestants.

Rapid change is a fact that families must acknowledge. Medical, pharmacological, and scientific advances, the growing emphasis on the civil and economic rights of minority groups, and the women's liberation movement are only a part of the cultural expansion of this century. Those who lack healthy emotional roots within their nuclear families, who have few or no kinship ties, who cannot adjust to rapid change, and who have little identity except as defined by job and income are more likely to become depressed, alcoholic, unfaithful to mate, or divorced[26]. Today's changing social environment makes it increasingly difficult for a parent to be certain of his identity. How, then, is he to provide emotional roots for the child?

American Childrearing Practices have no one traditional national pattern, only the general concern that children develop "normally." Parents are encouraged through culture, education, and the mass media to use whatever the dominant childrearing theory is at the time. At the turn of the century, the dominant theory reflected the prevailing scientific belief in the primacy of heredity in determining behavior. In the early decades of the twentieth century, child care emphasized the importance of environment, and by the mid-thirties Freudian psychoanalytic theory had gained ascendency. Presently neobehavioristic theories are prominent. With each new wave of "knowledge," parents are bombarded by conflicting reports and condemnation of previous practices. Often the change in theory-application occurs during the same parental generation, so that parents do not trust their own judgment and considerable inconsistency results. The inconsistency, rather than the theory, probably creates the main problems in childrearing. Sometimes parents strive not to rear their children as they were reared, but nevertheless do so unwittingly because of the permanency of enculturation. Children are often given approval and disapproval for their behavior and told they are "good" or "bad." This practice, along with inconsistency and other factors, contributes to competition and sibling rivalry.

Currently the importance of the father's role is being reconsidered, and he is more active in child care. Still, the mother is primarily responsible for the crying baby and young child care. The infant is often unconsciously trained in privacy, individualism, and independence by being left alone in his crib or playpen much of the time. There is still, unfortunately, the fear of "spoiling" the infant if he is held too much or responded to spontaneously. Thus the infant may develop behavioral extremes in order to get his needs met. He is being given the foundation to later stand out, push himself forward, to compete and achieve.

Then when the children are old enough to be out of the home, parents often strive to do things for their children and center their activities around their children's activities. Work responsibilities are not necessarily demanded, but there is subtle pressure for the children to repay by pleasing the parents through use of talents, organizational achievements, or honors won. Due to the small size of the nuclear family, the school-age child or adolescent may spend more time with peers than with family members. And because of the youth idealization of our culture, seniority does not invoke special respect for the older person (parent). The childrearing parent must offer more than age if he wants to maintain control.

A growing trend is for children to be cared for by babysitters or parent-surrogates; often these are not relatives. What happens if the mother and parent-surrogate differ greatly about childrearing practices? The child generally acknowledges the authority of his parents, or at least the mother, but parent-surrogates affect him nevertheless. Any adult who is with the child reinforces behavior in the child that conforms to the adult's own standard of behavior. The child conforms to the adult's desires in order to gain approval. If the parent-surrogate acts in a way contrary to the values of the parents, both parents and child are likely to be distressed[26].

CHANGING TRENDS IN THE FAMILY

The American family is in evolution. What about future trends?

Sex roles are increasingly blurred and sometimes reversed. The father is less authoritarian. Homes are increasingly democratic, with both partners sharing responsibility for home and child care and authority.

Besides the increasing acceptance of divorce because of weakening religious-moral influences, experimentation is beginning with other family forms. Perhaps because of widespread loneliness and alienation, communal families and group marriages are occurring in which several adults and their children band together to form a single family unit organized around mutual philosophical, religious, or other interests or needs. Also, with divorce more common, one sees "aggregate" families—families based on a divorced and remarried couple, so that the children of each couple become part of one big family. Further, the childless family is now better accepted since the new emphasis on zero population growth. And there is less condemnation when homosexuals live together, or when the occasional unmarried person, even a man, adopts a child. Polygamy may become more important in the future as an alternate family style, especially if women continue to live longer than men.

The current transiency and stress characterizing our society may place unprecedented strains on an already-strained institution. Some say the family is already dead except for the first two years of childraising. The impact of the new birth technology, including experiments with embryo implants and babies in laboratory jars, may alter orthodox ideas about the family and its responsibilities even further[35].

Not only do communes organize around adult interests and needs, they also organize around alternate childrearing methods. Initial observations reveal that childrearing in communes is a highly deliberate and self-conscious undertaking, for commune members have rejected much of their own upbringing and are painfully aware of the lasting impact of childhood socialization.

Parents in communes face a persistent dilemma. The dominant ideology is to let the child "do his own thing." But in doing so, adults cannot encourage conformity to valued practices or guide their children toward parental goals. Given this philosophy and the generally passive nature of recruitment to communal life, there is some doubt whether this form of alternative family life will persist.

Family life styles have always been changing, yet the basic concept, unit, and purposes of the family have remained. Perhaps disproportionate visibility has been given to recent alternate approaches, which are really a very small minority. A look at history shows that communal living and the ideals of the hippie movement had been espoused by sizeable numbers of people in various religious movements during the 1800s. Mateswapping, popular in the 1970s, was also popular in the 1920s. Eras of permissive childrearing have usually alternated with restrictive practices. For example, the period from the 1890s to about 1915 was a time of general permissiveness in dealing with children. In the 1920s and 1930s, with the emphasis on Watson's work in conditioning, which supported the theory that emotional expression is bad, parents became much more restrictive. Feedings were kept on a strict schedule; the child was not to be cuddled or "spoiled." Many parents after World War II, having been raised in a restrictive atmosphere and without many material advantages, became quite permissive in their childcare. They equated child needs with child wants[36]. As the next generation becomes parents, will they again become more restrictive? Or will the current trend toward smaller families, with their emphasis on individuality and independence, foster more permissiveness?

NURSING IMPLICATIONS

The family as the basic unit for the developing person cannot be taken for granted. Although family forms have changed and will continue to change, each person, in order to develop healthfully, needs some intimate surroundings of human concern. "No man is an island."

You will frequently encounter the entire family as your client in the health care system, regardless of the setting. You may be asked to do family-centered care, to nurse the patient and his family, or to do "family therapy." Yet you will not be able to carry out the nursing process with the family even minimally unless you understand the dynamics of family living presented in this chapter.

Rapid change, increasing demands on the person, technological progress, and other trends mentioned in this chapter seem to isolate people. A glance at one vanishing symbol of American family life—the front porch—can illustrate this point. What happened to the porch where the family used to gather? Where mother sat when the evening dishes were done? Where father rested after a day of work? Where toddlers rode their kiddie cars? Where Susie got her first kiss? Where neighbors stopped to chat? The porch has been converted into a private patio in the back of the house, and is used briefly when the family can force themselves to leave the air-conditioned comfort of indoors. Susie and her boyfriend are gone in his car. Father is absorbed in his television programs. Mother can't hear the toddler calling because the dishwasher, clothes washer, dryer, and garbage disposal block out all human sounds. The older children are car-pooled to separate activities.

You cannot call back the front-porch era. Nor do all families live with the above luxuries and isolated from each other. But you should understand that many families are not even aware of the forces that are pulling them apart. More than ever, they need one place in their living where they can act without self-consciousness, where the pretenses and roles demanded in jobs, school, or social situations can be put aside. The living center should be a place where communication takes place with ease; where each knows what to expect from the other; where a cohesiveness exists that is based on nonverbal messages more than verbal; and where a person is accepted for what he is. The family may need your help in becoming aware of disruptive forces, of their maladaptive patterns (such as those described in Chapter 8), and of ways to promote an accepting home atmosphere.

You can help families understand some of the processes and dynamics underlying interaction, so that they in turn learn to respect the uniqueness of the self and of each other. Certainly members in the family do not always have to agree with each other. Instead, they can learn to truly listen to the other person, about how he feels and why, accepting each person's impression as real for himself. This attitude becomes the basis for mutual respect, honest communication, encouragement of individual fulfillment, and freedom to be. There is then no need to prove or defend the self. As you help the family achieve positive feelings toward and interaction with one another, you can help them to achieve their tasks, roles, and functions[36].

The person's health problems, especially his emotional ones, may well be the result of the interaction patterns in his childhood or present family. Knowledge of the variables influencing family interaction—parents' self-esteem and upbringing, number of siblings, the person's ordinal position in the family, cultural norms, family rituals—all will help you assist the person in talking through feelings related to past and present conflicts. Sometimes helping the person understand the above variables in relation to the spouse's upbringing and behavior can be the first step in overcoming current marital problems.

You are a nurse, not a specialized family counselor, although with advanced preparation you could do family therapy. But you can often sense lack of communication in a family. Through use of an empathic relationship and effective communication, teaching, and crisis therapy, you can encourage family members to talk about their feelings with one another and assist in the resolution of their conflicts. Help them become aware of the necessity of working for family cohesiveness just as they would work at a job or important project. Refer them to a family counseling service if the problems are beyond your scope. Your work with them should also help them better use other community resources, such as private family or psychiatric counseling or family and children's services.

Your knowledge of the family life cycle, with developmental tasks to be performed at each stage, provides a foundation for learning the specifics of sequential development discussed in the companion text[27]. This combined knowledge will help you in assessing the status of the family and the individual person in planning care, in intervention, and in objectively evaluating your effectiveness.

One of the liabilities in working with families of various social classes and cultures may be *you*. For example, if you come from a middle-class American background, you will have your own opinions about what constitutes family life. Your attitude toward nonconforming families or unconventional living arrangements may interfere with your objectivity and thus with your ability to assist some families. You will have to go through your own maturation process of learning that your way is not always the best or only way. The process is difficult.

Your goal is health promotion and primary prevention. Your intervention early in the family life cycle may help establish a positive health trend in place of its negative counterpart. The care you give to young parents lays the foundation for their children's health.

REFERENCES

1. Ackerman, Nathan, *Psychodynamics of Family Life*. New York: Basic Books, Inc., 1958.

2. Adams, Bert, *The American Family: A Sociological Interpretation*. Chicago: Markham Publishing Company, 1971.

3. _____, and Thomas Weirath, eds., *Readings on the Sociology of the Family*. Chicago: Markham Publishing Company, 1971.

4. Anthony, E. James, and Therese Benedek, *Parenthood: Its Psychology and Psychopathology*. Boston: Little, Brown and Company, 1970.

5. Bell, Norman, and Ezra Vogel, eds., *The Family*. Glencoe: The Free Press of Glencoe, 1960.

6. Bigelow, Howard, "Money and Marriage," in *Marriage and the Family*, eds. Howard Becker and Reuben Hill. Boston: D. C. Heath and Company, pp. 382-86.

7. Blanch, Rubin, and Gertrude Blanch, *Marriage and Personal Development*. New York: Columbia University Press, 1968.

8. Bossard, James, and Eleanor Boll, *Sociology of Child Development* (4th ed.) New York: Harper & Row, 1960.

9. Cavan, Ruth, *The American Family*. New York: Thomas Y. Crowell Company, 1963.

10. Clark, Ann, "The Beginning Family," *American Journal of Nursing*, 66: No. 4 (1966), 802-5.

11. Coleman, Arthur, and Libby Coleman, *Pregnancy: The Psychological Experience*. New York: Herder and Herder, 1972.

12. Duvall, Evelyn, *Family Development* (4th ed.). Philadelphia: J. B. Lippincott Company, 1971.

13. Edwards, Margot, "Unattended Home Birth," *American Journal of Nursing*, 73: No. 8 (1973), 1332-35.

14. Erikson, Erik, *Childhood and Society* (2nd ed.). New York: W. W. Norton & Company, Inc., 1963.

15. Evans, Frances, *Psychosocial Nursing*, New York: The Macmillan Company, 1971, chapter 3.

16. Fitzpatrick, Elsie, S. Reeder, L. Mastroianni, *Maternity Nursing*. Philadelphia: J. B. Lippincott Company, 1970.

17. Gahman, Betsy, *Twins: Twice the Trouble; Twice the Fun*. Philadelphia: J. B. Lippincott Company, 1965.

18. Glick, Paul, *American Families*. New York: John Wiley & Sons, Inc., 1957.

19. Hadley, B. U., "The Dynamic Interactionist Concept of Role," *Journal of Nursing Education*, 6: No. 2 (1967), 5.

20. Kirkpatrick, E. L., et. al., *The Life Cycle of the Farm Family in Relation to Its Standard of Living*. Madison: University of Wisconsin, 1934.

21. Leichter, Hope, "Comments on the Robert Winch Paper," *Journal of Marriage and the Family*, 1: No. 2 (1970), 18-19.

22. LeMasters, E. E., "Parenthood as Crisis," in *Crisis Intervention: Selected Readings*, ed. Howard Parad. New York: Family Service Association of America, 1972.

23. Lidz, Theodore, *The Person: His Development Throughout the Life Cycle*. New York: Basic Books, Inc., 1968.

24. Lindberg, George, C. Schrag, and O. Larsen, *Sociology* (3rd ed.). New York: Harper & Row, Publishers, 1963.

25. Maier, Henry, ed., *Three Theories of Child Development*. New York: Harper & Row, Publishers, 1965.

26. Messer, Alfred, *The Individual in His Family: An Adaptational Study*. Springfield, Ill.: Charles C. Thomas, 1970.

27. Murray, Ruth, and Judith Zentner, *Nursing Assessment and Health Promotion through the Life Span*. Englewood Cliffs, N.J.: Prentice-Hall, Inc., 1975.

28. Parad, Howard, and Gerald Caplan, "A Framework for Studying Families in Crisis," in *Crisis Intervention: Selected Readings*, ed. H. Parad. New York: Family Service Association, 1969.

29. Rogers, Carl, *On Becoming A Person*. Boston: Houghton Mifflin Company, 1961.

30. Rubin, Reva, "Attainment of the Maternal Role, Part 1: Processes," *Nursing Research*, 16: No. 3 (1967), 237-45.

31. Schulz, David, *The Changing Family*. Englewood Cliffs, N.J.: Prentice-Hall, Inc., 1972.

32. Skolnick, Arlene, and Jerome Skolnick, *Family in Transition*. Boston: Little, Brown and Company, 1971.

33. Sobol, Evelyn, and Paulette Robischon, *Family Nursing: A Study Guide*. St. Louis: The C. V. Mosby Company, 1970.

34. Sorokin, P., C. Zimmerman, and C. Galpin, *A Systematic Source Book in Rural Sociology*. Minneapolis: University of Minnesota Press, 1931, 2:31.

35. Toffler, Alvin, *Future Shock*. New York: Random House, 1970.

36. Vincent, Clark, *The Family: Trends and Directions in the Seventies*. A speech to the Eleventh Annual Conference on Prevention and Community Mental Health, St. Louis, April 27, 1973.

37. _____, "An Open Letter to the 'Caught Generation,' " *Family Coordinator*, April 1972, pp. 143-50.

38. Winch, Robert, "Permanence and Change in the History of the American Family and Some Speculations as to Its Future," *Journal of Marriage and the Family*, 1: No. 2 (1970), 8-16.

Index

Upper class (*cont.*)
  definition, 332
  nurse's role, 343-344

Vaccine, 169
Value system, definition, 274
Variables affecting health:
  external, 7-9, 161, 165-167, 178, 229-230, 238, 250, 252-263, 278, 294-296, 341-342, 356, 366-367
  internal, 7, 9, 12, 161, 167-170, 186-188, 231-232, 238
Vegetarian, 305, 307
Verbal communication, 46, 47, 50

Visiting Nurse Association (*table*), 138
Voluntary agencies:
  contributions, 23, 138 (*table*)
  definition, 22
  organization, 24
  types of, 23, 138 (*table*)

Water pollution, 254-258
Wellness orientation, 7, 116, 137, 139
Workmen's Compensation, 33
World Health Organization, 6, 25

Zen Buddhism, 307
Zoonosis, 260